Cartographies *of* Disease

Maps, Mapping, and Medicine

Tom Koch

ESRI PRESS

REDLANDS, CALIFORNIA

ESRI Press, 380 New York Street, Redlands, California 92373-8100

All rights reserved. First edition 2005
10 09 08 07 06 05   1 2 3 4 5 6 7 8 9 10

Printed in the United States of America

Library of Congress Cataloging-in-Publication Data
Koch, Tom, 1949-
Cartographies of disease : maps, mapping, and medicine / Tom Koch.-- 1st ed.
       p.   cm.
   Includes bibliographical references and index.
     ISBN 1-58948-120-8 (pbk. : alk. paper)
     1. Medical mapping–History. 2. Medical geography–Maps–Data processing. 3. Public health–Geographic information systems.
4. Epidemiology–Statistical methods. 5. Medical geography–Methodology. I. Title.
     RA792.5.K63 2005
     614.4'2—dc22   2005005993

Ask for ESRI Press titles at your local bookstore or order by calling 1-800-447-9778. You can also shop online at www.esri.com/esripress. Outside the United States, contact your local ESRI distributor.

ESRI Press titles are distributed to the trade by the following:

In North America, South America, Asia, and Australia:
Independent Publishers Group (IPG)
Telephone (United States): 1-800-888-4741
Telephone (international): 312-337-0747
E-mail: frontdesk@ipgbook.com

In the United Kingdom, Europe, and the Middle East:
Transatlantic Publishers Group Ltd.
Telephone: 44 20 8849 8013
Fax: 44 20 8849 5556
E-mail: transatlantic.publishers@regusnet.com

Cover design by Savitri Brant
Book design and production by Savitri Brant
Copyediting by Tiffany Wilkerson
Print production by Cliff Crabbe
On the cover: A portion of a map by H. W. Acland showing the relation of
altitude to disease in three separate cholera epidemics in Oxford.
Source: Rare Books and Special Collections, University of British Columbia Library.

Contents

List of figures

Foreword

This is a book about maps.

It is not your usual book about maps. Your usual book about maps presents maps as a way of showing things. The world as known is taken for granted, and the maps give it to us in a graphic form we can hold in our hands. That's the usual take on maps.

Tom Koch has written a book about maps as a way of thinking about things. The world in Koch's book is invariably puzzling, and the maps are presented as a way that people grappling with the puzzle have for thinking about the world in a graphic form that can be reproduced and sent through the mail or over the Internet.

The maps Koch has written about are mostly maps of disease: yellow fever, cholera, influenza, measles, AIDS. Some of the maps are about death, and the puzzles have to do with why the dead died where they did. The maps propose answers to these puzzles. That is, the maps embody theories about disease causation and diffusion. In Koch's telling, the maps are a way that doctors and other researchers have had for thinking graphically about disease. Thus, maps are a kind of cognitive machine.

Koch's book is a history of the development of this machine. The book traces this development from a 1694 map of plague in Bari, Italy, to a 2004 map of AIDS in the United States. Along the way Koch presents us with a 1798 map of yellow fever in New York; an 1819 map of yellow fever in New York; an 1821 map of typhus or typhoid fever in New York; an 1832 map of cholera; an 1836 map of cholera in Hamburg; 1940 map of hernias in France; an 1841 map of sanitation in Dublin; an 1842 map of sanitation in Leeds; an 1849 map of cholera in Exeter; an 1850 map of cholera in London; 1854 map of cholera in South London; a handful of contending 1854–1855 maps of cholera in Soho (and another handful of twentieth century variants of one of them); an 1856 map of cholera in Oxford; an 1856 world map of health and disease; 1875 maps of cholera in New Orleans, Memphis, and Nashville, and United States as a whole; an 1876 map of cholera in East Africa; an 1878 map of offensive odors in Boston; a couple of 1885 maps of typhoid in Plymouth, Pennsylvania; an 1885 map of sewer outlets in Harrisburg, Pennsylvania; maps from Haviland's 1892 smallpox epidemic in Western Australia; maps from Sedgwick's 1901 *Principles of Sanitary Science and the Public Health*; a 1925 sandfly fever in Peshawar, India; maps from the *Welt Seuchen Atlas* of the 1950s; a 1960 map of cancer in Horrabridge, England; maps from May's 1961 *Studies in Disease Ecology*; 1960s maps of the death rate in England; a 1962 map of Burkitt lymphoma in Africa; a 1969 map of schistosomiasis in South America; 1971 maps of influenza in England; a 1972 map of bronchitis in Leeds; a 1977 map of hepatitis in Tasmania; a 1986 map of influenza in the United States; a 1988 map of malaria in India; a 1988 map of leukemia in England; a 1989 map of HIV in eastern Tennessee; maps of the late 1980s and early 1990s outbreak of AIDS in Ohio and the United States; a 2002 map of AIDS in Thailand; and a 2002 map of dengue fever in Pennathur, India, among others.

Through these maps, Koch gives us, for the first time, a history of cartography that takes it for granted that maps are a form of thinking that don't so much reveal knowledge as actively construct it. Since the knowledge of constructing was in many cases urgently needed, for Koch these maps become thought in graphic action, propelling changes in policy with effects on the lives of untold numbers. For this reason, these maps exemplify in a more straightforward fashion than many others the circuits of knowledge and power central to the concerns of Michel Foucault. Coming to Foucault second hand, through historians of science such as Andrew Pickering, Simon Schaffer, and Steven Shapin, Koch does not belabor the theoretic implications of his story. Yet behind most of Koch's maps lie facts that could only have been gathered by institutions operating under the authority and with the power of the state, increasingly as the story advances from the seventeenth to the twenty-first century. In turn, the maps constructed using these facts empowered the state and its institutions in myriad ways. Koch also examines the way these power-knowledge relationships have been naturalized, and the heart of his book is a deconstruction of myth so effective in this naturalization that has grown around John Snow, a man Koch greatly admires.

This deconstruction occupies three chapters, and each is critical. First, Koch takes pains to demolish the myth of John Snow as a solitary hero figure in a saga about the power of mapping to combat ignorance. In place of this lonely warrior, Koch presents a Victorian scientist thoroughly integrated into the scientific life of his time, a time that entertained competing theories about the nature, cause, and transmission of disease, as the dominant Galenic paradigm was giving way before the rise of modern medicine. Koch demonstrates Snow's dependence on well-established networks of both London mapmakers and collectors of social statistics, as well as on contemporary medical theory. By reproducing maps of cholera in Soho made at the same time as Snow's by Edmund Cooper and Henry Whitehead (and elsewhere in the generally contemporaneous work of H. W. Acland, Augustus Petermann, and others), Koch shows that mapping of cholera was commonplace, along with the mapping of other diseases.

Second, in place of an innovative mapping of disease that pointed inescapably to the causative effects of a pump, the removal of whose handle triumphantly ended the epidemic and proved the role of water in cholera's transmission, Koch gives us a theory of the disease's transmission pioneered by others such as Charles Coswell. Koch shows this outbreak was already on the wane by the time Snow removed the pump's handle, and a battle of the maps in which Snow's failed to carry the day. Nor was it simply that the maps of different researchers proved—as they saw it—different theories of the disease (generally miasmatic and involving foul odors and altitude), but that the maps could not ever agree about the facts—as their makers saw them—such as the location of a former plague pit. In Koch's reading, each of these maps is an argument over the nature of the world, particularly over the aspects or parts of the world that played roles in the theories about the nature, cause, and transmission of cholera that the maps articulated. These maps consist of evidence that supports theories that motivated the maps' construction and which in turn the maps were held to prove. That is, the maps were intentionally constructed to argue a point.

To conclude his deconstruction, Koch turns not to other maps of cholera, but to new versions of Snow's 1854 map of the Soho outbreak. As Koch shows, twenty years later the U.S. army surgeon, Ely McClellan, mapped the 1873 U.S. epidemic, which advanced distinctive graphic arguments and wrangled over the facts (including whether it was even cholera that caused the deaths). Indeed, the mapped debate continued well beyond Robert Koch's 1883 identification of the bacterium *Vibrio cholerae* as the cause of the disease. But then, as Tom Koch's book so convincingly demonstrates, maps are not presentations of facts but the graphic marshalling of selected propositions into arguments about the nature of reality. Maps are thought experiments with significant effects on our lives.

With the evolution of medical mapping into the later twentieth century, the advent of powerful, computer-based mapping technologies make these map experiments easier and easier to carry out. The painstaking labor that attended the creation of a single map by Filippo Arrieta in the seventeenth century has been replaced in the twenty-first by software that enables a mapper to rapidly create and review a map. In publication, the resulting maps may present themselves and appear as pictures of facts, but like the rest of the facts of experimental science, the mapped facts come into being as epistemic objects, more or less well-founded hypotheses, about things that might, or could, or should exist. As Koch's history demonstrates, their existence remains entirely provisional.

The tentative, exploratory, experimental nature of this process comes through in Koch's book most dramatically not in a description of computer mapping, but in Koch's recapitulation of Abraham Verghese's pencil-and-paper struggle to make sense of his HIV-infected patients in the late 1980s. Dr. Verghese practiced medicine in rural Tennessee. He and his colleagues were stunned when their practices became dominated by HIV-infected patients. What was this (then) urban problem doing in rural Tennessee? "There was a pattern in my HIV practice," Verghese wrote. "I kept feeling if I could concentrate hard enough, step back and look carefully, I could draw a kind of blueprint that explained what was happening here." One night he borrowed a map of the United States from his son's bedroom wall. On a sheet of paper laid on the map spread out on his living room floor, Verghese marked where his patients lived. He labeled this map "Domicile," but he could have labeled it "Birthplace" as well, for most of his patients were men who had come back home to Tennessee to die.

Verghese next mapped where his HIV patients had lived between 1979 and 1985, the time period when they presumably acquired the virus. The places on this "Acquisition" map circled the periphery of the United States and were mostly large cities. "As I neared the end, I could see a distinct pattern of dots emerging on the larger map of the USA. All evening I had been on the threshold of seeing. Now I fully understood." Through his mapping, Verghese had uncovered a circuitous voyage, a migration from home and a return ending in death. It was, Verghese had written, "the story of how a generation of young men, raised in self-hatred, had risen above the definition that their society and upbringings had used to define them. It was the story of hard and sometimes lonely journeys they took far from home into a world more complicated than they imagined. And far more dangerous than anyone could have known." As was the case with Snow's map, there were exceptions that on investigation only proved the rule. Patients who appeared on both maps were those who had had the virus delivered to their doorstep, hemophiliacs or blood transfusion recipients who had received tainted blood products.

The maps Verghese made that night on his living room floor might not be much to look at, but the thinking they enabled and embodied was rich. It is a process analogous to Verghese's, Koch implies, that lies behind and shines through each of the maps he has reproduced. Such an understanding is not novel with Koch. Martin J. S. Rudwick has mined a similar vein in his histories of geologic mapping, and a similar insight flowered in Jane Camerini's investigations of the role of mapping in the work of Charles Darwin and Alfred Russel Wallace. The inestimable novelty of Koch's book is to have traced the process across a three-hundred-year period from one disease to another, and to have brought the story up to the day before yesterday. Some may feel that Koch's unraveling of the myth of the genius crusader Snow has the effect of destroying an inspiration that might be drawn from such an example. But what could be more inspiring today than understanding that the maturation of science depends, as so patently in Snow's and the rest of the cases Koch presents, on elaborate networks of workers sharing resources? What could be more reassuring today than realizing that on the cutting edge, theories are always in competition? What could be more useful today than knowing that maps are not representations of "the truth," but cognitive machines for constructing and testing propositions about the nature of reality? In our elaborately networked age of interlocking specialization, doesn't it make it more exciting, isn't it a more powerful goad to have always been the state of the art? In this sense, Koch's book seems to me to be far more about the future than the past.

Like humans throughout history, we are cursed, or blessed, with the conviction that we finally understand the way things really are, that the maps we're making are maps of the way the world really is. With our molecular knowledge of viruses and our microbiological understanding of bacteria, we look back in amazement at the animalcules, at the infusoria, at the miasmas, vapors, and evil fates that animated earlier theories of disease. With our satellite imagery, GPS, and GIS, we imagine we can afford to smile at maps of the earth less complete or different than the maps we make today. But the lesson of history should instead be humbling, for each age, too, has imagined itself alone on the pinnacle of human knowledge. What may seem to be bizarre fantasies from the past next to the scientific images of the present day need instead to be read as templates for the way our own up-to-the-minute ideas will be thought about a hundred years or so in the future. Thirty years ago, in my doctorial dissertation, I argued that all maps were mental maps, forms of thought about the spatial relationships of things cast in a mode that facilitated their unambiguous communication. In *Cartographies of Disease*, Tom Koch has made this case in spades. What modern, computer-based mapping technologies have to offer is not more definitive representations of facts, but more efficient, effective communication of ever-more-powerful propositions about the nature, cause, and transmission of diseases. If we wrestle with these problems ferociously enough, Koch suggests, the day may dawn when we have made the last map of disease and only maps of health remain to be drawn.

Denis Wood

Acknowledgments

Writing is the least solitary of crafts. The hours at the word processor are individual. They serve, however, only as the end product of as many hours spent in association with others familiar with the subjects, the data that is built into the historical review. In research for this book on the history of medical mapping, a range of librarians, researchers, and editorial personnel have been unstinting in their time, generous in their assistance, and have ably assisted me.

I am particularly grateful to the many primary researchers willing to correspond and discuss elements of this history. Those whose work is described in chapter 11 include Dr. Jay Devasundaram, Dr. Scott Anderson, and Prof. Scott Orford. Joanna S. Gould, executor of the estate of Peter Gould, kindly permitted the use of her late husband's AIDS maps. Both Andrew Cliff and Peter Haggett, whose work has informed the field-at-large, were generous in their response to my e-mailed questions, as were John Snow scholars Michael Rip and Peter Vinten-Johansen of Michigan State University. Ralph R. Frerichs of UCLA, whose John Snow Web site was cited in an earlier chapter, was similarly generous with his time and insights.

It is less common, but no less important, to acknowledge the work of the many research librarians without whose assistance my work would have been slowed if not halted. I have been assisted by librarians at a daunting range of institutions, including, in alphabetical order, the Boston Public Library, British Library, Harvard University, London Metropolitan Archives, National Library of Medicine (NLM), Special Libraries Association (SLA), University of Toronto, and the Wellcome Trust.

At my home institution, the University of British Columbia (UBC), interlibrary loan personnel provided ready access to primary articles by a range of nineteenth and early twentieth century researches whose writings were only available at distant libraries. The library's media resource department photographed a number of maps from their collection to permit their use in this work. Rare Books and Special Collections librarian Ralph Stanton, whose charge is the preservation of UBC's historical collection, has been wonderfully supportive and generous in his permission to reproduce materials collected.

The personnel at two exceptional research libraries deserve special notice. In repeated visits to the New York Academy of Medicine, I learned from the assistance and advice of librarian Arlene Shaner, whose scholarship and professional expertise were an unexpected boon. At the College of Physicians of Philadelphia, archivist and curator Richard Fraser offered unflagging support and advice. I was fortunate to have their guidance. Staff at both libraries endured repeated visits and countless questions as I struggled both to find the original maps and their texts and then to obtain copies of the most important examples of the work.

Among my circle of friends and acquaintances, I am especially grateful to Denis Wood who helped me formulate a way to think about the maps as relational and the manner in which the history of mapping technology served as a tool of the transformation of knowledge across this history. Arthur Krim has been unstinting in his assistance uncovering early maps, reports, or issues. Elizabeth Leppman of St. Cloud State University kindly reviewed an early manuscript draft in an attempt to assure not simply its accuracy but also its relevancy to current themes in social science generally and geography specifically.

Most important, perhaps, has been the contribution of my long-time friend and sometime colleague, geographer Ken Denike of the University of British Columbia. This book's genesis lies in materials first developed with Ken for a course entitled *Spatial Data Analysis Using GIS*. Chapters on the relation between maps and statistics, and on the social context of epidemic disease, were first written to provide a context within which the GIS labs we developed could be best presented. As that teaching evolved into this book, his advise and encouragement remained constant supports.

Finally, it is a pleasure to recognize the assistance rendered by ESRI Press, whose personnel supported this work and saw it to publication. In almost thirty-five years of public writing in a range of venues—books, newspapers, magazines, monographs—I have worked with scores of editors and a number of publishers. Never before have I been given the editorial freedom, financial support, or personal encouragement provided by the ESRI Press editorial team. From the beginning, publisher Christian Harder and the team he assigned me of Gary Amdahl and Judith Hawkins shared an absolute commitment to this project, asking only what they might contribute to make it better. Also deserving of mention are others in the ESRI community, including *ArcUser*™ editor Monica Pratt, software prototype developer for health Tanya Costain, and ESRI's Bill Davenhall.

Finally, it is necessary to assert that every effort has been made both to assure the accuracy of the material presented and to credit the legitimate rights holders of the maps and illustrations that are at the heart of this book. Should any believe they have been inadvertently overlooked or their right to a specific image incorrectly assigned, both the publishers and I promise to correct the error in future editions.

Tom Koch

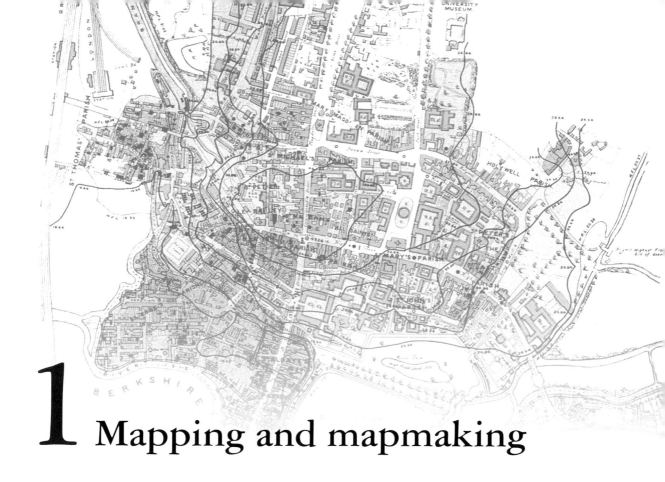

1 Mapping and mapmaking

Mapping is a way of thinking about abstract things in a graphic and practical way. In this book, the things thought about are the nature and diffusion of diseases, the ways viruses and bacteria spread through a neighborhood or around the world. The abstractions these maps consider are the ecologies advancing or impeding viral and bacterial introduction to human communities. The idea is not simply to use mapping descriptively to represent statistics to describe so many cases here or so many deaths there. That is important, but in itself insufficient. The real objective is to understand the *relation* between viral or bacterial communities, their human hosts, and the environment that inhibits or encourages their relationship. Typically, the hope is that by identifying elements of that relation, and then interfering with them, the intrusion of dangerous bacteria or viruses can be controlled and limited, if not eliminated.

The task seems increasingly urgent these days. In the late 1960s, U.S. health officials promised that "plagues will be banished forever from Earth" (Lederberg 2003). Why not? It was assumed that vaccination programs, the availability of effective antibiotics, and a generally improving standard of living had freed the developed world from the scourge of epidemic and pandemic killers. It was also assumed that other, poorer nations might be similarly advanced in only a matter of time. As officials declared victory over epidemic disease, however, the agents of those diseases were evolving in response to the changes then being made in society and in medical science. Today, we are in a new period of bacterial and viral evolution, the result of which has been a host of new diseases. These include AIDS/HIV, bovine spongiform encephalopathy (BSE, or mad cow disease), hantavirus pulmonary syndrome, Legionnaires' disease, Lyme disease, severe acute respiratory syndrome (SARS), West Nile virus, and the new antibiotic-resistant strains of diseases like tuberculosis and syphilis.

"Although these occurrences may appear inexplicable, rarely if ever do emerging infections appear without reason" (Morse 1999). Understanding those reasons has been a primary goal of medical mapping at least since the early nineteenth century. Even earlier, medical mapping was used to consider if not the nature of this or that disease, then both its patterns of diffusion and the methods by which it might be inhibited. Mapping was an approach employed both by the officials charged with responding to this or that disease incursion and the medical personnel who struggled to treat those afflicted. By contemporary standards, the techniques of mapping and mapmaking were as crude and limited as the science they presented. But that does not mean they were ineffective. Then as well as now, mapping served and serves the science of its day. The maps that result are traces of that science, evidence of both the brilliance and the limits of the medical thinking that informs and is informed by the mapping.

The emerging diseases of our age occur at a time when new techniques of mapping promise the potential of a better understanding of specific states of health, illness, and the conditions that promote one or the other. Geographic information systems (GIS)—computer not paper-based—share with traditional mapping an approach that is graphic and cartographic as well as statistical. Their power resides not only in the clarity of their presentation, but also in the manner in which the mapping process encourages our thinking about the relations between microscopic agents, human host populations, and the factors that encourage or inhibit their mutual relations. In this, mapping stands not independent of but in association with the other tools of epidemiology and public health that assist in our understanding of both the nature of human disease *in situ* and the potential for its containment.

The history of medical mapping is the history of an ecological perspective on the emergence and containment of states of disease because "mapping" refers to a way of thinking that is inherently ecological. It assigns relations between elements of one or more abstract sets in a manner that permits all to be considered together. In that assignment, mapping assumes at least one of the sets thus joined has a spatial component that provides a locational anchor (spatial coordinates) that is geographically descriptive. Regardless of whether a physical map results, the cognitive process of map thinking encourages a perspective that is relational and spatial at once. Mapmaking, on the other hand, refers to the process by which map thinking is transformed into a concrete two-dimensional artifact, a map (Wood 1993b).

Mapping is like story telling (Wood 2002; Kaiser, Wood, and Abramms 2005). Mapmaking is like story writing, indeed like publishing: it transforms the narrative into a form that can be reproduced and then shared. While distinct, the two are related. There is no mapmaking without map thinking. Map thinking inevitably invites a concrete result—a map artifact broadly sketched on paper, carefully drawn by hand or developed on a computer using a GIS program. How maps are made affects the mapping, transforming the way we understand the relation between the sets mapped. Methods of production and distribution together affect the conceptual process (what can we do and how can it be distributed?) that shapes the final artifact. Together, these related processes (thinking, mapping, making, and distributing) determine not only the map artifact, but also the process of map thinking, the way we first define and then address a particular problem in the context of a specific theoretical perspective.

Speaking, writing, publishing: each affects the other in myriad ways that uniquely contribute to the evolving story each attempts to tell. Mapping, mapmaking, and map publishing are similarly interdependent. But the root in mapping lies map *thinking*, the process through which elements of experience are abstracted, identified, joined, and then transformed into a common narrative.

Destinies

"In health care, destiny is geography" (*Dartmouth Atlas of Health Care* 1998, 21). Because both pathogen and host interact within an environment, understanding their relation means understanding the environment. This is first and foremost a geographic exercise in which elements encouraging or inhibiting the host/pathogen relation are located in place, in space at one or another scale. Both disease and its inverse, general health, are the result of a *pas de deux* danced in place by host and pathogen to a complex beat of local, regional, and global environmental elements. But it is also true that "overall disease burden is primarily a function of demography" (Gibson et al. 2002), the characteristics of human communities and the environments in which they exist. But demography is no less geographic, occurring in place and at various scales. And so, in thinking about health and disease we have to think simultaneously about demographic and geographic characteristics of host *and* pathogenic communities at various scales of interdependence, encouraging or inhibiting specific relations.

The challenge of mapping the complexities of an illness or the conditions promoting health is that both demand enormous specificity in the search for a general perspective. Each incidence must be carefully located, each factor precisely assigned. The greater the incidence of occurrence, the more potent the resulting map. For example, little can be said of two isolated incidences such as that of Isabella de Gracias, 19, or Mei Tang-Mu, 26, who each gave birth to a premature infant of 880 grams and 856 grams, respectively, at Women's and Children's Hospital in Vancouver, Canada, on June 16, 2003.[1] Certainly it is important to the families themselves, including the mothers, but as stated the incidents are disconnected, isolated factoids outside any meaningful context. That the first lived at 250 East

Hastings and the second nearby at 300 East Pender reveals only that both lived within a kilometer of each other in the downtown east side area of Vancouver. However, mapping all Vancouver's premature births by maternal residence may show that in 2003 women from the downtown east side were 24 percent more likely to have premature or low-weight births than were those from any other neighborhood in the greater Vancouver regional district.

The first question immediately becomes what contributes to the localized likelihood of premature and low-weight births? A number of factors have been identified, including the age of the woman, general health status, income, nutritional factors, number of prior births, likelihood of drug abuse, and the degree of prenatal medical care. Many of these correlate with income. In general, the poorer the mother, the less likely she is to have good nutrition, good healthcare, and so on. A quick look at income data by census tract identifies the Vancouver downtown east side, an area with a high proportion of immigrant and First Nations peoples, as among the poorest in Canada. Where women are relatively recent immigrants from developing countries, other data suggests that another level of risk is introduced.

In this way, we build from the specific to the general. Seeking means to address the problem, programs can be tailored to increase the likelihood of prenatal care for those individuals whose pregnancies are, by profile, most at risk. Maps invite locational responses (a clinic, a prenatal program) to locational problems (too many premature births in a neighborhood). Discussions of what services need to be offered, and where, become the concrete response to a general issue discovered in an aggregation of specific events (premature births in specific environments and their relation to variables—income and nutrition) at one or more scales of address.

The second, less frequently asked question is what is this phenomenon related to? To what extent may rate of low-birth-weight infants be an indicator of a more general context of illness, one of several health outcomes of socioeconomic or spatial factors? Here we find that in the United States at least the incidence of low-birth-weight infants correlates with incidence of tuberculosis (a disease of poverty), of HIV/AIDS, and of crime (Wallace, Huang, Gould, and Wallace 1997). All are outcomes of the environments we create and then impose upon those who live in areas that are socioeconomically deficient (Wallace and Wallace 1997).

Just as important, these urban zones of illness and crime are not contained, but in their turn become reservoirs by which disease radiates through the greater urban area. "Time incidence in the central city determines the incidence in the surrounding counties, as modulated by the area density of the community pattern" (Wallace and Wallace 1997, 1, 343). In building the maps of low-birth-weight infants and the socioeconomic characteristics that promote them (demographics, healthcare service levels, income, social service, and so on), we map not just a single problem but the context of a host of problems whose determinants are shared (Holling 1992; and Wallace et al. 1995). In this process, we also map reservoirs of ill health that affect not simply contained neighborhoods or specific populations, but the greater population as well.

This is the way mapping approaches the world. It thinks about classes of discrete events (people with diarrhea, respiratory distress, hernias, etc.) in the context of potentially relevant data (location, income, exposure to pathogen, etc.) in an attempt to demonstrate or disprove a causal relation. When events are aggregated at specific scales (neighborhood, city, state, nation, etc.) and in association with related classes of data (income, nutrition, family size, etc.), a graphically demonstrable conclusion matures that suggests potentially fruitful activities. At every step there is a balance between individual events within a class of occurrence and the context that enables or inhibits them. It is in the ecology, in understanding the relation of shared events (low-weight births) and their enablers (income, nutrition, etc.) that the hard thinking of mapping occurs.

Paradoxically, perhaps, mapping results as much from what is left out as what is included. "For a map to be readable, and useful, certain—in fact most—information needs to be excluded" (Heersink 2001, 136). The world is too full, the potential associations too numerous, to cover everything. From the start one therefore focuses, cuts, and defines the problem, then distills its elements in a way that permits what is left to be mapped. The question is always what elements are necessary to describe the determinants of this or that condition. How will these selections best describe the problem we have to consider?

These decisions are reflected in every map, each decision based on the intent of the mapper and the technologies available to the mapmaker. The intent of the mapper, who may or may not be the mapmaker, is crucial to the map that results. This should not be a surprise. All research reflects the intent of the researcher, who chooses to consider a limited set of data and then to present it in a particular fashion. Whether the data is argued in statistics, graphs, charts, or text, the nature of the task is always about the self-conscious selection and arrangement of data in the context of a hypothesis or theory.

Because maps are presumed to be representative of an objective world, however, the nature of that exclusion in service of a theory is sometimes obscured. It is therefore important to be clear that what the map is for determines everything that goes into it and all that is excluded from it. The mapped result typically will be a distillation of observed relations, not a representation; at least not in the way "representation" is typically used (Ingold 2000; Wood 1993a).[2] This is true because mapping is always the embodiment of a thesis, not a simple representation of an objective reality independent of that thesis. Medical mapping typically proposes a causal relation between selected fragments of a spatial ecology, not the ecology itself. Still, we often say a map is "a representation" (Robinson and Petchenik 1986), a two-dimensional picture of something happening in the four dimensions of our existence. This is how most people are taught to think of maps, just as they are taught to think of science as objective and, therefore, value free. It is this very objectivity, this representational ability, that some insist raises contemporary geographical information systems (GIS) mapping to the level of a "science"

(Schurmann 1999). But science is more complex than that (for example, see Lewontin 1992) and so is the process of mapping. So, too, are the maps that result.[3]

Mapping and mapmaking do not permit us to see the world in an objective fashion. Instead, they let us study interpretations of selected aspects of a spatially grounded, interrelated process. These interpretations are distilled in the abstractions we fashion as mappers, mapmakers, and as scientists. Mapping does not "provide the ability to imagine the world from 'outside'" (Hall 2003, 158), a necessity for the "objectivity" some cartographers promise. Rather, mapping puts us *inside* the world in a way that considers its constitutive relations. Nor do mapping or mapmaking "produce space" (Lefebvre 1974) in some magical way. Rather, they permit us to organize spatial events at scales that best articulate an understanding of the phenomena chosen for study. The outcome is an interpretation of the relation of things, of spatial relations between selected aspects of a dynamic ecology. The maps that result are neither the world nor an objective record of our worldly experience, but a means whereby we come to understand aspects of it. Maps embody the mapping, which is a way of making sense of health and disease in populations in the world. It is as simple and as hard as that.

Propositions

The authority of mapping resides in its relational perspective. Its power is derived from its grounded approach in which location is a principal attribute of the characterizing of events. It is as well a graphical way of thinking, in intention if not in fact, whose constituent propositions take the simple bidirectional form: "This is there" and "there is this" (Wood 2003). Mapping invites associations based on this bidirectionality: If these deaths (this) are clustered around that well (there), then that well (there) is central to these deaths (this).[4]

It is this equivalence that assures mapping presents the articulation of a relation or of relationships whose individual elements are necessarily spatial, transposed into locations (x,y) on the plane of the map. Isabella de Gracias and Mei Tang-Mu live at addresses whose coordinates locate their homes in proximity to each other in downtown east side Vancouver. The women are related locationally (geographically) by their proximity. They are related as well by their membership in the set of mothers who gave birth to low-weight babies. So, too, are other mothers living in Vancouver who gave birth to premature children in 2002 and who may be geographically related to de Gracias and Tang-Mu. When their home addresses relate them all, one to another, making of their individual experiences a range of experience, the "there" of mothers of low-birth-weight babies in the downtown east side blossoms categorically and geographically in the mapping.

The neighborhood they share is described both geographically and by attributes (physical and social) that may be contributing factors to their membership in the class of mothers of low-birth-weight babies. "There," the characteristics of the area, contribute to "this" problem that occurs within an area whose characteristics are known. The streets on which de Gracias, Tang-Mu, and the others live share common sources of water and power, a similar density of habitation, and a broadly similar general socioeconomic profile. Those qualities are part of the broader domain (the downtown east side) to which a specific range of events (premature birth of low-weight babies) is joined in an attempt to uncover causative relations. Range and domain are the "this" and "that" which are mutually defining.

What results is a "structural coupling" (Maturana and Varela 1992, 76–77) in which a history of recurrent interactions leads to a structural congruence between two or more parts of a system whose relations are identified through the process.[5] Mapping fuses the elements of these couplings in a mutually defining relationship, distills the relations within the structure, thereby reducing the mass of potentially relevant data in the search for pertinent associations. Perversely, the process embeds temporality and motility in a map that seems atemporal and motionless (Beck and Wood 1976, 214–215). In a map we may see the homes of women who gave birth to low-weight babies as if the locations were eternal, unmoving. But the women come from elsewhere, and the homes in which they now live are a base from which they travel in the greater community. Home is also a place they will leave, moving on to other apartments or homes (and perhaps other cities) across their life span. In the mapped aggregation of a time, that of these births, we ignore these facts and instead present a fiction of constancy, of a "this" and "there" that is frozen in time, as if nobody ever moved anywhere at all.

Similarly, while the map is a plane in which movement can only be suggested, motility, like time, is embedded as well. One may chart the progress of a disease around a nation or around the world in a map: West Nile virus was here in 1999, there in 2000, and moved on to that place in 2001. The travels of an individual are noted through different symbols representing movement along a mapped route. But the whole is itself out-of-time, a distillation of movement to be read as a whole in one glance. We take both the temporal and motile synchronicity for granted only at our peril. It is integral to the map's power and an element that contributes much to the map's utility in medical sciences.

When the process works, the result is transforming. The medical histories of Isabella de Gracias, Mei Tang-Mu, and fifty other women are distilled to a single class of events occurring within a specific time frame. That class is located within a domain (Vancouver's downtown east side) of city streets that is understood through a set of attributes (income, housing density, etc.) that may or may not help us understand the problem of low-weight births in that neighborhood. Mapped together, the range (this) and domain (there) are transformed into a single argument that relates the attributes of one to the characteristics of the other. The result is a testable proposition relating high incidence of low-birth-weight babies to characteristics of the downtown east side that simultaneously is defined as an area whose characteristics promote the risk of low-birth-weight infants. In other words, this is there, and there is this.

"There no longer can be any doubt that maps are propositions, that every map is an argument, and that maps shape our 'realities' in the same way those realities are influenced by conventional text" (Churchill and Slarsky 2004, 13). By arguing a relation of low-birth-weight babies and the downtown east side, one proposes a relation, at another level, between socioeconomic characteristics of the area as factors contributing to the incidence of occurrence in that area. If the maps shape our reality through the testing of relational propositions in this process of structural coupling, they do so only within a broader frame of the assumptions and suppositions of medical theories explaining disease and differing states of health. That is, propositions occur only within a theory of health and disease, which determine each proposition to be argued or the policy to be considered in addressing a disease outbreak.

Histories

The relation between theory and scientific proposition is generally accepted in medical history and sociology, but often ignored by those considering medical mapping. Those who promote mapping as a tool of discovery say that historically "mapping made scientific discovery available to all" (Jenkins 2001). They argue that the map's ability to analyze and articulate locational data in an easily comprehensible fashion facilitated a more popular understanding of complex issues of disease and health. But the importance of mapping to the process of scientific thinking, and especially medical thinking, is less commonly considered. The very accessibility of maps, some argue, came at the price of the statistical rigor that is the hallmark of contemporary medical science. Because of this, many assume the *real* thinking, the hard thinking about health and disease is not done by mapping but through statistical manipulation. Map*making* is just a way to display statistical interpretation of the relation between a pathogen and a host.

Nothing could be further from the truth. From their coterminous beginnings, medical mapping and medical statistics have always shared a common intellectual base. While many today think of mapping as no more than a way to illustrate statistical conclusions, the truth is that "the interplay between figures [maps] and texts is critical to the understanding of [scientific] papers. Each needs the other to tell the story" (Cockerill 2003, A2–3). Mapping and statistics both use graphic presentations: the map, the table, and the graph. Both seek to create categories of meaning from the sets of data they consider. Each in its own way proposes a relation between those sets and then tests the validity of that proposition. Statisticians may analyze mapped relations just as mappers may present statistical relations. Either way, the real question has always been *what* data is to be correlated and *how* they relate to elements that may encourage or discourage this or that phenomenon.

Medical mapping and medical statistics are both a part of the story of the slow progression of medical science and its struggle to understand the nature of disease and its presence within this or that society. Both developed not apart from, but within, the context of a broader medical science and the society that supported its attempt to confront the realities of endemic and epidemic disease. Mapping, statistics, and the sciences that they support grew not separate from, but as part of, the great transformation of a Hippocratic and Galenic medical tradition to one that defined states of disease and health in relatively modern terms.[6] One can't seek to understand the one without understanding the others.

The result is richer than the existing literature suggests and richer, too, than I expected when this project began in 2002. I then assumed, as does much of the literature, that medical mapping was a mid-nineteenth century phenomenon that arose almost spontaneously in the work of an adventurous, brilliant researcher or two. But genius is rarely fostered in a vacuum. The advances of nineteenth century medical mapping were real, but their reality was the continuation of a history that preceded them and prepared their way. Mapping did not arise full-blown in the nineteenth century any more than did bacteriology or virology in the twentieth century.

In struggling to understand the course of medical mapping through the range of maps that trace its history, the importance of mapping and printing technology is underscored. The history of medical mapping is the story not simply of medical progress but of progress in map*making* as well. Just as clinical medicine progressed through the introduction of specific instruments (the microscope, sphygmomanometer, stethoscope, thermometer, etc.), mapping developed through evolving technologies of production and distribution. Etched plates became copperplates that became lithographs. Hand presses became mechanized, their speed improved, and new printing technologies became ever-more capable of reproducing detailed graphics, first in black and white and then in color. More complex maps were produced and, just as important, could be shared.

Evolving computer technologies have permitted ever-more complex mapping and ever-more robust statistics not "out of time" but in time, within the history this book describes. They are twinned from the start, and the current "revolution" in Web-based data facilitating computer-based mapping is no more (but surely no less) than a next step in the conjoined evolution of mapping and statistics in service of medical knowledge.

But the real subject of this volume is not technological but conceptual. Its focus is the type of thinking that mapping promotes, and the ways of thinking that mapping brings to the study of disease. Because this book is about mapping as a way of thinking rather than simply a way of presenting, its lessons are generally rather than specifically applicable. Disease and health are my passion, my interest, and mapping is an approach I use in my work. But map *thinking* is a self-consciously intellectual approach to a startling congress of problems. To the extent this book serves its immediate subject, it offers a more general model informative to those whose interest may involve the potential of mapping in other areas. For this reason, the book is neither a simple primer in medical cartography nor an introduction to the epidemiology of infectious disease. It is for people in the health sciences interested in mapping and map thinking, and for those expert in maps and mapmaking interested in the study of health and disease.

The goal, therefore, is (there is no better way of saying this) to map the struggle to understand health and disease ecologies from the late 1600s to the present. Chapter by chapter a range of mapped events (plague, yellow fever, cholera, typhus, etc.) is considered within the concrete, interlocking domains of their occurrence. These are variously defined, study by study, as clinical, economic, geographic, scientific, and social. The general intellectual environment in which the resulting distillation occurred was the medical science of the day, a science that maps both presented and contributed to. What results is an understanding of disease and health as ecological outcomes in which we are always active and complicit.

While this promises to be a study of the cartographies of health *and* disease, the majority of its maps are disease-related. The reason is that for most of the last three hundred years the vast majority of maps made in service of medical knowledge have been of epidemic or pandemic conditions that were a signal threat to the lives and health of thousands, and in some cases millions of people. Indeed, where it has been considered as an independent state, health has historically been defined as the absence of chronic or acute disease. Thus, the promotion of health has typically been seen as the absence of conditions that create this or that disease, not a state whose own properties could be easily and independently defined.

Special attention is given here, as it is in most medical mapping textbooks, to the mapping of one disease: cholera. For a variety of reasons, this was the most frequently mapped scourge of the nineteenth century, the modeling of which became the paradigm for other, later disease studies. The central figure in this period was Dr. John Snow, whose mapping of cholera in 1854 London is typically described as the Archimedian point of medical mapping, and not coincidentally, of epidemiology and public health (Vinten-Johansen et al. 2003, 392–399). It is the point after which nothing was the same, a fulcrum balancing a medical prehistory (the old way) with what came afterward (our way). Seminal as it was, however, Snow's work was only an event within a series of events, a point on a timeline that preceded him and continued into our time. Because so much has been written about Snow and the epidemics he studied, the chapters on Snow serve to organize a great deal of the story of our knowing as told through maps of disease and health. The importance of his studies lies not in his maps alone but more precisely in the manner he mapped—conceptually and graphically—a typography of disease that was graphic, concrete, comprehensible, and scientific.

Previous authors have typically ordered their studies of mapping and historical mapping either cartographically or "thematically" (Robinson 1982). Cartographic maps locate the incidence of disease (or the locus of its vectors) with dot-like symbols (points), in networks of incidence and diffusion (lines), or within areas of administrative jurisdiction (polygons). Others have assumed a map's subject would serve a taxonomy clearly placing it in a single thematic category (maps of diffusion, location, jurisdiction, resource, etc.). These categories are too limiting and artificial, saying more about the researcher than the subject at hand.

Because maps are ecological and relational, most share a range of cartographic symbol sets: points, lines, and aereal markers. For example, the incidence of low-weight births (points) occur among people who live on streets (lines) they traverse daily across neighborhoods with socioeconomic profiles (polygons). To separate these elements is to sunder the relevant relations, the very tale the map seeks

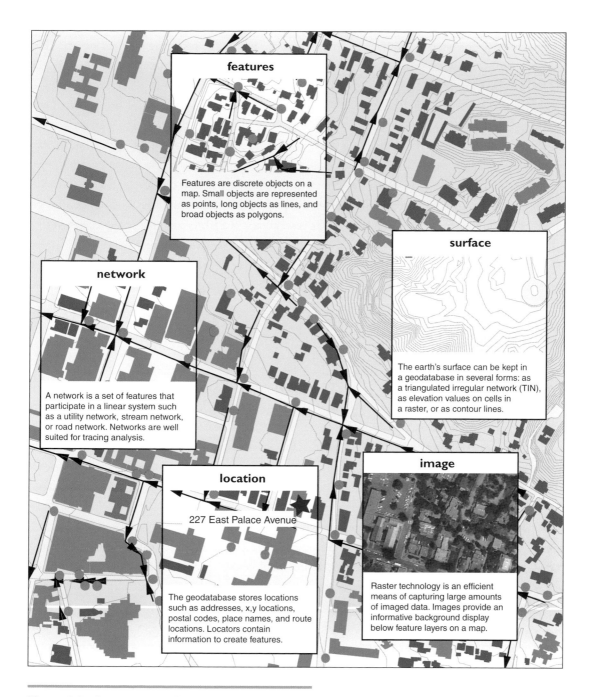

features

Features are discrete objects on a map. Small objects are represented as points, long objects as lines, and broad objects as polygons.

surface

The earth's surface can be kept in a geodatabase in several forms: as a triangulated irregular network (TIN), as elevation values on cells in a raster, or as contour lines.

network

A network is a set of features that participate in a linear system such as a utility network, stream network, or road network. Networks are well suited for tracing analysis.

location

227 East Palace Avenue

The geodatabase stores locations such as addresses, x,y locations, postal codes, place names, and route locations. Locators contain information to create features.

image

Raster technology is an efficient means of capturing large amounts of imaged data. Images provide an informative background display below feature layers on a map.

Figure 1.1 A taxonomy of mapped elements within a complex map environment. All work together to create a single argument, a proposition relating elements fused within an environment of connecting pathways that are cohesive and dynamic.

Source: Courtesy of the city of Santa Fe, New Mexico.

to tell. It is in the conjunction of locational feature, dynamic network, and general neighborhood that a map does all its work. To argue one to the exclusion of all others does no justice to the mapmaker's thinking or the resulting map itself.

It is not that symbolization and the specific content that symbols organize are not important. They are. So, too, is the general idea embedded in a thematic category, one that declares a researcher's specific topical concern. But symbolization and categorical choices are strategies of our knowing, not the knowing itself. The importance of medical mapping resides in the medicine being mapped, the relations being argued, and the thinking about states of disease and health the mapped result distills. And so this book is organized instead as a history ordered by the chronology of the slow advance of the medicine that individual maps served. This greater chronology asserts its own order upon the subject of both technologies of map distribution and production as well as the arguments individual maps present. And that, perhaps, is this project's most important lesson: mapping is important because it advances knowing. It is the science, and the way maps serve it, which should be our focus as new diseases and new health problems are confronted.

End notes

1. Isabella de Gracias and Mei Tang-Mu are fictitious examples used here for illustrative purposes. But the issue of low-birth-weight infants and the relation between economic status, age, parental history, etc., to the incidence of low-weight births is a real problem and one much discussed in the medical literature. And, of course, issues of socioeconomic disadvantage in Vancouver's downtown east side are similarly subjects of topical discussion and concern in Vancouver and its health provider organizations.

2. Against the traditional insistence by cartographers and geographers that mapping is representative is the work of the new or critical geographers (Lemann 2001), who in the 1990s were busy rewriting the history of mapping as a socially interpretative process. Details on the debate over mapping as a socially constructed rather than objectively representative process are best found in Tim Ingold (2000, 223–235) and in various writings in Denis Wood's oeuvre over the last fifteen years.

3. Whether mapping—whatever the technology—is a discipline, a tool, or a science depends, of course, on how one distinguishes science from other modes of knowing. For the flavor of the literature see, for example, Schurmann (1999); Wright, Goodchild, and Proctor (1997); Goodchild (1994); and Pickles (1997).

4. The idea of this equivalence and the propositional nature of mapping generally is based on work by Denis Wood (2003), especially work in collaboration with John Fels. Wood made available drafts of papers that advance their thesis but which at the time of this writing remained in review and not in press.

5. Maturana and Varela define history through an exploration of this process of structural coupling. Wood (2004a, 64–65) uses their phrase and more generally their approach to describe the manner and degree people are related in and through a shared environment—historical and modern—at every level.

6. This is a history told and retold by historians of science and of medicine. Those seeking popular, nontechnical, introductory texts in this area are referred to Porter's *The Greatest Benefit to Mankind* (1998) and Nuland's *Doctors: The Biography of Medicine* (1989).

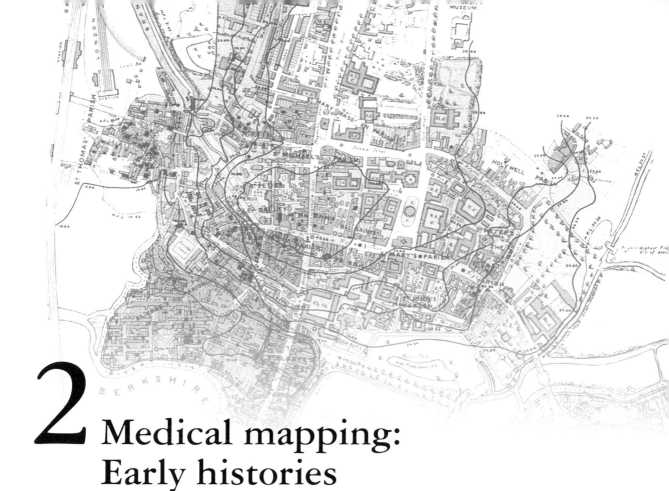

2 Medical mapping: Early histories

Epidemic disease

We are all double agents in the war against disease, encouraging its propagation while simultaneously fighting its diffusion. The communities we build, the technologies that enable them to function, and the commerce that sustains them assure environments favorable to the advance of our microbial friends and sometimes enemies. In a real way, medical science plays catch-up with the health problems we create in our evolving society; its advances are a response to the diseases we foster through economic, environmental, and social choices. It is no accident that medical mapping blossomed in the nineteenth century during a period of vastly increasing international trade and emigration, or that its renaissance began in the 1990s during a new era of globalization. In the early-to-mid-nineteenth and late twentieth centuries, similar elements coalesced to advance simultaneously a range of epidemic and chronic diseases as well as the mechanisms by which they might be understood. Medical mapping was a part of that process of understanding.

It is not simply that "multitudes of bacteria and viruses occupy our skin, our mucus membranes and our intestinal tracks, and we must learn to live with them in a 'truce' rather than victory" (Lederberg 2003, 20). That is true but insufficient. More centrally, new viruses and bacteria find our bodies habitable because of the lives we lead in cultures whose physical conditions are favorable to their generation, development, and diffusion. "Rarely, if ever, do emerging infections appear without reason" (Morse 1999, 39). What Morse calls the "microbial traffic" by which infectious agents transmit disease from animals to humans, or disseminate it into new populations, is well understood (McNeill 1976). These include a population density sufficient to support their growth, travel vectors permitting the agent to move to new populations, and environmental factors in those population areas that create a hospitable environment for microbial evolution.

"Travel and trade set the stage for mixing diverse genetic pools at rates and in combinations previously unknown" (Wilson 1999). In the late twentieth century, massive emigration and immigration fueled urbanization worldwide during a period of self-consciously intense globalization. Both goods and the people employed to create them traveled internationally at an ever-increasing rate. That exchange of goods and people contributed to a context that encouraged the evolution of a range of diseases for which human environments served as hospitable reservoirs.[1] It is no accident that "since the 1970s, there have been thirty-plus new diseases that have emerged. We also have old diseases that are reappearing where they've been eliminated, or appearing where they've never been before" (Dotto 2003, F7).

Something very similar occurred in the late eighteenth through the mid-nineteenth centuries. Massive migration by agricultural workers to the industrializing city and emigration from industrialized Europe (and later Asia) to the developing New World created an environment that favored the emergence and diffusion of a range of infectious diseases: cholera, syphilis, tuberculosis, typhoid, yellow fever, and others. In what is today called the "Great Migration," more than five million people moved from Europe to the Americas (Guillet 1963). In 1832 alone, decades before the migration peaked, more than fifty thousand emigrants—the majority from Great Britain—crossed the Atlantic to Canada and the United States (Hansen 1961).

It was, in Robert Boyd's memorable title, *The Coming of the Spirit of Pestilence* (Boyd 1999), that expanded the range of then local diseases to a global field of exchange. It was not simply that some ships traveled with people infected with a disease before they left their homeport for another. That happened, and when it did the results for passengers on those vessels were disastrous. As important, however, is the fact that nineteenth-century ships sailed with a cohort of fellow travelers—rats and insects—agents of a host of bacterial and parasitic diseases. Rodents, insects, and mites all found a welcome environment in first the emigrant ships and later the cities where their ships would eventually dock.

Greater and greater numbers of minimally paid workers poured into ever-more densely settled cities to operate the machines and staff the myriad jobs that made the cities work. There, emerging industrial centers typically bereft of even minimal standards of sanitation, protected water supplies, or adequate systems of sewage disposal assured that diseases that might otherwise have died for want of a hospitable environment would flourish. In this way, endemic diseases previously rooted in specific local communities became epidemic and sometimes pandemic.

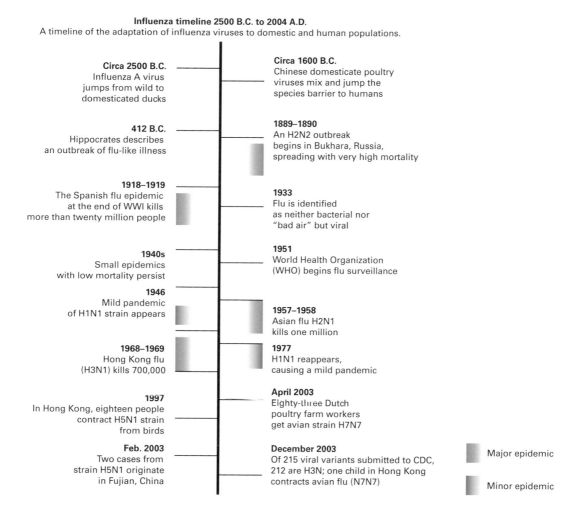

Influenza timeline 2500 B.C. to 2004 A.D.
A timeline of the adaptation of influenza viruses to domestic and human populations.

Circa 2500 B.C.
Influenza A virus
jumps from wild to
domesticated ducks

Circa 1600 B.C.
Chinese domesticate poultry
viruses mix and jump the
species barrier to humans

412 B.C.
Hippocrates describes
an outbreak of flu-like illness

1889–1890
An H2N2 outbreak
begins in Bukhara, Russia,
spreading with very high mortality

1918–1919
The Spanish flu epidemic
at the end of WWI kills
more than twenty million people

1933
Flu is identified
as neither bacterial nor
"bad air" but viral

1940s
Small epidemics
with low mortality persist

1951
World Health Organization
(WHO) begins flu surveillance

1946
Mild pandemic
of H1N1 strain appears

1957–1958
Asian flu H2N1
kills one million

1968–1969
Hong Kong flu
(H3N1) kills 700,000

1977
H1N1 reappears,
causing a mild pandemic

1997
In Hong Kong, eighteen people
contract H5N1 strain
from birds

April 2003
Eighty-three Dutch
poultry farm workers
get avian strain H7N7

Feb. 2003
Two cases from
strain H5N1 originate
in Fujian, China

December 2003
Of 215 viral variants submitted to CDC,
212 are H3N; one child in Hong Kong
contracts avian flu (N7N7)

Major epidemic

Minor epidemic

Figure 2.1 Influenza timeline.

Source: Adapted from Lewis (2004, 19).

The history of disease is one in which specific, environmental conditions give rise to reservoirs of evolving bacteria and viruses that diffuse along vectors of animal and human migration. Those reservoirs are typically urban, the unhealthy city where sufficient populations exist to permit a disease to first develop and from which it can then spread. This is an old story, one older than the maps in this volume, a tale as old as human settlement itself. Porter takes "the era of epidemics" back to 3000 B.C. and its populated cities (Babylon, for example) that rose in Mesopotamia and Egypt, in the Indus Valley, and in China in the valley of the Yangtze, the Yellow River. "Such settlements often maintained huge cattle herds, from which lethal pathogens, including smallpox, spread to humans, while originally zoognostic conditions—diptheria, influenza, chicken-pox, mumps—and other illnesses also had a devastating impact" (Porter, R. 1998, 22).

To take a single example, influenza is believed to have originated among domesticated fowl in China, mutating no later than 1600 B.C. into a strain that affected humans (Lewis 2004). The virus jumped from poultry to humans living in cities—China was the most urbanized nation of that age—and spread from there throughout the world. By 412 B.C. the disease was in the Mediterranean where Hippocrates described an epidemic outbreak. Influenza then slowly diffused with travelers along trade routes to lodge in other cities and towns where the population was sufficient to sustain it as an endemic disease. Over time it has evolved as our civilizations have matured, adapting to the environments we create.

From the start, cities meant density—of humans and the commingled animal species that sustain us—conditions ripe for the evolution of bacteria and viruses whose effect on humankind (and sometimes, animals, as well) could be disastrous. Human trade and travel—to the market, to the Crusades, or simply to another village—were the vectors by which the bacteria and viruses were transported to new populations. In the earliest histories, the diffusion of disease was limited by the paucity of environments

Mean pop.	Never infected (percentage)	Infected once (percentage)	Infected twice (percentage)	Infected three times (percentage)
92	80	20	0	0
257	51	32	17	0
352	50	33	14	0
603	31	32	32	5
784	21	39	35	5
1,059	15	34	46	2
1,465	7	25	61	7
2,373	5	15	64	15

Figure 2.2 Relationship between plague infection and population in India. Rows do not all total 100 percent because figures exclude percentage of population infected four or more times.

Source: Adapted from Twigg (1984, 186).

sufficiently large to serve as reservoirs, breeding grounds. As city sizes increased, and travel linked them, new opportunities for evolving diseases emerged.

The rate of infection and re-infection for plague in the Middle Ages, for example, was directly proportional to the size of a village or town's population: "Plague could maintain itself in towns but not to any extent in villages unless they were large" (Twigg 1984, 187). The shift from village to town and town to city in the nineteenth century assured that diseases that earlier would have occurred only sporadically, or been locally endemic, became epidemic, and in some cases, pandemic. Trade and migration that tied together the commerce of nations, were the vehicles that carried diseases between communities either by sea in sailing ships or over land by horse and horse-drawn carriage.

Plague: Bari, Naples, 1690–1692

It is appropriate that this history begins with a map of plague, a disease so pervasive and traumatic, so fearfully deadly that "it has transcended itself to become emblematic of something more invasive and apocalyptic than mere infection" (Marriott 2003, 10). In what is now thought of as its first pandemic, plague appeared first in China and then took almost a century to make its way through Asia and the Middle East to wreak havoc in the Mediterranean. The second pandemic occurred in the Middle Ages and may have appreciably hastened their conclusion. Again it was neither uniquely Asian nor European but pandemic, a global progression. The population of China was almost halved, dropping from 123 million people in 1200 to 65 million in 1239 (Marriott 2003, 10). In Europe the "Black Death," also called the "Oriental Plague" by some nineteenth-century medical researchers, was no less devastating. "Within a couple of years, plague killed around a quarter of Europe's population—and far more in some towns; the largest number of fatalities caused by a single epidemic disaster in the history of Europe. Thousands of villages were abandoned, and by 1427 Florence's population had plummeted by 60 percent from over 100,000 to about 38,000" (Porter, R. 1998, 123).

Plague returned in the 1600s when it again pervasively attacked much of Europe. While endemic, with localized outbreaks in cities like London every few decades (Tomalin 2002, 167), the greater pandemic of the mid-1600s was ferocious. Its devastating effect can be read in "Bills of Mortality" compiled in England by clerks who recorded the names and parishes of plague victims. For a grave to be registered, a parish scribe had to list a cause of death and the name, by local parish, of the deceased. In this way, the clerks created what might be thought of as the first official databases of disease incidence aggregated to an administrative unit.

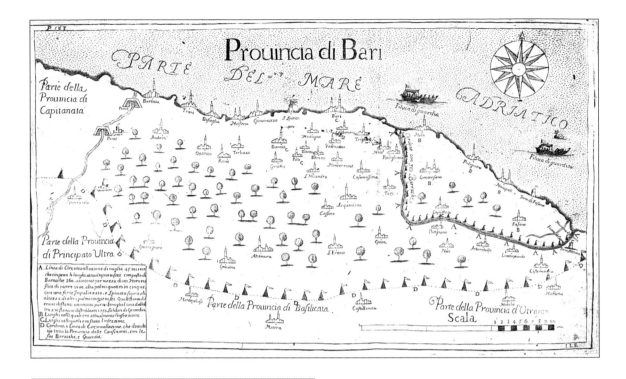

Figure 2.3 Map of the plague in 1690–1692 in the province of Bari, 1694, by Filippo Arrieta. The map shows areas most affected and the boundaries of a military quarantine imposed to prevent its spread to neighboring towns and other provinces.

Source: New York Academy of Medicine Library.

Nobody knew what caused the disease or sustained its diffusion. Sometimes an outbreak could be contained and sometimes, despite all efforts, the disease spread across provinces, countries, and continents. Some believed it a punishment on humankind for its multitude of sins; others insisted it resulted from the unfavorable conjunction of planets in the sky. Within the science of the day, steeped in the work of Hippocrates and Galen, there was a general assumption of a sickness in the air, a "pestitential atmosphere" arising from the effluvia of the city itself. Whatever plague was, what was known was that once it appeared it spread rapidly, decimating cities and towns, provinces and nations, almost beyond repair.

Two extraordinary maps of this period have survived in a single, book-length report on an outbreak of plague in the province of Bari in what was then the kingdom of Naples (Arrieta 1694). The author, Filippo Arrieta, was royal auditor for the province under the military governor of Bari and its neighboring provinces, Basilicata and Capitanata. Together the maps tell us much about the medicine and medical cartography of this period. They say a great deal as well about the assumptions and preconceptions of modern historians who have in recent years considered the mapping of this period.

In a seminal article on disease mapping and the beginnings of medical cartography, for example, Jarcho (1970, 131–142) considered the first map reproduced here as a predecessor of later and more rigorous disease maps. In it he identified two cordons, one forty-five miles in length and composed of 360 barracks enclosing the towns of Monopoli, Conversano, and Castellano where the infection was present and another, longer cordon (circumvallation) separating the province from its neighbors, Capitanata, Basilica, and Otranto. "Isolation was completed on the costal side by feluccas, two of which are shown on the map" (Jarcho 1970, 132).

For Jarcho, the map was a curiosity, an "interesting and attractive" example of medical mapping more notable for its survival—most maps of the seventeenth century have perished—than its content. And certainly, the quaintness of the hand-drawn symbols made it easy, perhaps too easy, to dismiss the artifact as intellectually trivial. This was especially true for those like Jarcho who assumed such maps were primitive representations rather than mapped distillations of complex processes. Thus, he sees the two feluccas as representations of specific coastal ships—"two of which are shown on the map"—rather than symbols of a naval blockade symbolized generically.

It is an understandable if unfortunate mistake. To a modern cartographer the map suggested a crude and undeveloped mapmaking that should be disdained for anything but its quaintness. The symbols (churches, hospitals, trees, boats) were drawn in childish profile while the coastline and boundaries were rotated and oblique (Wood 1992a, 174–178). Towns and cities were symbolized by drawings of simplified buildings, churches (with a cross), or hospitals (without) where the ill were typically taken for treatment or burial. A "C" distinguished towns where the outbreak had occurred but was passed from those "B" towns where the infection was active. Between the towns, trees symbolized if not rural then non-urban areas of the province.[2]

Despite the crudeness of its symbology, the map was more involved—intellectually and graphically—than Jarcho realized. Within it can be seen a complex series of four levels of containment designed to prevent the spread of the plague. The coastal patrol symbolized by the feluccas (*feluca di guardio*) served both to contain the area of active disease and to prevent shipping to more westerly towns where the plague had been active. On land, a dark wall with the repeated letter "A" along a *linea di circonvallazione* separated the area of active plague from western neighbors (noted by a "C") where the plague had been active, and from southerly areas where it had yet to appear. On top of the wall are tents symbolizing the location of troops stationed at quarter-mile intervals to enforce the quarantine.

Within the district of active plague was a third containment level that was ten miles in circumference, marked with a "B," and described in the legend but not symbolized in the map. These individual districts separated towns free of plague but susceptible to it (Mola, Polignano, Fasno, etc.) from others in the district where plague was active or had recently been active. These inner cordons were enforced by the deployment of 250 soldiers from fifty barracks, troops living in the town and charged with their protection. Finally, the map included a general, provincial cordon "D" separating Bari province from its neighbors. Here, too, the quarantine was enforced by troops whose tents are used to symbolize their presence. The military cost of deploying 1,750 troops stationed at 350 barracks was considerable, as Arrieta's text makes clear.

The map distills the details of a major military operation designed to halt or at least slow the spread of plague, one that reflects a real understanding of the disease's typical pattern of diffusion. Levels of containment separated the province from its neighbors ("D"), districts where plague had been ("C") from those where outbreaks were active, and insulated individual towns still plague-free from those where it was evident ("B"). The map reflects a surprisingly modern approach to disease containment.

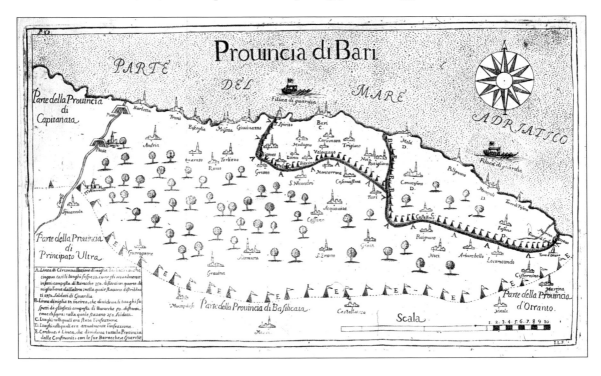

Figure 2.4 Map of plague containment zones in 1690–1692 in the province of Bari, Italy, 1694. Tents represent troop deployments on provincial borders, zones of active plague and those where plague had already occurred.

Source: New York Academy of Medicine Library.

This modern approach is clearer in a second map (figure 2.4), one not discussed by Jarcho (1970). In this second map there are two walled areas, one around the north central area of the province where the plague was active ("D"), and a second ("C") around Bari and nearby towns where the disease had earlier appeared. The broader containment area ("E") is province wide, one separating Bari from its provincial neighbors. In modern terms (Haggett 2000, 98–103), the whole map describes an interlocking series of quarantine buffers designed to separate areas of infection and thus slow the rate of plague's progression. Inherent in the map is a theory of the disease, one based on its past activity, contemporary pattern of occurrence, and known potential for diffusion.

In 1694, medicine in the Hippocratic tradition was about observing nature, not probing for its secrets (Barry 2004, 16). Plague (like other diseases) just was, its periodic outbreaks a fearsome given whose cause was acceptably unknown. The science of the day was capable of various explanations of its nature but incapable of a means either to effectively treat or to prevent its occurrence. What health and administrative officials had was a knowledge of past outbreaks—where they had occurred, the pattern of their diffusion, and the damage they had caused—and a conviction that containment might halt or at least slow plague's progression through the province and kingdom. Embedded in the map is a tight argument linking the history of plague's previous occurrences (the basis for containment), the limits of medical science (no treatment but a general etiology), and the social structure of the greater community (civil, military, medical, and religious). Containment strategies were conceived and carried out with attention to all.

That Arrieta's maps of plague in Bari are a rare example of seventeenth century medical mapping does not mean such mapping was a rarity in that age. Nothing in his text trumpets the map as an innovation. Indeed, the maps are included as commonplace distillations of the administrative program, the *cordon sanitaire* for which troops were carefully deployed. The provincial coastline and boundaries were administrative familiars; the map's symbolization presents a sense not of the new but of the commonplace. It is not simply the scale bar and the compass rose but the legend, too, that insists the map was an accepted analytic approach to disease containment studies for Arrieta and his contemporaries. The symbolization—feluccas for coastal patrol, tents for the army deployed, trees for the countryside, and churches or large buildings for the town—were not cartographic experiments but regular and accepted symbols of the cartographic age.

It is worth noting that the approach to disease containment argued in these two maps was thoroughly modern. Into the twentieth century, officials faced with any number of epidemic outbreaks would struggle with the idea of quarantine and how it might best be carried out. Where attempted in the nineteenth century, quarantines of towns and regions were typically half-hearted, attempted with either a simple roadblock or the isolation of an infected ship in a harbor. The idea of a system of multiple buffers separating affected from at-risk areas was an idea that eventually reemerged, in a more sophisticated form, only after World War II with modern studies of disease diffusion (Haggett 2000, 99–102).

With the appearance of first Legionnaires' disease, human immunodeficiency (HIV) in the 1980s, and bovine spongiform encephalopathy (BSE) in the 1990s, issues and protocols of quarantine again became a subject of national and international debate. These became more heated with the appearance of severe acute respiratory system (SARS) and avian flu outbreaks in 2003 and 2004. Those experiences give Arrieta's maps and writing a contemporary pertinence they lacked for Jarcho, for whom the maps were of a solely antiquarian interest.

But then, in the late 1960s, many administrators and medical researchers believed infectious diseases were largely controlled; therefore, there was little interest in historical approaches to epidemic outbreaks. Infectious disease studies were a relatively unpopular specialty in medical schools where the assumption was that, unlike other times in human history, "in the battle of man against microbe, man was winning" (Verghese 1995, 26). The conclusion that we therefore had little to learn from past battles (the war metaphors abound here) colored the interpretation of the historical maps and the thinking embedded in them. In an era in which epidemic disease is again an acknowledged threat, this early example of the mapping of disease incidence and containment takes on a new import that is thoroughly modern.

Eighteenth century

Almost surely other maps were drawn in the seventeenth and early eighteenth centuries. There are records of some, reports and descriptions, but the maps themselves have not survived. Most that were topical appear to have been drawn, as were the Bari province maps, at a local or regional scale. But then, trade and political responsibility in those days was typically regional—market area to market area—rather than continental or international. The scale of the map reflects the scale of the society it describes. An exception reflecting the first stirrings of internationalism (and international trade) was Leonhard Ludwig Finke's 1792 "Nosological Map of the World" drawn for but not published in his three-volume *Versuch einer allgemeinen medicinisch-praktischen Geographie....* The more complete, if still somewhat abridged, title translates as "Notes on General Practical Medical Geography... Dealing with the History of Medical Science and Pharmacology of the Indigenous Population of the Varying States of Germany." An ambitious work, it attempted to describe a broad topography of disease relating a taxonomy of observed diseases and the pharmacology of their treatment to the peoples affected by them. This was, perhaps, the first use of the phrase "medical geography," one advanced by Finke in this way: "When one brings together all which is worth knowing with regard to the medical status of any country, then no one can deny that such a work describes the name of a 'medical geography'" (Howe 1961, 9).

Leonhard Ludwig Finke,

der Arzeney-Gelahrtheit Doctor und Profeſſor zu Lingen,

Verſuch

einer allgemeinen mediciniſch-praktiſchen

Geographie,

worin

der hiſtoriſche Theil der einheimiſchen

Völker- und Staaten-Arzeneykunde

vorgetragen wird.

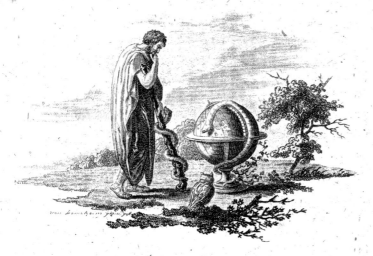

Erſter Band,

welcher die Länder enthält, die ſich vom 45ten Grade, ſo wohl
nördlicher als ſüdlicher Breite, bis zur Linie erſtrecken.

Leipzig,

in der Weidmannſchen Buchhandlung, 1792.

Figure 2.5 Front page of Finke's *Medical Geography*, 1792.

Source: Wellcome Library, London.

Unfortunately, the map is lost if, in fact, it ever existed. Finke wrote that while he made the map, it was not included in the original text "because I was afraid that the work would become too expensive" (Barrett 2000b, 917). At the end of the seventeenth century the cost of textual production was relatively high. The cost of graphic reproduction was, for Finke, simply prohibitive. "I do have it ready but have not sent it to be printed and I think it will not be printed soon" (Barrett 2000b, 917). It would be a century before new printing technologies reduced the onerous expense of including even the most basic map in a private publication, and decades more before it could be done inexpensively. By the time that occurred there would be new diseases to study, new epidemics to fear.

Much of the thinking about disease in this era assumed a type of environmental determinism that was geographically specific. The general assumption was, as the German physician Hoffman put it in 1746, that endemic diseases were the result of "a fixed and static cause essential to the country, and that they therefore remain in the country without change and variation for many years" (Howe 1963, 8). The problem was that with the stirrings of colonialism and international trade, those distant, presumably static diseases were to become mobile and dynamic. British troops stationed in the evolving empire would be subject to illnesses not seen before at home, diseases that some would transport back to England when their tours were ended.

Thus, as early as 1771, British physicians were turning their attention to conditions that, while unknown in England, were endemic in nations like India where British subjects were garrisoned and to which British ships sailed. In the United States, at the founding of the Philadelphia College of Physicians in 1787, home of the then new nation's first medical library, the goal was the advancement of the science of medicine through "investigating the diseases and remedies which are peculiar to our country; by observing the effects of different seasons, climates, and situation upon the human body" (Mitman and Numbers 2003, 393). Within a decade, Philadelphia researchers like Samuel Latham Mitchell, founder and editor of the *Medical Repository*, a critical medical journal of the day, would be writing explicitly about a "medical geography" that, like Finke's, linked place and health together (Mitman and Numbers 2003, 393). In this period, mapping became a tool that considered the relation between the environmental conditions that might be generative of this or that illness and the incidence of disease itself (Howe 1963, 9).[3] It did this through the mapped consideration of the "situation upon the body" of those made ill by epidemic or endemic diseases assumed to be generated by specific local conditions whose origins could also be mapped.

Yellow fever

One of the first diseases to begin the march from its locus "there" to a mercantile nation's "here" was yellow fever. In the late 1700s, eastern U.S. cities were struck with ferocious epidemics that killed thousands of citizens. In 1793, approximately 10 percent of Philadelphia's population perished in an epidemic; in 1798, more than three thousand people died from the disease in a four-month period in that city (Shannon 1981). Thousands more succumbed in cities like Baltimore and New York City. Because these outbreaks typically occurred in the vicinity of city docks, some assumed the disease somehow was imported on ships. In the language of the day they were "anticontagionists" who thought humans somehow transmitted the illness interpersonally. The theory required that disease be perceived as something unseen but distinct, an "animalcule" but undetectable and presumably living microscopic agent specific to a disease and responsible for transmitting it from person to person. It was this invisible agent that visitors carried to the city from foreign parts, anticontagionists believed, an import accompanying the increase of trade in sailing ships.

This was a radical, minority view that flew in the face of classical medical theories, the Hippocratic and Galenic vision that had served medicine for centuries. It was, after all, Hippocrates who, in a translation by Adams still cited in the 1960s by Howe (1963, 7), directed "whoever wishes to investigate medicine properly" to proceed "first, to consider the season in which a disease occurs" and "then the winds, the hot and the cold, especially such as are common to all countries, and then such as are peculiar to each locality." It was in the local climate and the winds, the water and the very air, Hippocrates said, that the conditions permitting a specific illness might be found. The good news, most believed, was this meant that diseases were static, anchored to the local winds and airs, not independent and portable.

People were therefore susceptible to different illnesses at different times of the year. Everyone knew, for example, that colds and flu were rampant in the damp winter, fevers in the summer. Why not assume the seasonably cold and warm airs, those that were wet or damp, were at least partially responsible? Opposed to this perspective, one supported by tradition and theory that seemed experientially self-evident, the anticontagionists labored under a significant burden. There was no visible evidence to support their theory of causation by an unseen, invisible agent. In the absence of a microscope of sufficient power, the advance of invisible and malevolent animalcules as a causative agent was perceived by most as fanciful, and those who advanced the argument were treated as fanatics.[4]

In the late eighteenth century, the majority of medical personnel believed in the established wisdom that foul air, "miasms," arising from excrement, decaying vegetable matter, marshy soils or stagnant water" gave rise to disease (Forry 1841, 39; Mitman and Numbers 2003, 393). "It was accepted that these emanations were more preponderant and dangerous in some geographical areas than others," with lowland, swamp, and marsh more odiferous and, therefore, more dangerous than elevated areas where the smell was more pristine (Bhattacharya 2003, 299). In the evolving port city aggressively dedicated to trade, good air was typically found on higher ground away from the harbor while foul airs were assumed to congregate at dockside, where urban refuse fermented on the local riverbanks.

Once bad air was inhaled, it brought the disease into the body either through the processes of "exhalation" or "contagion" (Shannon 1981).[5] The former was the product of the stench of rotting vegetables and animal materials that when inhaled at a distance of three hundred to four hundred yards gave rise to disease. Contagion described infection from foul airs at closer proximity. In closed spaces, the smell of many bodies and no sanitation was equally severe, a potent explanation for the many deaths that often occurred in the tenements of the urban poor. For evidence there was the stench itself, a clearly unhealthy and unpleasant odor, that everyone could perceive. "The 'sense of smelling,' as the noted Philadelphia physician Benjamin Rush termed it in 1805, 'was thus a powerful tool in understanding and interpreting human relationship to the environment' (Valenčius, 2000, 136), and of the environment to disease.

All this seemed to explain the yellow fever epidemic nicely and without reference to anticontagionist theories. Medical investigators pointed to another hard piece of evidence for those who found the evidence of their own senses insufficient. The incidence of yellow fever was proximate to the observed source of the noxious odors. For contagionists, demonstration of that relationship in space was a clear triumph of the science of their day, mapped proof of the workings of the traditional theory of disease arising from foul air that pollutes both home and neighborhood.

Yellow fever was a fearsome disease, and the panic it caused is understandable, even today. "The illness begins with fever, chills, and muscle pain so intense it can feel as if a leg or an arm has been broken in two" (Spielman and D'Antonio 2001, 58). Blood oozes from the mouth and nose as internal hemorrhaging sends blood into the stomach, the cause of the telltale black vomit. Death typically followed. A fatal, mysterious, ugly, violent disease, yellow fever was the logical focus of medical investigation, and Philadelphia, the new nation's busiest port and arguably its more important city, the logical place for those studies to be undertaken.

Valentine Seaman, a surgeon at New York Hospital and a pioneer in nursing education, investigated the yellow fever outbreak in his city (Stevenson 1965). In a fifty-two-page monograph (1796a), an article in the then new journal, *Medical Repository* (1798), and another in a book on "bilious fevers" by Noah Webster (Seaman 1796b), Seaman argued the origin of the city's disease outbreak was the smell that arose from the city's garbage and sewage that accumulated in the harbor area. As he put it: "In the city there appears to be an intimate and inseparable connection between the prevalence of yellow fever and the existence of putrid effluvia" (Seaman 1798, 324–325).[6] He made the argument in part through maps in the *Medical Repository* article that remains the most frequently cited and perhaps most concise of his statements. Seaman's map splendidly distilled the contagionist argument in an attempt to prove that, as he put it in his journal article, "no yellow fever can spread, but by the influence of putrid effluvia." Yellow fever, in other words, was static, not dynamic, a creature of localized foul smells of urban waste.

The argument was not new, simply particularized to the New York outbreak using the best techniques of science and cartography then available. In 1763, William Hillary published a book on the "changes of the air and the concomitant epidemical diseases in the island of Barbados." To this was added a "treatise on the putrid bilious fever, commonly called the yellow fever, and such other disease

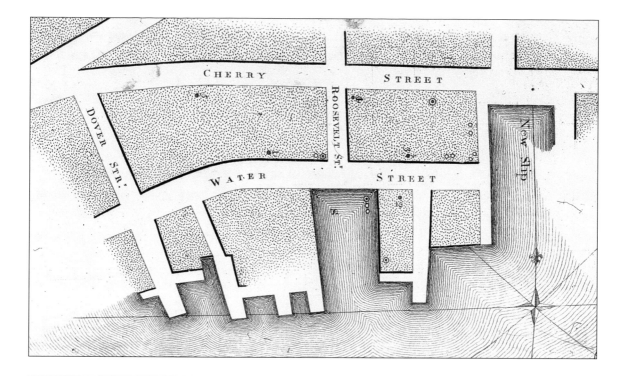

Figure 2.6 Seaman's 1798 general map of yellow fever outbreak in the Roosevelt Street basin area, New York. Fatalities are numbered sequentially. Near-fatal deaths are symbolized by an "E," cases whose diagnosis is uncertain were symbolized by an "o".

Source: National Library of Medicine.

as are indigenous or endemic in the West India Islands, or the torrid zone" (Hillary 1763). The climatology was assumed to be generative of the "bilious fever" and an example of a natural reservoir, the torrid zone, for fevers and illness generally. What Seaman did was consider the precise relation of foul air in temperate climates to putrid disease, arguing that the proximity of yellow fever cases to areas of smelly urban waste proved an environmental relationship.

In his first map, Seaman located ten fatal cases of cholera occurring in a 1797 outbreak that "appear to have originated in East George Street," all but two of the deaths occurring "within the small compass of seventeen houses, in the lower part of the street." The map included the index case of the outbreak, assigning number one to a seaman taken sick in East George Street who had recently arrived in the sloop *Polly* from South Carolina on which one crewman had died (presumably of yellow fever) on the passage northward. Seaman considered and then rejected the ship as a possible source of the infection. While it was possible that the deceased brought the disease with him on the *Polly*, Seaman admitted (Stevenson 1965, 236), it was clearly the local conditions in New York City that gave the fever its deadly effect. "It may be," he wrote, "that a partial principle of death lurked in his [the seaman's} system, during the whole time after the death of his comrade, and most likely, never would have seriously acted upon him had he not immersed himself in this or some such like furry-fostering miasmata."

The general cause of yellow fever appeared to be "the junction of certain matters emitted from the human body, labouring under such a disease, with the effluvia arising from animal and vegetable substances in a state of putrification" (Seaman 1798, 331). One could do little about the "matters emitted from the human body, labouring under such a disease" (Seaman 1798, 331), but one might be able to do a great deal about the effluvia that sustained and supported the disease itself. The real culprit, Seaman argued, or at least the one within human reach of repair, was therefore the environment itself, the dockland terminus of the Roosevelt Street drain (not shown on the map below) into which poured city waste "in addition to the other putrid matters that such places are always collecting." Daily, ebb tide exposed perhaps eight hundred square yards of rotting, perishable materials (everything that a household or small business would throw out) and "putrid matters," human and animal waste washed down to the port from the city's open sewers. The smell was foul and the proximity of this odiferous waste area to the yellow fever outbreak manifest.

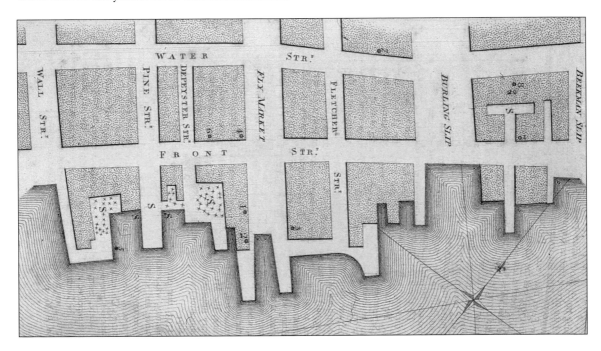

Figure 2.7 Seaman's 1798 detailed map of the 1795 yellow fever outbreak in the Market Street area. Fatal cases are numbered sequentially. Slips, puddles, filth, and garbage are marked by an "S." An "x" was used to indicate common convenience.

Source: National Library of Medicine.

Seaman hammered the point home in a second map in which he etched, or had etched, a greater but still limited range of yellow fever deaths on the greater domain of waste depots in the urban neighborhood. To do this, he included an "S" to symbolize slips, puddles, filth, and garbage, and an "x" to locate areas of convenience, concentrations of human waste washed down the city's streets in open sewers to ferment on the tidal flatland of the docklands. In this way, Seaman fused the range of deaths to the domain of smells emanating from the rotting urban waste in an urban environment of streets and commerce (homes and docklands).

What resulted was a map of odors and their origins joined to one of many incidences of yellow fever that attempted to demonstrate a cause and effect relationship. The result was a proposition equating areas of incidence with those of odiferous waste on the basis of proximity. Seaman's intent was to demonstrate to "every unprejudiced mind that in the city there appears to be an intimate and inseparable connection between the prevalence of yellow fever and the existence of putrid effluvia" (Seaman 1798, 324–325). Of course there was a relation between the locus of foul odors and the incidence of the disease he studied. It just was not the one he thought he had proven.

The odiferous dockside area was also a breeding ground for mosquitoes "never before known, by the oldest inhabitants, to have been so numerous as at this season" Seaman wrote. It seemed obvious to him on the evidence that both yellow fever and the plague of mosquitoes were spontaneous, generated in the fouled, urban air. "The rise of putrid miasmata equally favor the generation of these insects," Seaman concluded. The mosquitoes were not yet perceived as a vector of the disease but instead as a secondary and annoying but less deadly effect of the miasmatic, foul odors that were the root cause of the fever.

Seaman did not draw the maps he used. Rather, he drew or had drawn symbols of disease incidence and of the location of the effluvial sites onto an existing copperplate map of the city, adapting existing plates for his work. The process of etching a copperplate for printing was a complex, expensive, specialized, and time-consuming process. It was a task requiring skills and training that Seaman, a physician, was unlikely to possess. Nor was there a need for a new plate to be made; in 1789, and again in the 1790s, copperplate city maps were commercially produced and sold to New Yorkers. A bustling, growing city, "in the late eighteenth century the city of New York was frequently charted for the benefit of its citizens, its visitors, and its government" (Stevenson 1965, 237).

It was Seaman's genius to adapt these to his purpose, to make of the city map an integrated argument on disease location and generation. The maps gave his work an immediacy and accessibility that an article without the maps would not have had. His mapping was as carefully considered as his medical casebook, as detailed as the texts of the articles he wrote. The result was not a simple "disease map" but a mapped argument about disease incidence and the environment that promoted it. The city streets are neither a frame nor a "basemap" on which the deaths and waste sites sit but an active agent.

That language, while common among cartographers, suggests a separation between disease data and environmental data that violates the thinking Seaman's map distills.

Afflicted inhabitants of the Docklands lived in streets that urban wastes washed down until they pooled where the stench gave rise to the furry miasmata. Yellow fever is located here (and here, and here), the map said, in the city whose effluvium is there (and there, and there) in the city. The waste smells and the foul odors cause disease. See the odiferous sites and their proximity to where yellow fever has been rampant. Note how the streets run down to the water, carrying the wastes here, and here, and here, spawning disease. The scale of the maps served both Seaman's description of the outbreak and his theory of its cause. "In 1795 that part of the town that bore the chief burthen [sic] of our calamity, was remarkably distinguished by the peculiarity of circumstances and situation (aided by the singular regularity of our rains), seemingly well calculated for the accumulation and decomposition of all kinds of perishable animal and vegetable substances" (Seaman 1798, 331).

For Seaman the argument was unassailable. What was required, he concluded, was for the city to undertake programs that would clean up the refuse and thus the air that bred disease. The mapped relation suggested, indeed, *demanded* this response. The mapped incidence of disease pointed to an area where the wastes congregated and caused those incidents. If the proximity of waste was generative of the disease that was killing New Yorkers, then the obvious way to stop the disease was to clean up the effluvial sites and thus free the city from the potential for another yellow fever attack. Take away the generative area of waste, he argued, and illness proximate to it will disappear.

This study of a specific disease had, for Seaman and for others, a more general applicability. He was a late eighteenth-century sanitarian; one who believed the health of humans was directly related to the environment in which they lived. The critical environmental factor was atmospheric: the miasmatic airs that smelled fair (healthy) or foul (unhealthy) depending on local conditions. But yellow fever was only an example of a broader argument relating disease in general to the foul airs of the developing city. Into the twentieth century, sanitarians would argue time and again that cleaning up sewage and wastes would generally promote health through the elimination of environmental conditions that caused foul airs that were generally complicit in ill-health.

Seaman's mapping, his fusion of suspected cause and disease incidence on a plane representing the study site, was nothing short of brilliant. In his mapmaking he was hampered, however, by a technology of production that was expensive and difficult to manipulate. He documented many more cases but only mapped ten, he explained, because he was unable to find a way to include the others in his map (Seaman 1798, 317). Had he included all the cases he had recorded, the result would have been dense to the point of illegibility. In his mapping he was also constrained by the paucity of symbols at his disposal. He lamented "the want of proper marks to identify [the disease] where it is slight." He lacked an easily interpretable symbol by which he could distinguish between mortality and morbidity, for example, between slight and deathly severe cases. Despite these limits, his map admirably advanced a thoroughly ecological argument in which the epicenter of the outbreak was shown to be proximate to areas of foul, odiferous airs generated by rotting sewage that the science of the day argued were generative.

The growing prevalence of printed maps in the city in the 1790s made the mapping of his argument and his study, while innovative, also somehow natural and appropriate.[7] As Stevenson put it (1965), "Taken together, the New York penchant for drawing municipal maps for all sorts of purposes and the medical and sanitarian penchant for sketching out disease maps verbally seem to point to an inevitable conjunction—the actual drawing of an epidemiological map of disease."

Seaman's map grafted onto the growing "penchant" for city and regional maps the habit of mapping, trying to join specific elements into a chain of cause and effect on the basis of density (of occurrence) and proximate location. Through mapping Seaman made the connection graphic and thus stable, evidence anyone could understand. In this manner he began to transpose the telling to the mapping, the narrative to the graphic, in a way that would, by the mid-nineteenth century, become common, taken for granted.

And Seaman was correct. The waste congregated in the city's docklands *did* hold a critical epidemiological relation to the incidence of yellow fever in the city. That it was with factors favorable to the breeding of *Aëdes aegypti*, yellow fever's actual vector, rather than the miasmatic odors themselves was an easy mistake to make. What Seaman did not understand, what the science of the day did not predict, was that the foul, miasmatic airs were not themselves generative but instead a product of conditions that signaled a habitat favorable to mosquitoes, imported on sailing ships, that carried yellow fever to the city population. In the 1790s, there was no way of knowing that the proliferation of mosquitoes was more than an incidental side effect of the odiferous airs.

Horizontal versus vertical

Modern researchers typically distinguish between "horizontal," health-related studies of factors that may generally promote health or retard disease, and "vertical," disease-specific programs independent of the rest of the healthcare systems (Tan, Upshur, Ross, and Ford 2003). We do this today as a way of organizing our knowledge of the vectors of specific diseases and our understanding of their viral or bacterial nature. That social and environmental factors contribute to them is not in doubt. It is simply easier to categorize the mass of potentially available data in this way. As a result, general and specific have been to a great extent separated into allied fields of contemporary study.

In Seaman's day, the cause of specific diseases was unclear and their relation to general environmental conditions only guessed at within then prevailing theories of disease generation. It is therefore no surprise that his work, and that of his successors into the nineteenth century, conflated vertical and horizontal approaches. Seaman's study of this outbreak occurred within a broader, intellectual frame of sanitarian concern for the urban environment as a health determinate that was at once horizontal and vertical. Improving sewage disposal, water quality control, and waste removal services would not simply diminish the likelihood of new yellow fever attacks. Sanitarians believed an improved sanitary infrastructure would benefit health generally, limiting the progression of illness in general. Seaman's study thus served on two levels simultaneously. It was both the study of a specific outbreak as well as an example of the sanitarian argument in which foul urban airs and disease were generally associated.

Pascalis

Another example of this conflation of horizontal and vertical research perspectives is evident in the work of Felix Pascalis, who in 1819 mapped another of New York harbor's recurrent yellow fever outbreaks "in an effort to establish the outbreak's causative factors" (Stevenson 1965, 243–244). Yellow fever as a miasmatic disease was a long-standing interest of his. As early as 1796, he had written an essay on the properties of the effluvia of contagion in the 1795 epidemic of New York (Pascalis 1796). The 1819 outbreak was only the latest effort in Pascalis's continuing research into urban waste and odors as a source of illness in the evolving city.

Facilities for mapping had improved considerably since Seaman's day. Pascalis therefore was able to find a better solution to the problem of graphic case reportage. On his map, Pascalis assigned fatal incidents of yellow fever at the level of city blocks in a manner similar to early urban tax maps of residential location. Each death was numbered to reflect its order of occurrence. The result looks like a land parcel map with numbers reflecting the order of deaths rather than tax roll locators.

Again, mapping showed that the highest concentration of deaths occurred in an area that was overflowing with "perishing and fermenting materials," whose result was "an offensive smell and, no doubt also, deleterious miasmata" (Pascalis 1819, 19).[8] The location of the smell was described textually but not graphically. Unlike Seaman, Pascalis did not map the effluvial sites detailed in his text, the open sewers that flowed into the area and into the harbor. Still, the map was a critical part of his argument that "yellow fever is produced by impure and deleterious exhalations from putrid substances" (Pascalis 1819, 17).

Perhaps because he was able to map a far greater number of cases, a denser range than had Seaman, or perhaps because he was more demographically inclined, in the body of his report Pascalis attempted a simple quantification of the density of the outbreak:

It will be seen, by the annexed diagram, that in the vicinity of Old Slip, out of 57 cases, the enormous proportion of 34 or 35 originated from that single block . . . ten persons, out of the number of 83 sent to Fort Richmond, the greater part from that block, shortly after sickened with the malignant fever, and three of them died in the Marine Hospital (Pascalis 1819, 241).

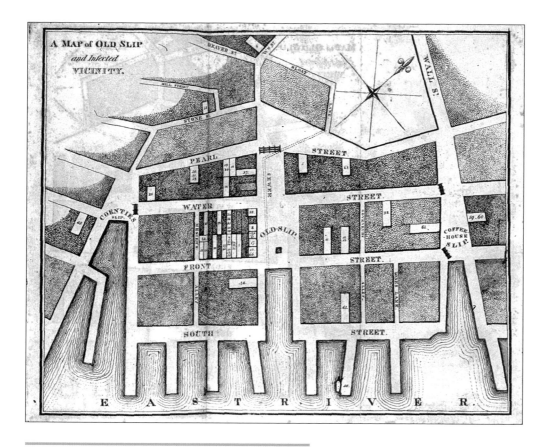

Figure 2.8a   Pascalis's map of yellow fever cases near Old Slip, New York City, 1819.
Fatal cases are numbered sequentially by time of death.

Source: New York Academy of Medicine Library.

While he believed such outbreaks were "engendered by domestic causes," foul airs that pervaded certain areas, he recognized that others believed them to be "communicated by human contagion from foreign ports." The battle between contagionist and anticontagionist theories of disease was heating up, and Pascalis saw his study as a way of deciding the issue between them. The long title of his monograph makes his interests clear:

> *A statement of the occurrences during a malignant yellow fever, in the city of New-York, in the summer and autumnal months of 1819; and of the check given to its progress, by the measures adopted by the Board of Health. With a list of cases and names of sick persons; and a map of their places of residence within the infected and proscribed limits: with a view of ascertaining, by comparative arguments, whether the distemper was engendered by domestic causes, or communicated by human contagion from foreign ports.*

In arguing a "domestic" (contagionist) theory of disease causation, Pascalis had in mind a horizontal perspective on general health more than a vertical concern with yellow fever alone. If the outbreak were an example of a class of miasmatic illnesses, general sanitation would be seen as more important than if the disease were imposed from other locations. Were the contagionist argument correct and the "furry-fostering miasmata" the culprit, then more epidemics surely would occur if the filth of the city, its open sewers and dumps, were not cleaned up. But were the disease introduced by travelers and commerce, the impetus to urban hygiene would be diminished and the quarantine of cargo and passenger ships (or closure of the port) the logical response. Thus, his argument focused on showing not that foul airs *conveyed* disease but rather that they *caused* it in every instance. The broader goal was political and social, proof of the need of an urban sanitarian infrastructure, as well as scientific.

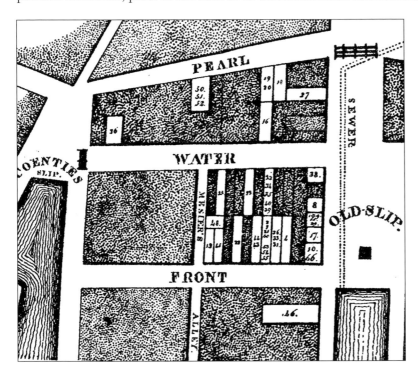

Figure 2.8b Detail in black and white of Pascalis's map of yellow fever cases near Old Slip, New York, 1819. Fatal cases are numbered sequentially by time of death.

Source: New York Academy of Medicine Library.

This perspective materially affected the data he collected, the mapping he did, and the map artifact that resulted. For him, the dockside outbreak necessarily had little to do with the port and its business. The presence of ships in the harbor was incidental to the foul-smelling urban wastes concentrated in the area. He therefore did not include on his map the cases of those who sickened onboard ships in the harbor. Even though the inclusion of shipboard cases would have increased the incidence of mapped occurrence and thus strengthened numerically the correspondence he argued, they were literally out of mind and "off the map."

The map that resulted admirably summarized Pascalis's argument and correctly mapped the range of urban cases, implicating the sources of foul, miasmatic air that any reader could him or herself locate in the map. The map distilled in a single image the argument carried in the accompanying text. A cluster of yellow fever cases occurred near urban waste sites whose foul odors were, in the miasmatic theory of the day, assumed to be the cause of the outbreak. Not for the last time, the assumption was that congruence equals causation, that simple proximity is proof of a cause-and-effect relationship. Alas, proximity indicates only the likelihood of an association that may in fact result from intervening but unknown, and thus unmapped, variables.

Data and statistics

One other map of this period needs at least brief mention. In 1821, the New York Board of Health mapped nine sites at which occurred an estimated 150 deaths from a disease called the "black vomit," probably typhus but which at the time some believed might be yellow fever. Although the excretion was different—the former's dark and the latter's bilious yellow—the nature of the disease was unclear to treating physicians. As part of an investigation into the outbreak, a map on which cases were aggregated to the buildings in which those affected lived was used to consider the demographics of the disease.

Because it was believed that African-Americans were somehow protected racially from yellow fever (Spielman and D'Antonio 2001, 64), it was important to distinguish between cases affecting African-American and White citizens as a tool in disease identification. If both were affected equally, or if more African-American than Whites were affected, the assumption was that the disease could not be yellow fever. But if those dying from the disease were all White, even where they lived with African-Americans, then at least circumstantial proof of yellow fever could be inferred.

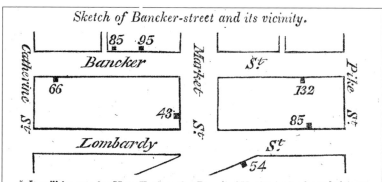

Figure 2.9 Bancker Street map of an epidemic outbreak of an unknown disease, perhaps typhus or typhoid fever, New York, 1821. Numbers refer to lots in which patients died.

Source: New York Academy of Medicine Library.

The written report in which the map was embedded was at some pains to provide the analysis the map lacked. "On the lot 95-Bancker-street, 34 blacks and 9 whites were sick of the fever, and on the lot 66 Bancker-street, 8 blacks were sick, and on the lot 85 Lombardy-street, 9 blacks" (New York Board of Health 1821, 181). The investigators did not symbolize the racial distinctions made in the text, either because of a paucity of symbol types or because it did not occur to them to try. The text itself gives no hint. Either way, the map only locates the houses of those affected by the unknown disease, leaving the density at an individual location, and the racial data of those who lived there, to be described in the text. What is notable about this work was its attempt to determine the nature of a disease outbreak through the addition of a type of demographic data to the map surface in a manner that would be clinically significant.

Here were the first stirrings of the statistical argument that would become critical over the next few decades, one that grew not independent from but in relation to a mapped approach to studies of disease and health. As methods of not only data accumulation but also representation improved, new ways of handling health-related data would develop. The Bancker Street map is an early example of the attempt to represent not only the incidence of disease within an undifferentiated population but to do so with reference to specific, demographic data in a manner permitting variable effects on subpopulations to be analyzed. As the next chapter attempts to make clear, this growing interest in statistical rigor grew within an intellectual environment that simultaneously encouraged increasingly capacious mapped consideration of health-related data. The movement for better statistical and graphic analysis culminated in a series of extraordinary studies of cholera outbreaks in the 1850s. They must be seen as examples of a greater change in the study of health and disease that struggled, as did Seaman and Pascalis, between a horizontal focus on general conditions promoting health and narrower, vertical studies of specific disease outbreaks.

Conclusion

Seaman, Pascalis, and the New York Board of Health researchers were first-rate investigators who knew how to formulate a hypothesis based on the available evidence within the context of an established scientific theory. The result was studies in which datasets were chosen, correlations sought, and the result then summarized at a specific scale. To understand specific outbreaks, they mapped disease occurrence in their cities and sought a causative agent that was proximate to the outbreak area. The maps that resulted from this approach were distillations of studies whose conclusions seemed both scientifically and experientially true. One could smell the sickening foulness generated by effluvia and garbage across the dockside areas in which these epidemic outbreaks occurred. Where the smell was strongest, people fell ill. The relation between disease and suspected cause was argued and mapped. Within the conceptual frame of the day, the result seemed to bolster a miasmatic theory of disease. It would take another century of science and advances in microscopy to provide the missing link that completed the perceived connection between the incidents of yellow fever and the unsanitary effluvial sites of urban waste. Understanding that the mosquitoes that also congregated amid the garbage were in fact the vectors of the disease agent rather than innocuous, if annoying, artifacts of the smell would require a different theory of disease.

Endnotes

1. The epidemiology of any disease is specific to its individual pathogen, but the process of its appearance and diffusion can be described in general terms. In broad strokes, dense populations of humans present a potential reservoir for new virus or bacteria that evolve either in response to human action (the over-use of antibiotics, for example) or the bringing together of animal species that are reservoirs of viruses or bacteria that may jump the species barrier. The diffusion of these new microbial agents is facilitated by both human migration and the transmission of cargo. Processes specific to individual conditions is what the long, slow study of medicine and epidemiology is about.

2. The only existing copy of these maps that I know of and have seen are at the New York Academy of Medicine Library, whose staff assisted in the photographing of the image and translation of the classical Italian in the maps' legends. Both for her general assistance and her translation of the legends, I am indebted to New York Academy of Medicine Library librarian, Arlene Shaner.

3. Howe here cites Lind's *An Essay on Diseases Incidental to Europeans in Hot Climates,* noting the climatic determinism that assumed that tropical heat and humidity were themselves inimical to health and industry. Into the twentieth century a belief would exist that tropical climates were inimical to health and that the cooler, northern altitudes were necessarily superior and healthier. Thus, mapping in the later nineteenth century often attempted to correlate altitude and moisture with the incidence of individual diseases. Because I have yet to find a copy of Lind's essay, it is not cited or quoted here.

4. Weed (1942) describes the then powerful resistance to an animalcular theory of disease in the early nineteenth century in his review of the life and writings of Baltimore physician, John Crawford (1756–1813). Even a decade after Pasteur's and Koch's definitive studies, criticism of the bacterial theory of disease generation continued.

5. Much has been written on the history of miasmatic disease. There are the early classics of Hippocrates and Galen, for example, and then the voluminous writing of eighteenth- and nineteenth-century medical researchers and theorists. A useful recent review of nineteenth-century debates over disease can be found in Vinten-Johansen et al. (2003, 172–185).

6. All three examples of Seaman's writings are preserved at the National Institute of Medicine in Bethesda, Maryland. The *Medical Repository* article is the one that included maps, however, and the source most typically cited in detailing Seaman's medicine. That practice is continued here, with the observation that a close textual comparison of all three sources would be instructive.

7. A parallel history of urban maps has grown without reference to medical uses. Krieger and Cobb (2001), for example, present a detailed history of that city through their maps. A review of the work by Krim (2002) presents a useful companion to the work.

8. Pascalis is sometimes cited under his birth name, Pascalis-Ouvière, Felix, or on occasion as "Ouvière, Felix Pascalis." The confusion arises from the Anglicization of his name midway through his career. His "Statement of Occurrences" is variously credited both as a *Medical Repository* article (1820) and as an independent pamphlet published in 1819 (Shannon 1981). To avoid confusion, only the *Medical Repository* article is quoted here.

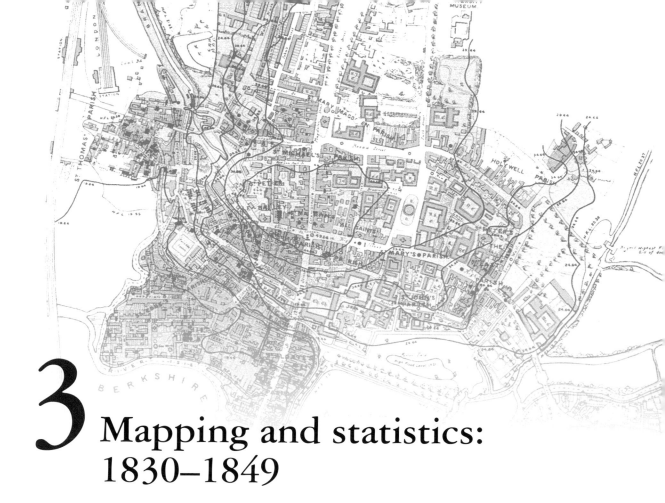

3 Mapping and statistics: 1830–1849

Historians, at least cartographic historians, typically assume that, as Robinson (1982, 156) put it, "medical mapping in Europe burgeoned in the 1830s when cholera first appeared." The implication is that its utility was so rapidly recognized that medical mapping grew independent of all other factors as a response to the first cholera pandemic. Certainly, a number of increasingly complex maps were generated in the 1830s; even more were made in the 1840s. But it was not a case of spontaneous generation; the mapping of disease did not emerge as a result of the cholera epidemic. Rather, it grew out of the earlier work of researchers like Seaman and Pascalis and decades of attention to the increasing number of infectious diseases. Medical mapping evolved with a host of new approaches and techniques in science generally and in medicine specifically.

From 1830 to 1850 new medical theories and new ways of arguing their validity were being generated. New printing technologies, especially the transition from copperplate to lithography, resulted in techniques of mapmaking that were increasingly more able to distill these new arguments. Finally, more cost-efficient systems of production permitted an ever-greater number of public and professional journals to be published at a time when the mail that carried them to subscribers was becoming an efficient and profitable international enterprise.[1] The bibliographic tendencies of the age and the libraries they spawned preserved many of the reports and journals whose maps are presented in this chapter.

The history of this period of mapping and mapmaking in service of specific scientific goals—identifying the nature and cause of infectious disease generally and cholera specifically—is linked as well to the distinct but simultaneously evolving history of medical science itself. Across the mid-nineteenth century, medical science struggled with its Hippocratic and Galenic roots, inching toward a broader theory of disease that would finally emerge only with microscopy in the 1880s. As part of this struggle, contagionist and anticontagonist theories of epidemic disease continued to vie for supremacy in an age in which epidemic disease was a constant fear.

Social reformers seeking to address issues of the unhealthy city selected elements of the disease debates, using them to advance their cause. Medical mapping thus occurred within a complex ecology (scientific, social, and technological) whose components together conspired to promote its development.[2] In this ecology a single disease—cholera—took a preeminent place in the minds of medical researchers, medical mappers, and the public. Indeed, into the 1880s, cholera was *the* disease, a metaphor not simply of illness but of deathly epidemics, the general "kingdom of the sick" (Sontag 1978), and the urban reservoirs that promoted them.

Britain and cholera

On October 23, 1831, a Saturday, Sunderland Keelman William Sproat "became violently ill, had a severe shivering fit and giddiness, cramps of the stomach and violent vomiting and purging" (Morris 1976, 11). Sproat's physician consulted two other doctors, one of whom had encountered cholera in the 1820s while stationed in Mauritius with the 82nd regiment. On Sunday, they diagnosed the illness as Asiatic cholera as opposed to English, or endemic, cholera, a common diarrheic intestinal disorder. On

Year	Cholera deaths	Pandemics
1831–1832	31,474	First pandemic
1848	1,908	Second pandemic
1849	53,293	
1853	4,419	Third pandemic
1854	20,097	
1866	14,378	Fourth pandemic

Figure 3.1 Cholera deaths in England, Scotland, and Wales, 1831–1866.

Source: Adapted from Morris (1976, 13).

Cartographies of Disease

Wednesday Sproat died, the first of more than one hundred thousand British citizens who would perish from the disease in four pandemics that raged in 1831–1833, 1848–1850, 1853–1854, and 1866.

Across those years the mortality rate for cholera patients was typically between 20 and 25 percent (Morris 1976, 13). While this sounds severe, it must be perceived in the context of the times. During the cholera years between 309,000 and 400,000 people died per year in England from all causes. Only once did deaths from cholera ever climb above fifty thousand people, and in most years the number was far less. So while cholera was a significant health event, it was not catastrophic in the way, bubonic plague, with its extreme mortality rates, had been.

Cholera's arrival in Britain in 1831 was not unexpected. Indeed, it had been anticipated for several years. Called *cholera morbus,* or more popularly Asiatic cholera, it killed thousands of Indian citizens in Calcutta in 1781–1782 and more than twenty thousand pilgrims at Hurdwar in 1783–1784. However, British officials only became concerned, when it killed not just indigenous persons, but also British troops in Jessor, India, in August 1817. In that year, three thousand members of the ten-thousand-man British army then stationed in India under the Marquis of Hastings died of the disease.

That got the attention of Foreign Office officials who then tracked the disease's progress from India across Asia (Ceylon and Borneo in 1821, China and Japan in 1822), the Middle East and into Russia in 1823 where its progress stalled. In that year, a new epidemic began in India, killing thousands more. This outbreak again spread along established trade routes to Tehran, Astrakhan, and from there up the Volga. In 1829, it again reached Russia with undiminished vigor. At that point British officials realized that "nothing could prevent it spreading over Europe" (Morris 1976, 23).

"Its occurrence in St. Petersberg, during the early part of 1831, forcibly arrested public attention and the government of [England] was induced to send thither Dr. Russell and Dr. Barry to watch the progress of the disease, and acquaint themselves with its details" (Shapter 1849, 2). Trade between Russia and Western Europe, between Russia and Great Britain, and between Europe and Great Britain made Sproat's death, and those of other cholera victims, inevitable. Not coincidentally, it also assured the diffusion of the disease from England to its worldwide trading partners, including Canada where, in 1832 its effect would be severe (Godfrey 1968).

Clinical and social concerns

While other diseases were greater killers, cholera became *the* epidemic disease of the nineteenth century, a public terror especially feared. It was, one journal of the day shrilled, "one of the most terrible pestilences which have ever desolated the earth" (*Quarterly Review* 1832, 170, quoted in Morris 1976, 14). The journal editors' concerns were not simply with the deaths that resulted but the effect of cholera upon the nation's balance sheet, on patterns of trade and commerce. Violent outbreaks killed the workers whose labor was essential to the mills and shops of industrializing England. It created a class of widows and orphans who were left without any clear means of nongovernmental support. Wealthier citizens fled the city during an outbreak in an attempt to escape the disease, further affecting the business of the city and the nation. Commerce was therefore restricted where it did not come to a halt. And, of course, the cost of the illness included the necessity of at least minimal care for the victims of the epidemic who overloaded existing hospitals, workhouses, and other social institutions. The economic burden of the epidemic disease became a principal subject of official and general public concern.

Clinically, cholera was marked by violent diarrhea with a "rice water" stool whose characteristic white flecks were not rice but the epithelial lining of the intestine. Death from dehydration typically occurred in twenty-four to forty-eight hours. The corpses of those affected typically took on a dark-hued appearance.[3] That nobody knew what caused the disease, and therefore how to prevent or treat it, made the epidemic more horrible still. Theories on causation ranged, as they had for yellow fever, from the influence of comets to poisonous exhalations from the earth's crust (Godfrey 1968). Whatever its cause, the relative speed of its diffusion, and the weeks-long duration of its outbreaks in major cities, were terrifying. From the miasmatic perspective it was like a deadly weather system, a killer low-pressure cell that moved across the land leaving disaster in its wake.

Other, nonclinical factors contributed to public panic and official concern. Beginning with the 1831 outbreak, cholera had an unusually public face, one written about in a range of new and rapidly developing daily journals and weekly magazines (Morris 1976, 14–15).[4] By the early 1830s, advances in printing technology created an evolving and populist "penny press" whose broadsheet papers were generally affordable to the majority of working-class citizens (Monmonier 1999). Religious periodicals, medical journals, broadsheet newspapers, household magazines, and scientific journals all wrote about cholera, its possible causes, and suggestions for the treatment of its symptoms (rhubarb was considered an efficacious treatment by most medical experts).

Medicostatistical mapping

The explosion of public and professional writing about both the social effect and clinical face of an epidemic disease was a new phenomenon. Simultaneously, maps were becoming increasingly popular adjuncts to official reports on commerce, trade, population change, and of course, disease (Robinson 1982, chapters 5 and 6). Maps of cholera incidence—and medical mapping generally—were thus an outgrowth of the more general acceptance of and demand for maps in official and scientific documents. They are therefore examples of the map's growing general acceptance rather than an exclusive response to the epidemic itself. The assumption that medical mapping grew as a response primarily to the epidemic puts the cart before the horse.

That many of those maps have survived is testimony to improved modes of production using better paper for longer print runs, thus enhancing the chance of the survival of at least some pages of each article or report. It also reflects the development of various institutions whose bureaucrats commissioned studies and then stored the result in official and public libraries. Vinten-Johansen and his colleagues (2003, 325–326) list twenty-two "examples of cholera maps published between 1832 and 1855." Jarcho (1970), with a more ecumenical definition of what constituted a cholera map, counts forty-four cholera-related maps published between the years 1820 and 1838. Jarcho's catalog of cholera maps includes several from the earlier Indian outbreak as well as maps of cholera incidence in other non-European countries. A small class of Jarcho's maps attempted to describe not the density of national outbreaks but the disease's progress internationally over time.

If studies of cholera were a beneficiary of the general advance in printing and publishing, mapping benefited as well from a growing partnership with statistical forms of investigation anticipated by the Bancker Street map of the 1820s. In the 1830s, the numerical analysis of social and medical phenomena was becoming an increasingly accepted method of both social and scientific study in a way that was increasingly rigorous and meaningful. It was at this time that population statistics, the aggregation of incidence by population size, first began to be popularly used. Called "moral statistics" in 1833 by Andre-Michel Guerry (Robinson 1982, 156–158), it was used to quantify a range of phenomena (criminal incidence, education levels, income assessments, medical events, etc.). More generally, the increasing use of statistics led to what some medical historians now call the "Paris School" (Porter 1998, 406–408), a *méthode numerique* in which a range of clinical phenomena was analyzed using elementary statistics to describe incidence as a function of population.

Many if not most of the maps that resulted used a choropleth technique to show variations in the incidence of disease by parish or regional district. Areas of greater intensity were shaded using a darker stippling than areas in which it was less prevalent. Data was increasingly aggregated at the jurisdictional level most directly responsible for citizen health and welfare.

A leader in this movement to mapped statistics was Malgaigne, whose experiments in what Jarcho (1974) calls "medicostatistical" mapping investigated a range of phenomena, including the number and location of surgical operations at Paris hospitals, and in another study, the location of the incidence of fractures. In 1839, he created a map, published the next year in a then-new journal of public health (*Annales d'Hygiène Publique et de Médecine Légale*), exploring the incidence of hernia in France based on the population of French political districts.

Along both sides of his map are a *tableau des hernieux* listing incidence by administrative department. His data was based on the physical examination of military recruits as a way to sample the greater French population. The result created a generally comparable range of occurrence in which incidence was normalized by department population. Variations in incidence were summarized not only in the tables, included in the map, but also through lighter and darker stippling representing lesser and greater incidence of hernia in the choropleth mapping itself.

The resulting map joins the range of hernia incidence with the characteristics of a domain (population of political departments) to create a surface that makes spatially explicit the data by population and administrative district Malgaigne presented in his table. The result served not only to make

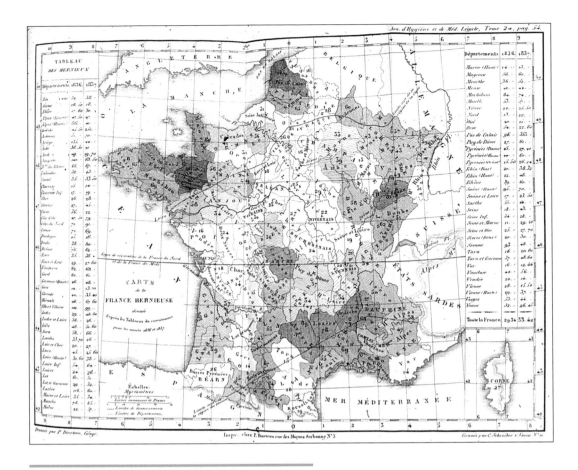

Figure 3.2 Malgaigne's 1840 map of the incidence of hernia in France. An early example of the "Paris School" of medical statistics, the map itself was used to test various hypotheses about the potential cause of hernias.

Source: New York Academy of Medicine Library.

variations in incidence clear but also permitted a series of propositions to be framed and tested. Each proposition tested the relation between unusually high hernia incidence and a local feature of the areas in which it was observed.

Some believed the use of olive oil rather than butter in cooking favored the development of hernias, for example. The map therefore included a line representing the boundary separating southern districts, where olive oil was most frequently used in cooking, and northern districts where it was not. If this affected hernia rates, one would expect to find more hernias below rather than above the line. Similarly, to test the proposition that hernias might be more Mediterranean than northern, a disease favoring one region over another, a line was drawn at latitude 46° north to test for gross regional differences. Could a statistical difference be observed between areas above and below the line of latitude? A third line was employed to distinguish the northern limits of grape cultivation in France to determine if those areas where wine was more commonly drunk than cider had, as Malgaigne himself believed, a greater incidence of herniation.

These lines of hypothesis were imposed on the landscape not because they represented objective data, "real world things" observable in the landscape, but because they presented ideas that could be spatially articulated and graphically considered. They were artifacts of the researcher's thinking rather than obviously pertinent elements of the landscape. Each line framed an if/then proposition, each proposition representing a theory of hernia causation based upon regional differences. The result was a significant tool of investigation distinct from, but related to, that of statistical analysis.

Why make the map if detailed statistical tables would carry the same results? The answer for Malgaigne was that they did not. Spatial questions demanded a spatial response that mapping provided in a way purely numerical consideration could not. The ability to create a surface in which variations at the departmental level served as the domain for specific experimental ranges (north versus south, olive oil versus butter, wine versus cider, and so on) was uniquely useful. It was both easily interpreted and, at least by the standards of the day, acceptably rigorous. For Malgaigne, the utility of the technique was demonstrable. That it disproved theories of herniation—or conversely, proved the null hypothesis—in no way detracted from its value. "We had here a direct means of testing the validity of this assertion," Malgaigne wrote. "Now it must be recognized clearly that the totality of our investigations distinctly contradicts it" (trans. Jarcho 1974, 97).

Others shared Malgaigne's delight in the ability of maps to distill complexity and test propositions in a comprehensive and rigorous fashion. Several years later, Augustus Petermann, for example, explained in similar terms the map's advantages as an analytic tool. Another pioneer in combining statistical and mapped analyses (Robinson 1982, 180–181; Gilbert 1958, 177–178), Petermann's concern was the mapping of cholera, not hernias. But what he said held generally true for all those using mapping as an analytic approach to disease investigations:

> The object, therefore, in constructing cholera maps is to obtain a view of the geographical extent of the ravages of this disease, and to discover the local conditions that might influence its progress and its degree of fatality.
>
> For such a purpose, geographical delineation is of utmost value, and even indispensable; for while the symbols of the masses of statistical data in figures, however clearly they might be arranged in systematic tables, present but a uniform appearance, the same data, embodied in a map, will convey at once, the relative bearing and proportion of the single data together with their position, extent, and distance, and thus, a map will make visible to the eye the development and nature of any phenomenon in regard to its geographical distribution (Petermann 1848).[5]

That had it in a nutshell. Maps made overt the geographic distribution of phenomena that were being progressively and ever-more rigorously defined by the evolving statistics of the age. They permitted ranges of data (disease incidence, population, etc.) to be joined in a way that encouraged hypotheses to be framed as propositions and then explored both graphically and statistically. The resulting maps were not mere addenda to reports but central exhibits in which propositions relating potential cause and observed incidence were tested. They made "visible to the eye" the science whose components were intellectual, constructions distilled from data informed by theory. As an 1850 British parliamentary report including maps would emphasize, maps made clear in a way raw statistics might not "the predominating influence of locality over the progress of the disease" (Grainger 1850, 199).

The concern with relative proximity and the density of an outbreak present in the work of Seaman and Pascalis became, in the 1830s and 1840s, increasingly central concerns, an ever-more closely considered element of medical investigation mapped *in situ*. At the same time that some were quantifying population data and mapping its relation to specific medical conditions, others were writing and mapping more general "medical topographies," detailed descriptions of the elements of a specific district or region that at least potentially promoted health or invited disease. Hennen's 1830 *Sketches of the Medical Topography of the Mediterranean* is one example. Another produced at the same time in England offered detailed, health-related descriptions of districts like Cornwall and Brighton (Howe 1961, 10). These early medical topographies were the logical successors to the earlier studies of Pascalis and Seaman, whose interest was locally sanitarian and related to a specific disease, yellow fever.

Topographies of disease

"Topography" meant something very different in those days than it does today, more than a century after Cantor developed his theory of sets (circa 1880). While the term first gained popularity in the 1820s, its origins lay in thinking about the relation between disease and environment that stretched back into the seventeenth century (Harrison 2000, 55). In general, it referred to an analysis situs, an analysis of relative positions defined by proximity or distance generally (Firby and Gardiner 1982, 11). In this case, those relations were between disease incidence and potentially contributing environmental conditions, especially those that were odiferous. It was geographic, geometric, and propositional, relating the location of "x" to "y" in a causative manner. The work of both Seaman and Pascalis was therefore topographic, as was the work of Finke's successors in an evolving medical geography relating conditions of climate and geology to the incidence of specific diseases. It was in service of this topographic approach to disease incidence that, in 1818, the U.S. Surgeon General Joseph Lovell ordered army surgeons "to note everything of importance relating to the medical topography of his station, including the weather" but not excluding other sources of miasmatic odors, of course (Mitman and Numbers 2003, 394).[6]

In both the evolving school of medical statistics and that of medical topography, mapping was indispensable. An example is Thomas Shapter's frontispiece map of *The History of Cholera in 1832 in Exeter*. Published in 1849 on the eve of the second cholera pandemic, the map "showing the location where the deaths caused by pestilential cholera occurred in 1832–1834" is important. It sought to describe, in the words of a *Lancet* reviewer (*Lancet* 1849, 317), a "city close, confined, badly drained, and still worse supplied with water" (Vinten-Johansen et al. 2003, 324). Its careful attention both to the incidence of the disease and the environment in which it proliferated is still an evocative description

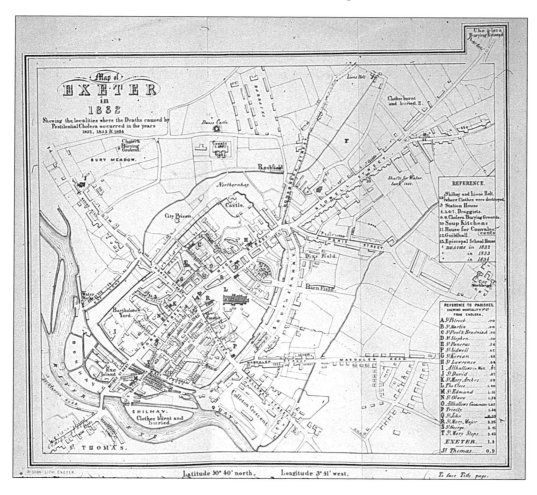

Figure 3.3a Shapter's map of cholera in Exeter, 1832, published in 1849. The map includes a statistical table of deaths by parish population and incidence of disease by parish in the years 1832–1834.

Source: New York Academy of Medicine Library.

of a historical epidemic. Reduced and transposed to these pages, denuded of the text in which it was embedded, the power of the map to its original readers is hard to perceive. And yet, for Shapter and his contemporaries the map carried a powerful argument for a zymotic variant of the miasmatic theory of disease.[7]

Shapter's map served his general miasmatic thesis in several ways, not the least of them a descriptive function familiarizing readers in the late 1840s with Exeter itself and its response to the first pandemic. On the map are locations—convalescent homes, burial grounds, soup kitchens, and sites for the disposal of the clothes of the infected, and so on—that signaled the city's response to the epidemic. During the bubonic plague pandemic of the 1600s special burial pits for the victims of epidemics had been created; special locations for the cleansing of their clothes (often with lye) were instituted. In the cholera epidemic of 1831, these old protocols were returned, the evidence of them embedded in the map.

The map is a topography of Exeter and the relation between its geography and the incidence of disease. Shapter used it to test the then-current miasmatic proposition that bad air in lowland areas near

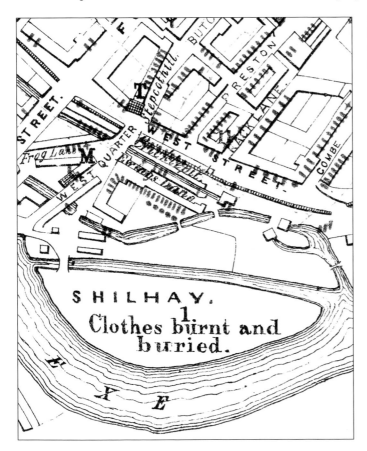

Figure 3.3b Detail of Shapter's map of cholera in Exeter, 1832.

Source: New York Academy of Medicine Library.

effluvial sites was responsible for the epidemic outbreak. The map thus includes two legends *(figure 3.3a)* whose respective elements list the constituents of the if/then proposition. The first identifies pertinent locations (the burial ground, for example) and the second the incidence of cholera by percentage of parish population. In the map, Shapter presents evidence of relative intensity both through his symbolization of individual cases, year by year, and through the legend's aggregation of case data at the parish level. What he found was that there were "a few isolated spots in which a remarkable and undue amount of mortality took place" (Shapter 1849, 24). These occurred in relatively low-lying areas of dense habitation near the river, areas of poor drainage and effluvial build-up that resulted in the type of odiferous, miasmatic airs that Pascalis and Seaman had earlier described as generative of the disease.

For Shapter, the result was irrefutable. Cholera was a miasmatic condition generated by the bad airs of low-lying lands. The evidence was in the map. A reader might look at the index and find the districts with the greatest incidence of cholera, St. Thomas and St. Mary Steps, for example, and see they are in the low-lying areas near the river. There, too, the reader can count the marks indicating the plethora of cholera cases occurring in each year.

Implicit in the map and its accompanying text was a social history of the city (here were the workhouses, there the churches) and of its approach to disease control and containment. To the map's extreme east, between the two legends, exists the "city workhouse" where nineteen people died of cholera in 1834. In the city center, north of the 1831 and 1832 epicenter, stands the historic guildhall. Charitable soup kitchens were on Sidwell Street toward the edge of town. At the north end of the street was a "cholera burying ground," balanced by a second in the Bury Meadow (so named after a previous plague epidemic) at the map's northwest. Two depots for the burning and burial of clothing were set first at the end of Sidwell Street and second in Lion's Holt to its immediate northwest, both in areas inhabited by the poor rather than the city's well-to-do.

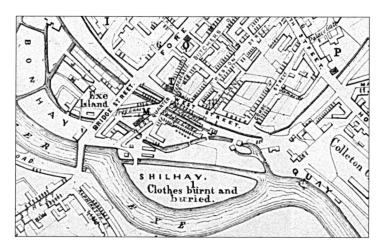

Figure 3.3c Detail of Shapter's map of cholera in Exeter showing the horizontal bars (1832), diamonds (1833), and dots (1834) used to signify the location of fatal cholera cases in the city in those three years.

Source: New York Academy of Medicine Library.

The richness of data reflects the efforts of the local board of health, which was created in response to Parliament's Cholera Prevention Act of 1831 (Shapter 1849, 44–45). In preparation for the epidemic that it knew was inevitable, Parliament ordered every town to constitute a local health board to oversee a local response to the anticipated epidemic. To assure accurate data and a correct assessment of the severity of the epidemic, the Exeter board created a series of forms to assure proper data collection. The most basic forms were records of those who died (name, residence, parish, sex, occupation, date of onset, etc.), while other forms were used to aggregate that specific data by week and month. It was these that Shapter drew upon in his study and the crafting of his tables and map.

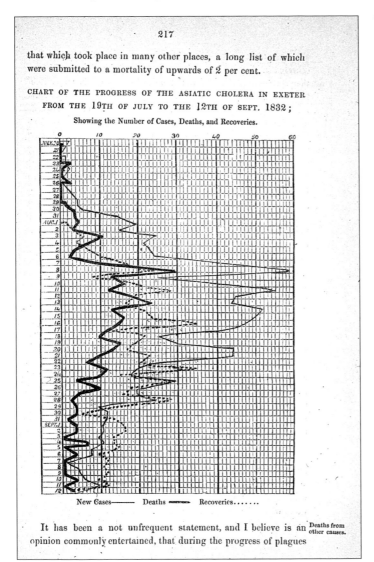

Shapter used this data to profile the general progress of the disease over time, to create a "fever chart" of the epidemic's progress. After all, physicians knew a febrile disease began with a light fever that continued until the patient was in crisis and then, if he or she was to live, "broke" and resolved. Why not assume a similar pattern for the epidemic itself? Shapter therefore charted the number of new cases reported each day, noting which were fatal and which were not, from July 19 to September 12, 1832. The result was the now-familiar, bell-shaped pattern of an epidemic that begins slowly, grows rapidly over weeks to a peak rate of occurrence and then diminishes for a roughly equal number of weeks until the epidemic subsides. Others would independently confirm a similar pattern elsewhere. Some would attempt to fit the bell-shaped curve to geographical data (wind, rainfall, temperature, etc.) in an attempt to test the relation of incidence to physical determinants that were thought to fuel the epidemic itself.

The scale of the map is sufficiently fine to permit individual deaths, summed by date in the chart, to be mapped and data at the parish level to be suggested but not otherwise distinguished. In larger urban studies, like Malgaigne's study of French districts, the tendency was to use choropleth techniques to describe relative incidence at a coarser scale. An example of this approach, one in which individual cases are only aggregated, is a map of the 1832 cholera outbreak in Hamburg, Germany.

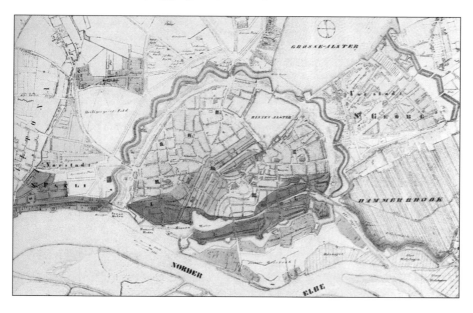

Figure 3.5 Map of the 1832 cholera outbreak in Hamburg, Germany, 1836, near Rothenburg. This map was later included in the Grainger report on cholera to the British Parliament in 1850.

Source: British Library.

First published in 1836, it was later redrawn for inclusion in an 1850 British parliamentary report on cholera (Robinson 1982, 180-181). The hand-tinted map joined incidence of disease mortality to city region through a system of lighter and darker choropleth coloration. The administrative domain was thus fused to tables of local incidence in a manner that better presents relative intensity of occurrence at the scale of a larger, industrial city. The result is the same, again emphasizing the apparently persistent predilection of cholera to occur in low-lying areas near rivers—in one case the Exeter and in the other the North Elbe—rather than in areas of greater altitude.

The conclusions, graphic and statistical, also supported an anticontagionist argument for disease transmission by the ships that plied the river, carrying goods across the nation. The trick, once a pattern appears, is to interpret the results. In most cases, that determination was not as easy as Malgaigne's simple lines on his map to distinguish between French regions might suggest. Here the map could have been used for either argument but, because the contagionist theory was ascendant, the idea that the map might implicate river traffic itself was largely ignored. Like Seaman and Pascalis, the mapper created a map that served his purpose within the context of a general disease theory, albeit a map in which support for a wholly different, anticontagionist argument was embedded.

The Exeter and Hamburg maps are notable not for their uniqueness but for their typicality. At this time, a number of similar maps were being drawn both on the continent and in England, arguing a host of relations pertinent to cholera and other illnesses. In 1840, for example, Robert Cowan used a similar approach to show a relationship between fever and overcrowding. Increasing mortality, he argued, was due to "excessive immigration without any corresponding increase in housing" (Melnick 2002, 2). Dr. Robert Perry mapped a six-fold difference in the rate of fevers in different Glasgow neighborhoods. In the map of a typhus outbreak, he located the individual homes of those with typhus on a map (Melnick 2002), and in 1844, drew a Hamburg-style map as part of his study of the 1832 cholera epidemic outbreak in Glasgow (Robinson 1982, 183–84).

What perhaps is most significant about the Hamburg map is its inclusion in a British parliamentary report on the incidence of the disease. Its reproduction there emphasizes both the international nature of the cholera experience and the international manner in which scientists of this era attempted to address it. Two generations before it would have been unlikely for a map by Pascalis, or even earlier, Seaman, to have been redrawn and reprinted in an official British or German report. But by 1850, an increasingly efficient international mail system and faster, less-expensive printing technologies combined to create an international medium for the exchange of data about the incidence of disease. Maps were critical to the medicostatistical analytic approach that blossomed in the 1830s, and by the time of the second cholera pandemic, evolving technologies or production and distribution assured researchers in the Americas, Britain, and Europe would have access to each other's work.

Medical mapping served not only analytic and documentary functions but another whose importance in the internationalization of medicine is too often ignored. The map's graphic nature was an indisputable asset to those who read other languages only with difficulty. One did not need to be a linguist to translate Norden Elbe for the north arm of the Elbe River. One could read the map without understanding the German text because the relative proximity of the river to the city districts with the greatest incidence of cholera was clear. Mapping provided both a universal tool and a graphic *lingua franca* for researchers interested in international reports but without any real facility in the languages of their production.[8]

Health, poverty, and wealth

The maps of cholera in cities like Hamburg, and those seeking to establish patterns of occurrence for less serious conditions like hernias, were fundamentally vertical studies whose narrow focus was a specific disease or health burden. At the same time others were using similar techniques to consider the general, horizontal determinants of health at the scale of the city, the political region, and the nation. These two approaches to mortality and morbidity, so clearly joined in the early work of Pascalis and Seaman, began to separate during the 1830s as individual investigators sought to focus their studies more narrowly. Cholera was one health problem among the many that sanitarians had long believed resulted from the unhealthy conditions of the growing city. Thus, cholera was only one of a number of disease subjects being mapped and considered. "With or without cholera, the appalling living conditions of the poor, who made up a very large segment of the population, could not escape notice, and various aspects of housing, land use, and population characteristics began to be mapped" (Robinson 1982, 156). It thus is necessary to detour temporarily from the story of the mapping of cholera to a more general consideration of the contemporaneous mapping of broader social and economic determinants of health and disease.

Edmund Chadwick

As a class, sanitarian maps presented an argument that in the evolving industrial city specific conditions created areas predisposed to ill health rather than arguments about the causes of a specific illness. An early example of this work is in Edmund Chadwick's famous *Report on the Sanitary Conditions of the Labouring Population of Great Britain to the Poor Law Commissioners* (Chadwick 1842, 160), a "forceful indictment of unsanitary living conditions in the industrial slums, as well as a severe criticism of physicians ignorant of the causes of contagion and of the moribund local health boards" (Melosi 2000, 46). Well researched and well argued, the report included a host of tables and the map "A Sanitary Map of the Town of Leeds." In it the "least cleansed" and typically most impoverished districts (those most conducive to ill health) were mapped in a darker color than more sanitary, wealthier, and, in the end, healthier districts.

When he headed the London Board of Health in the 1840s, Chadwick had hoped literally to clean or "flush out the city" by hooking up house drains to the public sewers. It was his goal to abolish cesspits

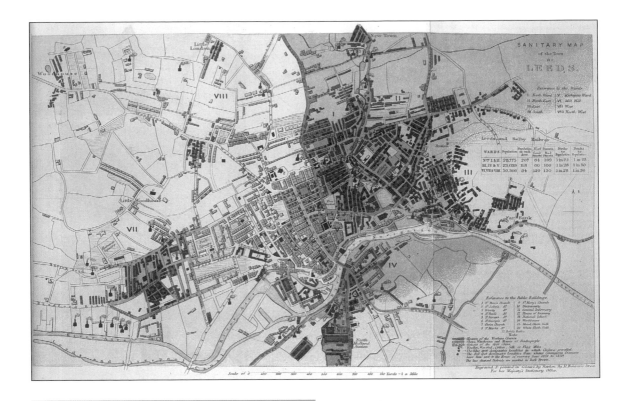

Figure 3.6a Sanitary map of Leeds, 1832, used by Chadwick in an 1842 report to Parliament on the British Poor Laws. Darker brown colors indicate less cleansed areas, lighter brown colors indicate cleaner areas.

Source: The Wellcome Library, London.

and cesspools, localized sources of London's foul, miasmatic odors. Alas, he failed to gain the necessary legislative support to carry out his plan to collect and divert all the runoff of the city's effluvia into an integrated sewer system. Nobody doubted the general merit of the plan, but the expense, at the time, was assumed to be prohibitive. The result by the late 1850s, after the third cholera pandemic, would be that "the [Thames] river was receiving some 260 tonnes per day through seventy-one main sewer outlets" (Porter, R. 1998, 56).

The importance of Chadwick's map, for our purposes, lies in part in its prominent inclusion in his report, the most detailed and most widely distributed of its time. Its argument that the evolving city housed unsanitary pockets in which disease might fester was fundamental. No less significantly, it argued implicitly for a mapped approach to health-related issues, and for mapping as an investigative as well as a descriptive tool. Chadwick did this to draw attention to economic class, embedding into the map symbolization of employment categories, disease incidence, and general wellness. The houses of the working class are on streets shaded with a gray hatching and distinguished from those of the first class on streets that contain a diamond-style pattern.

Across the city, the "less cleansed" areas are shaded a darker brown and these, not surprisingly, are areas largely inhabited by working-class rather than wealthier families. Blue spots are hand inked onto the map to indicate "localities in which cholera prevailed," while red spots are used to identify residences from which people with "contagious disease have been sent to the house of recovery from 1834 to 1839." Finally, the ratio of good (healthy) to bad streets by parish district was calculated based on deaths by population as well as a density measure of population per acre. The message is clear: increasing density of population per acre correlates positively with mortality and negatively with births. In the map, and in the text, increasing density of population similarly correlates with the blue and red dots that symbolize where cholera and other contagious diseases occurred in the city. Population density correlates with increased disease and is, therefore, a cause of increased mortality. Understood in the text but unmapped was the relation between increasing density and poverty: poor folk lived in dense quarters unlike the well-to-do and rich whose homes were large and whose neighborhoods relatively sparsely populated.

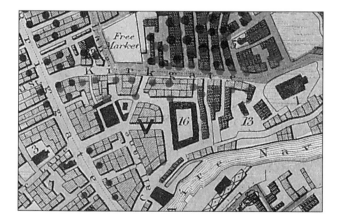

Figure 3.6b Detail of Chadwick's map showing incidence of cholera (dark blue spots) and of other contagious diseases (red spots) within the study area.

Source: The Wellcome Library, London.

Here the horizontal concerns with health and disease complemented—methodologically and conceptually—the vertical study of specific diseases like cholera, typhoid, and yellow fever. Mortality and morbidity are positively related to population density that is shown on the map to relate to class. The statistical key relating births and deaths by district, and density (population and disease indicators) to those figures, emphasizes the manner in which the general coloration of the map was determined and the essentially statistical nature of the data Chadwick so carefully distilled in this and other maps. The argument was profoundly graphic and statistical simultaneously, the distillation of a sophisticated and profoundly social perspective of the relation of class and place to the incidence of health and disease.

A barrister and former secretary to economist and social theorist Jeremy Bentham, Chadwick had earlier authored the British Poor Law that created public workhouses where the environments were self-consciously vile. The assumption had been that they would encourage shiftless, lazy people to return to socially profitable work. What he discovered, however, was that what kept many people from employment was neither laziness nor the lack of good work habits (which the workhouse in theory would teach) but that they were often too sick to be employable. Chadwick's interest therefore shifted to issues of public health and sanitation. The result was a socioeconomic perspective informed by a miasmatic theory of disease that would hold it was less expensive to prevent disease (by promoting a healthier, less odiferous environment) than it was to live in an unhealthy city that promoted disease.

The concern of Benthamites like Chadwick was not primarily humanitarian but economic. They worried that the sickliness of the poor was a potential barrier to the realization of a government's legitimate economic objectives. A diminished workforce would be insufficiently productive and the private businesses that government advantaged would suffer as a result. In this way health becomes an issue of economic infrastructure, not a good in its own right. Both the failure of sanitary infrastructure and the high density of habitation in evolving slums, rooms whose air was dank and close, pervaded with the odors of the poor inhabitants, contributed to the problem of foul airs. The first was the source of the "exhalation" of rotting effluvia in the city contaminating the general air. The second assured transmission by "contagion," the close-quarter scale of disease inhalation in miasmatic theory (Shannon 1981, 222).

Bentham and his followers also believed both in science and good records, "a compilation of statistics on a national scale would illuminate the precise relationship between poverty and illness" (Vinten-Johansen et. al. 2003, 171–172). Chadwick, like others of this school, therefore embraced statistical and mapped analyses as a way of identifying environmental sources predisposing a population to unprofitable ill health. His report "skillfully wove statistics, example, and lurid descriptions into a warrant for government intervention into the urban environment. He dramatized the need for pollution abatement, waste removal, and clean water supply" (Porter, D. H. 1998, 58). He included mapped arguments because, as Petermann said, mapping made "visible to the eye the development and nature of any phenomenon in regard to its geographical distribution."

It is worth noting how experimental this perspective was and how sophisticated the result. Attempting to correlate income and class with population density and the incidence of disease or health remains a fundamental challenge of epidemiologists and social scientists today. In the first half of the nineteenth century, a period in which hand-colored lithography created severe limits on the number and type of symbolizations a map might carry, the practical challenges were extreme. Similarly, at that time the statistics with which mortality and morbidity by district might be analyzed—deaths per population per acre—were almost as new as the understanding of class and its relation to density and income, health and disease.

Simply, there were few conventions and no hard and fast rules to this work. Chadwick pioneered the grand study and struggled with the questions of both statistical analysis and graphic distillation. His map of mortality and class in 1838 Bethnal Green, to take another example, attempted to relate mortality to classes of more prosperous tradesmen and shopkeepers compared to tradesmen and weavers. The streets of the more prosperous tradesmen and shopkeepers were signified by short, parallel dashes while those of weavers and laborers by a gray, diagonal hatching. Deaths from any of four categories (contagious disease, epidemic disease, disease of the brain or nerves, pulmonary or digestive disorders) were symbolized by a cross (+) when at least five deaths occurred in 1838 in that street block.

Visually, the result is that streets where the lower class resided are more embedded with those crosses than those where the tradesmen and shopkeepers resided. Here the issue is principally mortality

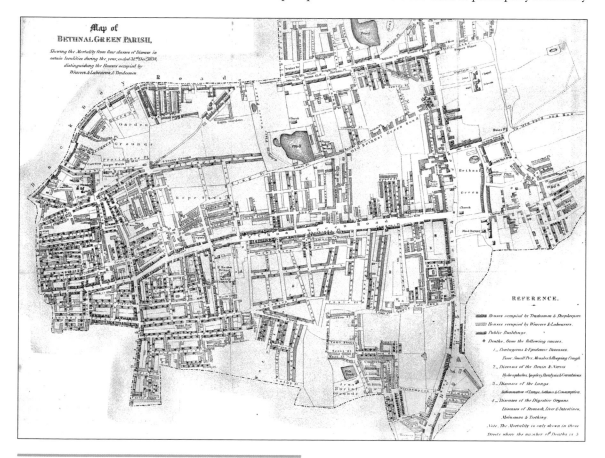

Figure 3.7 Chadwick's map of the relation of mortality to class in Bethnal Green. A cross (+) symbolizes mortality by street address. A gray, diagonal hatching symbolizes the streets of trades people, laborers, and weavers.

Source: Wellcome Trust.

as a function of class, the statistics more covert than in the more famous Leeds map. The argument, however, is fundamentally the same even if the graphic argument is somewhat less spectacular in black and white. In the Bethnal Green map, as in the Leeds map, the proposition is one of relation between mortality and class rather than mortality and, as it was in the Pascalis and Seaman maps, a waste site from which disease was assumed to diffuse.

Another, quite extraordinary example of this thinking, and a more modern approach to coloration, is presented in W. R. Wilde's 1841 *Sanitary Map of Dublin* (Robinson 1982, 185). The context of the map, and its publication with the tables of the data it summarized, is at least as significant as the quite radical argument it presented. In an official census report on mortality in Ireland, Wilde mapped the city's streets by economic class. The intent was to describe the city not by district but by street and residence, to show the relation by mortality and income (class) at a scale more specific than that of the parish district choropleth map. Unlike Chadwick, Wilde was not interested in arguing propositions of mortality and morbidity directly, but only those of class and location in the city.

In the hand-tinted map, Wilde was able to differentiate six categories of street ranging from first-class, private streets of privileged residence to third-class streets inhabited by the poorest populations. Each was assigned a different color to create a network of economic disparity. The result was detailed, and in the greater context of an official census of mortality replete with supporting statistical tables, damning. The map was not criticized for its findings. They were unassailable, fully supported by the report's voluminous statistics presented in tabular form.

The map was panned instead for its clarity and ease of comprehension, something that some feared would cause "infinite discord" among the poor. "The blue streets [upper-class houses] may remain on terms of cold acquaintanceship with the crimson [second-class shops and dwellings]," warned editors of *The Athenaeum,* a well-read London publication (*Athenaeum* 1844, 29). "It will then be blue and crimson against all other hues . . . we may confidently anticipate a rupture of all social relations." Of course, that assumed contented relations in fact existed between members of the various classes who lived in the different streets, and further, that mapping the observed divisions (and then publishing the resulting map) would itself create a newfound and profoundly alienating awareness of economic difference and its consequences.[9]

The critics were concerned principally with the map's communicative power, its ability to distill the report's numeric argument in a way that anyone could understand. They argued it was the map's ability to present the argument in a manner easily interpreted rather than the fact of economic differentiation itself that was a danger to the public weal. Not for the first time, and certainly not for the last, critics sought to dismiss a map not for its argument but for its ability to distill complex arguments in a comprehensive way. To do otherwise would have required they acknowledge an unpleasant social reality that was, if not hidden, then certainly not obvious in the tables whose data the map presented graphically.

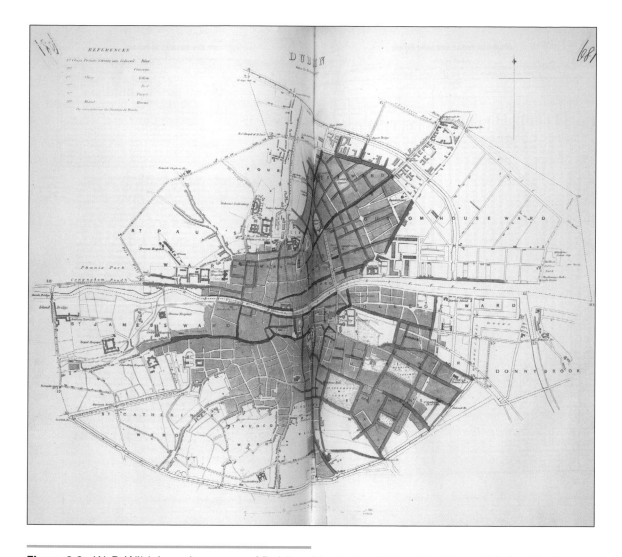

Figure 3.8 W. R. Wilde's sanitary map of Dublin with streets distinguished by social class in the 1841 report of the census of Ireland. Hand-tinted copperplate engraving.

Source: British Library.

The map distilled three entwined arguments that together were perceived as threatening. In the first, it argued systematic social and economic inequalities existed street by street, and in some cases, block by block. Second, and no less important, in the context of the greater report on mortality, the map related these differences to mortal results. The result concluded that economics, location, and the poverty that was their mapped conjunction affected states of disease and health. The result distilled the whole in a way that was graphic, powerful, intuitive, and therefore presumably explosive.

Charles Booth

The horizontal study of health determinants suggested by first Chadwick's and then Wilde's maps expanded the general, sanitarian concern into the horizontal realm of socioeconomic realities. The extremes of wealth and poverty that were mapped were objects of concern not for egalitarian reasons but because they represented conditions that were assumed to breed social unrest and, more importantly, illness. It was in these maps that the idea of "social determinants of health," much discussed in our time, were perhaps first considered. The nineteenth-century endpoint of this thinking that began in the 1830s and 1840s was Charles Booth's extraordinary mapping of poverty in London. Booth's monumental study, published in a series of volumes between 1889 and 1903, stands today as one of the most comprehensive pieces of social and environmental research conceived and carried out by a single investigator.

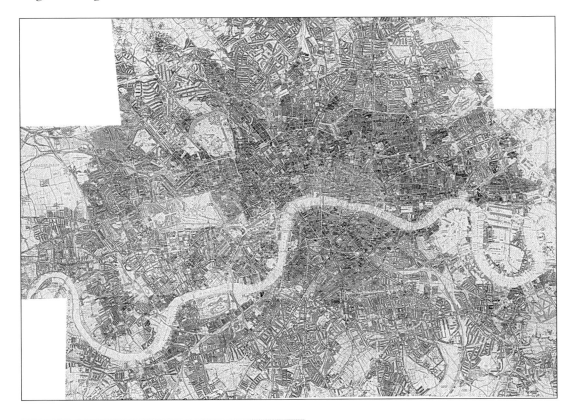

Figure 3.9a Booth's poverty map of London with the Thames river running through it. A uniquely comprehensive index of poverty was used to create a comprehensive portrait of London poverty on a block-by-block, building-by-building basis.

Source: By permission of the Library of the London School of Economics and Political Science.

Unsatisfied with then-current official definitions of poverty and the work of earlier, popular social investigators like Mayhew (Yeo and Thompson 1971), Booth created his own index of poverty based not on a house-to-house survey—the task would have been impossibly massive—but through interviews with London officials, and especially those of the school board who he believed had the most detailed knowledge of social conditions, especially poverty (Orford et al. 2002).[10] With the introduction of compulsory education in London in 1871, a means test had been devised for those families unable to pay their children's fees. This required, in turn, school officials to collect data on family income, occupation, rent, and other factors, data that Booth used to create a comprehensive and sophisticated index of poverty. He used the resulting data to create an income map of London based on the index. The result was a socioeconomic portrait of London that owes much to both Wilde and Chadwick's earlier work. A recently created Web site permits Booth's study and his mapping to be considered in detail (*booth.lse.ac.uk*).

The most famous of Booth's maps, his "Descriptive Map of London Poverty," is daunting in its detail. The whole of London is mapped by household in terms of the degree of poverty recorded, street-by-street, for each house. Six classes were used to distinguish the poorest from the wealthiest along a color ramp of lighter to darker red. The map's range is the economic status of London homes based on Booth's poverty index. Its domain is the physical city—its streets and its shops—at least those that were by then included in the comprehensive city maps that had become a common element of late-nineteenth-century industrialized cities.

Booth worked on a commercial map whose congress of specific urban landmarks—the railway yards, the open-space commons, and churches—emphasized the map's authority in its presentation of a broad economic and social topography. To separate the general structural components of the map (streets, houses, shops, parks, etc.) from the economic data fused to it is to do violence to the result. The brilliance of Booth's map is that it presents an integrated surface on which relative poverty or affluence defines the city by house, block, and parish, permitting each to be seen in terms of the poverty that distinguished some homes (and blocks or neighborhoods) from others. The result joins the detail of Wilde's map to the broad sweep of the choropleth map of Chadwick's early efforts.

Booth's map fused sophisticated statistics, born in the social and medical demographics of the 1820s and 1830s, with the advanced mapmaking (and printing) skills that were available to researchers at the end of the nineteenth century. As important, it advanced both the sanitarian perspective of early medical investigators and that of social reformers like Chadwick. By mapping the relative poverty of London, Booth did not also map disease incidence but chose instead to identify the areas where disease would be more likely and (expensive) health care less available as a function of income inequality.

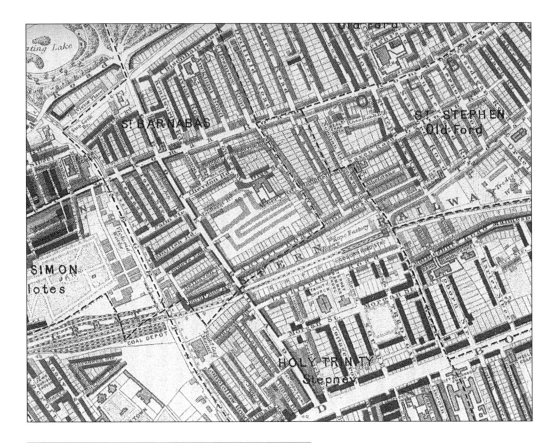

Figure 3.9b Detail of an East London section of Booth's poverty map showing variations in poverty and wealth by street.

Source: By permission of the Library of the London School of Economics and Political Science.

National and global scales

The majority of the maps discussed in this section are drawn at the scale of the city and city-district where diseases like cholera and yellow fever most directly affected citizens. Even Booth's map, occurring later than the others, is based on data organized at the scale of the parish district and the built environment within it. Other maps, the one of hernia incidence, for example, mapped phenomena at a national scale. National maps were almost always choropleth distillations whose focus was a specific health-related subject (cholera, urban waste, yellow fever, etc.) occurring within a relatively limited time frame and in a specific geographic domain. These works assumed that "physical causes lie at the bottom of whatever differences the maladies of different portions of the earth may present" (Drake 1850, 1) and that mapping the physical and climatic conditions of specific regions with the diseases that occurred in them would describe a causal relation between climatology and geology on the one hand, and disease incidence on the other.

It was this work that the newly founded American Medical Association (AMA) meant when in 1855 it voted to establish a committee on medical topography that would establish a relation between locality and epidemic disease for each state and territory. As the annual report of the AMA put it, "Few subjects of greater interest and importance could be presented to the consideration of the American Medical Association" (American Medical Association 1855, 6; Mitman and Numbers 2003, 395–396). Some of this work was based on the reports of military physicians posted across the expanding nation. In 1842, for example, Samuel Forry drew upon some four thousand quarterly sick reports submitted from across the continent by military physicians to produce his landmark *The Climate of the United States and Its Endemic Influences,* work previewed in a journal article the previous year on "Statistical Researchers Elucidating the Climate of the United States and Its Relation with Diseases of Malarial Origin, Based on the Records of the Medical Department and the Adjutant General's Office" (Forry 1841; Mitman and Numbers 2003, 394). Finke would have been proud.

There was another class of maps emerging in the decades of the early-to-mid nineteenth century that sought to understand disease, and especially pandemic disease, at a national and international scale. Their principal concern was not the cause of a disease—anticontagionist or contagionist did not matter—but its progression from a specific city or nation to other cities and nations. They were, in effect, the first of a class of maps that studied the diffusion of disease rather than charting its incidence. As such, they represented a distinct form of mapping that would blossom only in the second half of the twentieth century.

An early example of thinking at this scale can be found in Brigham's 1832 *A Treatise on epidemic cholera* (also see Jarcho 1970, 155–156).[11] Brigham's map fused cholera's temporal progress to a domain of countries reporting the disease internationally. A line that begins in India, where the disease was endemic and from which it spread, snakes around the world both over land and by sea route. The map used the Mercator projection employed in nautical maps and maps of international travel and trade routes. The lines drawn to connect countries internationally resemble those that were used to chart commercial sea and over-land routes of the day. Indeed, to us, the map is one of commercial land and sea routes on which the progress of cholera is mapped internationally.

Brigham was also neither unique in his scale of address nor in his method of mapping. In 1832, a "geographical and statistical account of the epidemic of cholera from its commencement in India to its entrance to the United States" was published in the United States. Its frontispiece was a large (51 x 44.5 cm) cholera map of the world, also using a Mercator projection, in which cholera's imposition is shown as a line of sea travel from England (Jarcho 1970, 136). As early as 1824, others had mapped cholera's regional progress across grid maps of India's geographical features (mountains, rivers, coasts)

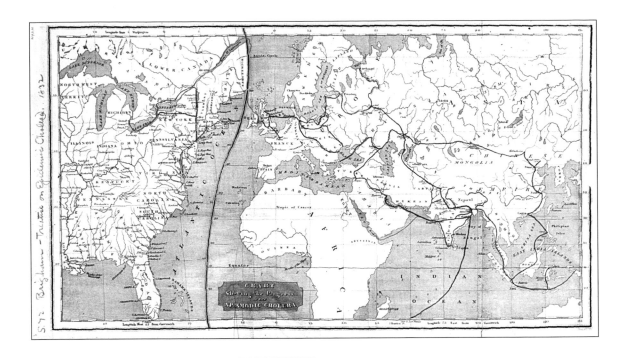

Figure 3.10a Brigham's world map of the progress of cholera in 1832. The hand-drawn line represents cholera's progress around the world, the lines closely following existing trade routes.

Source: New York Academy of Medicine Library.

as it moved from city to city (Jarcho 1970, 134). In 1831, Schnurrer used a 10-degree rectangular grid of Europe to illustrate the movement of cholera at a continental scale in his *Die Cholera Morbus*.

In these examples one sees the temporal and motile synchronicity that some believe is a characteristic of mapping generally (Beck and Wood 1976), and is certainly a principal characteristic of these maps of disease diffusion. Distilled in the map are benchmarks of more than a decade of cholera's progress along then-prominent commercial routes of trade. The lines on the map symbolize the travels of hundreds of ships sailing established sea corridors over years and of an unknown number of cargo vehicles traveling by land over similarly familiar roads. This long history of motion and travel over time is visible at a glance, in the mapped instant, as it were.

For modern researchers the whole describes a "relocation" pattern of diffusion, one in which a disease moves like some peripatetic traveler staying in one place for a time before moving to another, and then another, until it has ended its journey (Haggett 2000, 2–4). The metaphor is inexact, however, as metaphors tend to be. Cholera after all is not a person but a bacterium that exists through replication and dispersal in favorable environments. It may remain embedded in a place for years, as it was in India, while cascading more rapidly through other nations (Turkistan, Russia, and England) in an

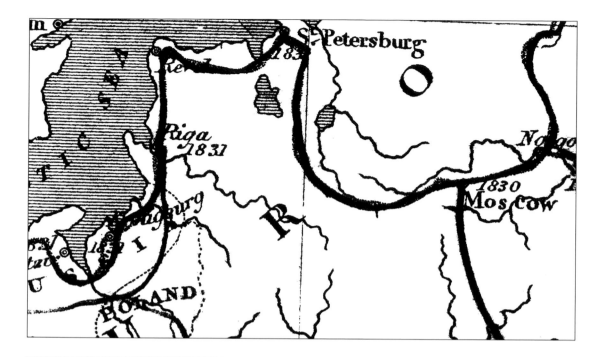

Figure 3.10b Black-and-white detail of Brigham's world map of the progress of cholera in 1832. The hand-drawn line represents cholera's progress with dates of outbreaks beside individual towns.

Source: New York Academy of Medicine Library.

almost syncopated manner, rooted in one city for months while it simultaneously spread from that city to surrounding towns via a local transportation system. It was in the port and also in the countryside, moving from entry ports to smaller, secondary areas as a person whose infection had yet to manifest carried the bacillus from an infected area elsewhere, to home or to market.

The map's synchronicity, its ability to distill the disease's international course, did not come at the cost of all specificity. Because it mapped the disease by nation and city, the map also said, "Here is where British soldiers died in India in 1918. There are the deaths of Moscow and St. Petersberg in 1831, and the outbreak in Riga in 1831." It is not simply that "in *these* cities occurred cholera at *those* times." More importantly, the map demands we see the progress of the disease as the sum of its specific visitations, each segment of its travel a line between occurrences in one city and then another, the sum of the lines a biography of cholera's progression. Britain's line segments begin in Sunderland and continue from there into other areas of England, and afterward to the New World with which it traded. The result was a distillation of choleric history, international in scope but plastic in its scale. The track of the disease included the cities whose populations were affected in its course among the trading nations of the world.

In the 1850s, Heinrich and Hermann Berghaus created even more impressive maps of both endemic and epidemic disease in their *Physikalischer Atlas*. Besides a dedicated map of cholera, the atlas included an ambitious world map of the geographic distribution of human diseases (Jarcho 1969), one of four sheets in its "Anthropography" section (Camerini 2000, 193–194) with inserts identifying characteristic diseases of, for example, North America and the West Indies. Areas of greater incidence are stippled to create a darker area. Within the greater context of the whole atlas, and its sections on clothing, occupation, and religion, "a recognition of disease as an intimate part of the total human and social experience," is implied (Jarcho 1969, 414). As important, perhaps, maps of trade routes made the implicit link of disease as an export that traveled established trade routes with other, more desirable goods of expanding, international commerce.

"The Brigham and Berghaus maps of disease in a true sense verge on the ecological, since they are accompanied by isotherms, tables of altitude, and similar significant data" as inserts on the map (Jarcho 1969, 414). This is, however, a bit optimistic. But more cautiously, and correctly, one can say that for the first time the broad relation of endemic and epidemic disease to location, and some of the geographic elements defining those locations, was explored systematically and graphically.

Perhaps the best map of this global vision of health and disease is A. K. Johnston's 1856 *The Physical Atlas of Natural Phenomena*. In its map "The Geographical Distribution of Health and Disease in Connection chiefly with Natural Phenomena," the oceanic trade routes by which cholera traveled are mapped like graceful, curving roads across the ocean, the 1832 diffusion to North America highlighted in red. The endemic disease afflicting each nation and region are included; they are, in effect, jurisdictions of health and disease. The bottom of the map is full of charts summarizing the relative mortality of consumption by population, rheumatism among troops stationed around the globe, and a "value of life" index based on rates of national mortality by age. A companion chart focuses the index for principal cities embedded in the larger map.

A. K. Johnston owes an obvious cartographic debt to Berghaus who, with his brother William, published four of Berghaus's maps as part of an 1843 National Atlas before becoming a mapmaker in his own right (Camerini 2000, 198–199). While he learned much from that experience, this map is clearly his own, an almost encyclopedic compendium of cartographic and statistical techniques fused in a manner that strengthened the mapped result (Howe 1961). Lines chart the progress of disease (by time and type) between countries distinguished by general states of specific illness or relative health. The names of each disease are noted in areas of endemic occurrence. The result defines a landscape of disease districts (the province of goiter, the state of catarrh, the city of leprosy) across each country. The effect of these diseases is summarized in the value of life charts on the map's lower right side that compare life quality and disease incidence for specific populations, nation by nation and city by city. The charts sum the locational argument that the map distills both for specific conditions (consumption and

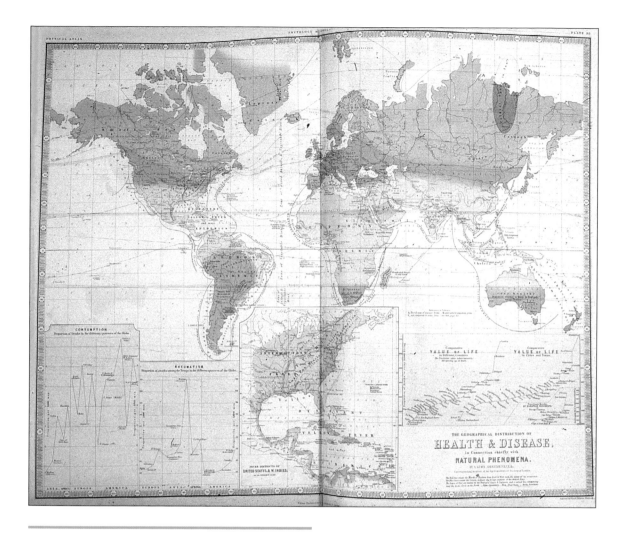

Figure 3.11a A. K. Johnston's map, *The Geographical Distribution of Health and Disease in Connection Chiefly with Natural Phenomena,* 1856.

Source: National Library of Medicine.

rheumatism) and as general indicators of life expectancy, or as the mapmakers thought of it, the "value of life" indexes.

Here was Finke's dream come true, a map of known disease at a scale and with detail he could not have dreamed of in 1792. Its use of a Mercator projection, complete with lines of latitude and longitude, reflected cartographic techniques more typically used in those days to map global oceanic trade routes. Nor is this surprising. It was the need to map mercantile routes and the cities they served that

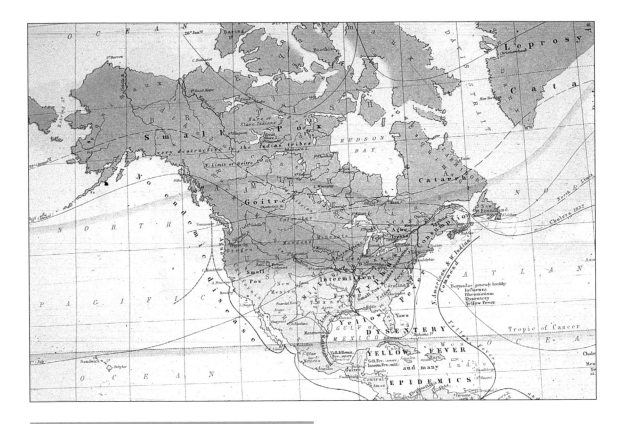

Figure 3.11b Detail of A. K. Johnston's 1856 map, The Geographical Distribution of Health and Disease in Connection Chiefly with Natural Phenomena, from his *Physical Atlas of Natural Phenomena,* showing North and Central America

Source: National Library of Medicine.

first gave impetus to the atlas in the 1500s (Binding 2003). Cartography developed during the mercantile era as more of the world's harbors were charted and the routes between them mapped.

These were increasingly collected in atlases that served both sailors and the merchants whose goods they carried around the world. In the 1800s, the form of the atlas with its many maps was married to the needs of an evolving medical science faced with increasingly global pandemics and a slowly dawning recognition that disease itself was a challenge of modernity, a fact of life encountered by every trading vessel and continental train that hauled goods and people across the continents where traders lived.

To get a sense of the detail of the map, the specificity contained in its global panoramic, consider the map section that includes North America and the Caribbean. Isobars for temperature wave across the map that shows a relatively complete set of oceanic transit routes. On land are major towns (even Vancouver, Canada, and San Diego, California, are included) as well as the principle landscape features, mountains and rivers. For each region, the endemic diseases are listed, with goiter in Canada's western provinces and catarrh in the northeastern region. Bermuda is generally healthy, but the western Caribbean is listed as a frequent site for epidemic yellow fever and cholera. And so it goes, the world of disease linked by transportation routes that here detail the chronological march of cholera, tying the whole together.

It is common today to talk about how the world has shrunk, about the manner in which ever-more rapid means of transportation and communication have conquered the distance that separates us. It is the arrogance of modernity to assume we are privileged in a way our ancestors were not. Johnston's map reminds us how much modernity's advance is one of degree rather than kind. Compare the scale of knowledge of Seaman and Pascalis, or the almost touchingly local concerns of Arrieta, with the sweep of the world Johnston distills. Here was an international portrait of mortality and potential morbidity pertinent to all the trading nations and regions of the mercantile world of the day.

The world had not shrunk from that of Seaman or Finke. Indeed, it had grown impossibly more vast, the complexity of regions contributing to an interrelated global vision in which real distinctions of locality were to be seen within the broad patterns of exchanges between the trading peoples of the world. The course of the world we know today—one vast and complex and yet intimately related—is here presented, reflected in a mature if not wholly modern map.

With these maps, the distillation of knowledge is also a summation, the addition of literally hundreds of local studies and the reports of thousands of local health agencies. It was in the commonality of disease and its international progression, mapped in city after city of nation after nation, that an international perspective on disease transmission would grow in the 1970s.

Conclusion

Jarcho suggests the classical period of medical mapping ends around 1840 "since it can be fairly asserted that by then the mapping of disease had gained permanent acceptance among medical writers" (Jarcho 1970, 131). That almost certainly overstates the case. Even today, some health experts see medical mapping as at best an illustrative adjunct to the hard work of more rigorous professionals. To these critics, those who employ mapping as an analytic tool are largely amateurs who see themselves "as rushing out into the real world to save real lives while the stodgy, plodding scientists fussily demand more evidence before they are willing to act" (Vinten-Johansen et al. 2003, 397).

This assumes a necessary division between the mapping amateur and the rigorous (if stodgy) professional that is denied in this brief history. Medical mapping developed as a way of thinking about disease. In the late 1600s, the Bari plague map identified the pattern of disease diffusion and the methods of its address. In the work of first Seaman and then Pascalis, mapping was a way for researchers to think about both the nature of a disease and the environments that promoted it. In the 1830s, with the development of medical and social statistics, mapping was a full partner in the aggregation of individual cases in a manner that could be shown to be significant. By the 1840s, it had become almost impossible to think about incidences of disease and potentially causative factors without mapping in one way or another.

It is tempting to think about this early period of medical mapping of disease in a condescending manner. As Lee (2002) put it in another context, "Nice maps, shame about the theory." The idea of a potent miasma or simple geographical determinism seems quaint to us. The theories of early medicostatistical researchers—that incidence of hernia perhaps was related to the use of cooking oil, for example—are amusing. But it is important to remember how many theories and hypothesis have been generated, presented, tested, and then proven, only to be discarded later (sometimes much later), as our understanding of the determinants of health and disease changed. To dismiss as curiosities the work of Berghaus, Malgaigne, Pascalis, Seaman, et al. because they endorsed a disease theory later proved incorrect is to miss the point. They were pioneers not simply in mapping of disease but in medical science. They developed hypotheses based on the best medical and social theories of their time and then attempted to test those theories with all the tools available at their command. The mapped propositions that resulted at once distilled and advanced arguments that, while inadequate from our perspective, were critical to the process by which we today have reached our own level of understanding.

Endnotes

1. The 1840s saw the birth of national and international mail services supported by the sale of postage stamps by governments. A system of mail carriers and mail delivery provided a structure by which the mass of new publications could be disseminated nationally and internationally. Newspapers, for example, could be posted for free in England if they were mailed within eight days to subscribers. It was therefore not unusual by the mid 1850s for British researchers to be aware of the work of their counterparts in the Americas and around Europe, and for Americans to be aware of the work by British, German, French, and other like-minded investigators around the world (Koch 2003).

2. It is here that the work of historians like Shapin and Schaffer (1985) and Pickering (1995) demands application to the history of not medical mapping but the more general field of cartography. The direction one might take from the perspective of their works, based on the rigorous understanding of the history of medical mapping, is only hinted at or suggested. Subsequent works hopefully will expand upon the application of their understanding of technologies, in the first case, and the "mangle of practice" in the second, to this history.

3. The cholera epidemics of the nineteenth century have become fodder for social historians. O'Connor for example, argues that "Asiatic cholera staged a traumatic transformation of white, working-class flesh into worthless black-stuff—in medicine and popular journalism the dark, dehydrated corpse of the cholera victim is liked to tar, coal, pitch, even feces" (O'Connor 2000, 11). Perhaps, but the ferocity of its onset, its robust rates of mortality, and the frequency of its occurrence mid-century were also sufficient causes for fear.

4. Pamphlets and papers for the edification of the emerging literate classes were frequent in the mid-1600s, although costs of production kept weekly or daily journals from being common (Tomalin 2002, xxxvi–xxxvii). Censorship laws introduced by Charles II effectively ended this period of privately printed, public argument. During the 1800s, improved printing technologies and burgeoning, increasingly literate, trade and middle classes created both an expanding market of interested readers and the technology to satisfy their interest.

5. Gilbert (1958, 178) gives the source of this quotation as Petermann's 1852 "Statistical Notes" accompanying his map of cholera. Robinson (1982), a far more precise researcher, cites the map and the statistical notes as being published in 1848. Gilbert used mostly secondary sources rather than the originals from which Robinson worked. For that reason, the latter's reference is used here.

6. Mitman's and Numbers's 2003 article on miasma as a theory and medical geography in general provides an enormous wealth of information and the beginning of a critical review of nineteenth and early twentieth century thinking. I am indebted to John Kerry for bringing it to my attention.

7. The basis for this disease theory rested upon early ideas of fermentation and the idea that, just as nonliving yeast was an "exciter" that in the proper fluid was capable of replacing itself, diseases were the result of "exciters" entering the body and the blood. It was through the analogy with fermentation that experts assumed nonliving agents specific to individual diseases (cholerine for cholera, for example) found in the blood were a fertile field for some type of propogation. The idea held "until investigations in the collaterial sciences could uncover the specific nature of the [disease] causative agents" (Vinten-Johansen et al. 2003, 182–183).

8. The internationalization of medical research into cholera is clearly detailed in John Snow's reports of 1854 and 1855 where, in arguing an anticontagionist view, he critiques studies written by researchers in Great Britain, various European countries, and India. Many, but not all, of the researchers he quoted used maps.

9. The Irish were well aware of the social divisions of their society and its effect on working-class members. Rebellion in the 1790s, crop failures in the early 1800s, and political unrest throughout this era make clear the degree to which economic disparities and political inequalities ran rampant across the Irish landscape (Hansen 1961; Koch 2003, 75–76).

10. Researchers using contemporary GIS technologies have recently recreated Booth's map, linked the data to contemporary boundaries, and recalculated the index of relative poverty for modern times. The result presents a comparison of both mapping techniques, then and now, and the constancy of the poverty that nineteenth century authors—Charles Dickens, Charles Mayhew, John Snow, etc.—documented so carefully. See Orford et al. 2002.

11. Jarcho (1970, 136–137) describes five different copies of this map, all of which he reviewed. They included versions in the New York Academy of Medicine, the U.S. National Library of Medicine, Yale Medical Library, a copy in his own collection, and one "in possession of a book dealer in New York." In all the maps a stippled line over which a red ink line was then drawn indicated cholera's worldwide diffusion.

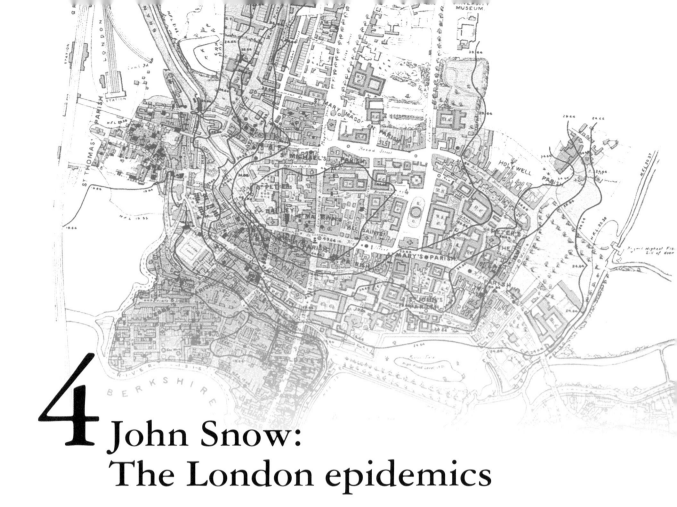

4 John Snow: The London epidemics

While William Sproat lay dying in Sunderland in the fall of 1831, John Snow was working as a medical apprentice in Newcastle upon Tyne (Winterton 1980). He soon became busier. In 1827, he was indentured to William Hardcastle, a surgeon-apothecary whose practice extended beyond the town and into the local mining communities.[1] By the time cholera arrived in England, Snow was a senior apprentice capable of unsupervised care under the broad guidance of his superior. On December 7, Newcastle's first cases of cholera were confirmed and through 1832 outbreaks occurred in varying areas within Hardcastle's medical jurisdiction. As his assistant, Snow was responsible for the treatment of patients in Killingworth, a mining community hard hit by the epidemic. In addition, he almost certainly saw cases both in the town of Newcastle and elsewhere in the region, wherever he was sent as Hardcastle's surrogate (Vinten-Johansen et al. 2003).

Later, when cholera returned to England at the end of the 1840s, Snow would remember his experience in the Newcastle area during the first epidemic. The son of a Yorkshire farmer, he was perhaps more attuned than many of his medical contemporaries whose births were more privileged and whose concern for the poor less personal. Almost certainly, his experiences in the Newcastle area contributed to both his general sanitarian perspective, one that would have done Seaman and Pascalis proud, and his linking of sanitary conditions to the spread of cholera.

One assumption in the 1830s was that cholera required contact either with a sick person or with the "fomites from infected bedding and clothing" (Vinten-Johansen et al. 2003, 166). How this transfer occurred was uncertain, however, and the contagionist perspective, one that answered a more traditionally miasmatic view of airborne and air-generated disease, dominated medical thinking into the 1880s. For Snow, the severity of the cholera he treated in the early 1830s was directly related to the abysmal sanitary conditions of the poor, especially those in the mines. In an 1849 essay, for example, he wrote: "The mining population of this country has suffered more from cholera than any other, and there is a reason for this. There are no privies in the coal pits and I believe this is true of other mines: as the workers stay down the pit about eight hours at a time, they take food down with them which they eat, of course, with unwashed hands, as soon as one pitman gets the cholera, there must be great liability of others . . . to get their hands contaminated, and to acquire the malady" (Snow 1849a).

As the 1830s epidemic ran its course, Snow left Newcastle upon Tyne in 1833 to take up an assistantship with a nearby rural apothecary, John Watson. Under Hardcastle he had learned the basics of a general surgical and medical practice. With Watson his apprenticeship was again general—apothecaries were the general practitioners of the day—with an emphasis on pharmacology. His association with Watson was unsatisfactory, however, and the next year he took up a post as assistant to another, more agreeable senior, West Yorkshire apothecary John Warburton. There his responsibilities again were for a generally rural population. "Warburton took charge of patients in town and supervised Joseph, Jr., his son and [primary] apprentice. Snow was responsible for patients in the rural parishes" (Vinten-Johansen et al. 2003, 46). The whole gave Snow a diverse and varied clinical background that covered town and country, deep mines and broadly agricultural communities.

The division between surgeon, apothecary, and physician (MD) was important. In those days, surgeons were the general workers of medicine, performing a range of diagnostic and general procedures (bone setting, blood-letting, suturing, etc.). Apothecaries dispensed drugs in general, nonsurgical practices. It was common for a young man like Snow to train in both fields and seek qualification as a surgeon-apothecary, a general medical consultant. Only university-recognized physicians carried the MD after their name, however. They were at the top of the heap, both as researchers and in the care of complex internal complaints as well as performance of complicated surgeries.

In 1836, Snow moved to London to complete his training as a surgeon-apothecary, taking his surgical examination in the spring of 1838 and his apothecary examination in the fall of that year. Formally qualified, he set up practice on Firth Street in the Soho area of London, a courageous act for a young apothecary and surgeon without family connections. On a street with at least four or five other medical persons—and in an area with at least half a dozen more within a mile radius—his general practice was never grandly lucrative. Fortunately, Snow's life style was abstemious. A teetotaler and a vegetarian, he was neither a dandy nor a bon vivant. A central London practice, even a modest one, provided the money for his studies at Hunterian School of Medicine on Great Windmill Street, near Haymarket in Westminster, a short walk from his home and practice. In 1843, he sat the formal examination and earned the right to put an MD after his name.

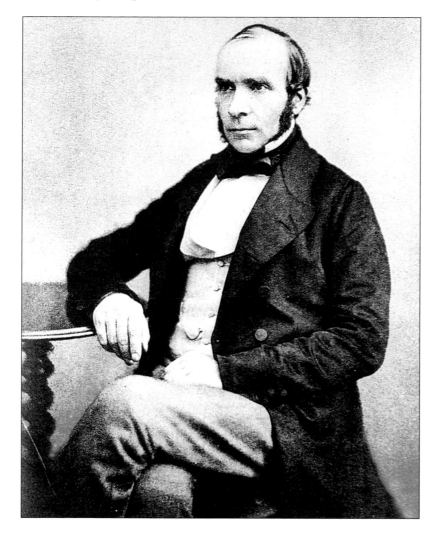

Figure 4.1 Photograph of Dr. John Snow taken in 1857, a year before his death.

Source: British Library.

As important, residence in London gained him access to local medical societies where members read reports on their research and critiqued the reports of others. The Westminster Medical Society, for example, where he was an active member, met on a weekly basis to hear and discuss the researches and cases of its members. These societies, whose numbers grew through the 1850s, were a sign of a growing interest in research by medical professionals, and a growing scientism in medicine generally. For Snow, they presented a forum where he could hone his critical skills in the discussion of the work of others, and ever more frequently, present his own ideas in a collegial forum. These were the days in which began the now common practice of presenting research lectures that would later be written up and submitted to journals, some of which were closely allied with particular societies.

All this occurred within the greater context of the publishing revolution that, in the 1840s, was in full swing. Faster presses, and a nationally regulated system of mail delivery, meant opportunities for an increasing congress of publishers who sought to more profitably and efficiently use their equipment through the production of an increasing number of general and specialized publications (Koch 2003). The new, faster printing technologies permitted decreased costs of production and the potential to print more—and better illustrated—publications. An increasingly reliable, relatively inexpensive national and international mail meant an ever-greater national and international audience for the publications that resulted. As costs of production dropped and demand grew—people were coming to *expect* a literature in fields of science—new journals were the result. In addition, within the more popular press, the world of broadsheets and general magazines, interest in medicine was increasing. By the late 1840s, it was not uncommon for daily journalists to attend the meetings of medical societies (and, later, university medical lectures), writing up reports on new techniques and procedures and ideas.

It was in this environment that John Snow, MD, developed three interrelated careers simultaneously. First, he built and maintained a general medical practice treating the plethora of daily ailments that are a general practitioner's stock-in-trade. Secondly, he launched a career as a medical researcher whose papers were presented at the local societies, and later, published in medical journals. From 1838 to 1842, he published at least seven papers in the *Lancet* (whose first edition premiered in 1838) and the *London Medical Gazette*. Finally, John Snow became a specialist.

Soon after the first London demonstration of ether as an anesthetic in late 1846, Snow turned his attention to the problem of anesthesia. By September 1847, Snow had published a clinical textbook called *On the Inhalation of the Vapour of Ether in Surgical Operations*. It was an impressive feat. In less than a year Snow had studied and, by the standards of the day, mastered the problem of dosage, developed an inhaler that permitted the drug to be more reliably administered, and with his textbook advanced himself as a leading clinical specialist in the field. The subtitle of his text announced as its basis "a statement of the result of nearly eighty operations in which ether has been employed." In the first nine months of 1847, he administered anesthetic in fifty-two cases at St. George's Hospital and, between May and September, to another twenty-three patients at University College Hospital (Vinten-Johansen et al. 2003, 115).

John Snow had arrived. He had become a primary practitioner in a new medical specialty, an authority whose writings were read and seriously considered. That the new approach to painless surgery was widely reported in the newspapers and news magazines of the day hurt neither his reputation nor his practice. The 1840s were an increasingly public age, and those who worked at the cutting edge of science were increasingly in the public eye.

Mapping: Public examples

The mid-nineteenth century was also an era in which mapping was becoming an accepted element of official studies of everything from agricultural production to shipping practices (Robinson 1982). At the same time, a new generation of popular journals used maps both as illustrations accompanying articles and as statements in their own right. In England, *Punch,* or the *London Charivari,* founded in the early 1840s, was an early devotee of the mapped argument. Its reputation rested upon both the excellence of its writing, acerbic and fractious by turns, and its groundbreaking use of illustrations, including maps.

In 1846, for example, *Punch* published a sketch map of dense traffic on the Thames River and on its bridges.[2] In it, private coaches jam the bridges. Steam trains whose stations were at their south end line up one after another, and a fleet of ships steams up and down a river overcrowded with boat traffic. A few birds fly near the westernmost bridge, almost lost in the general confusion. The caption describes the map as a "sketch taken from the top of the monument by an enthusiastic follower of high art, showing the ex-urban progress of the various locomotives, steamers, and vehicles along the roads, the rails and the river" (*Punch* 1846, 32).

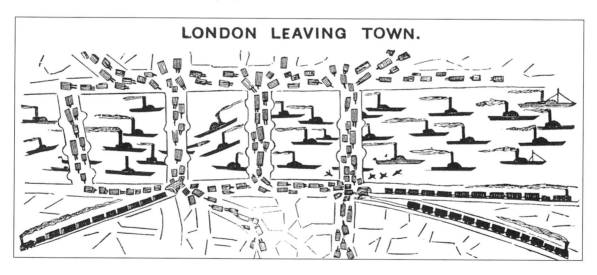

Figure 4.2 "London Leaving Town," urban traffic on central bridges in London during the summer in 1846. It was an attempt to "catch as they fly the various moving machines that take the metropolis beyond itself."

Source: *Punch* (1846, 32).

The result presented in the map the sheer intensity of transportation and the various methods of travel in the inner city. It may be the first map of a traffic jam, of the overwhelming intensity of weekend, rush-hour travel as it overburdens the capacity of routes in and out of the city center. This was more than simple illustration, however. It was an argument in which sheer density of occurrence in an intermodal urban network argued issues of capacity and delay. Comparing the sketch map to a *Punch* pen and ink illustration that addressed increasing urban density in another way emphasizes the difference between map and illustration.

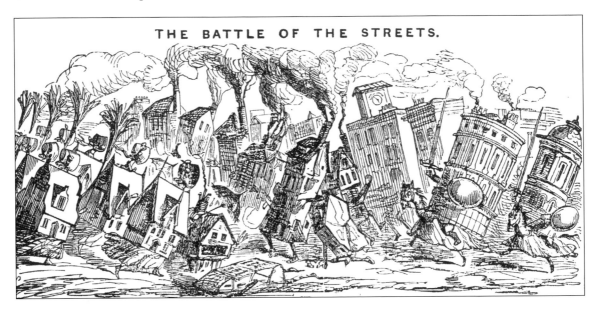

THE BATTLE OF THE STREETS.

Figure 4.3 "The Battle of the Streets." A *Punch* illustration showing the effect of street widening on the city as "the old brick and tile order" were transformed to accommodate increased traffic. Comparing this with the sketch map of traffic congestion illustrates the difference between mapped argument and graphic illustration .

Source: *Punch* (1845, 64).

In 1845, "The Battle of the Streets" was used to describe "the contest between the broad and the narrow," the city that resulted as narrow lines unable to handle increasing traffic were widened to accommodate both new businesses and the volume of travelers it generated. Here the sense is of a city collapsing upon itself in the transformation of its buildings and roads, an impressionistic image of London in the midst of change, parts falling upon each other, a city in which "the old brick and tile order will be utterly superseded by the modern stuccoite" (*Punch* 1845, 64).

Mapping and illustrative graphics were sometimes combined in a way that, while not geographically representative (scale of address and relation of elements are self-consciously incorrect) powerfully

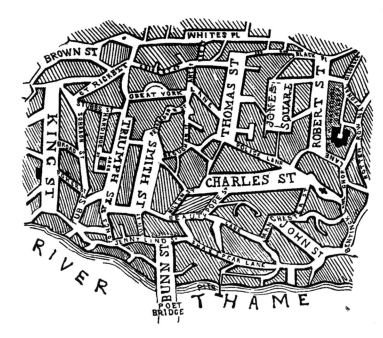

Figure 4.4 "Modern Streetology."
Map of Central London showing
streets that were being widened
and more traditional, narrow roads.

Source: *Punch* (1847, 265).

summarized an argument. In 1847, for example, *Punch* published a very different map of urban growth and congestion. Here the focus was not the traffic itself but the street network on which it flowed. To accommodate new businesses, London streets were widened unsystematically in an attempt to accommodate the increase in urban traffic volume. The resulting "Modern Streetology" concluded that "we get plenty of streets, but no thoroughfares; for every new way of any extent or importance is remarkable for its beginning at a place from which no one ever comes, and ending in a quarter to which no one is ever going" (*Punch* 1847, 265).

What resulted was a network notable not for its capacity and connectivity but for its impediments to travel. To make its point the map uses two sizes for city streets, very broad lines and a larger lettered font to contrast those that had been widened with narrower lines and a lighter, smaller font for those streets that were unchanged. By mapping the range of street width onto the domain of the central city—the National Gallery and Poet Bridge are added to identify the area to readers—the choke points where traffic necessarily would back-up was argued. Off King Street on the map's west side can be seen Broad Street, later famous as the site of the 1854 cholera outbreak that John Snow would map.

These maps here serve to underscore the growing ubiquity of maps and map-like graphics in popular as well as official documents, the general context for what was to become Snow's most famous work, his map of the Soho-area cholera outbreak in St. James Parish in 1854. Certainly, these maps support the development of the myth of John Snow as a lone, cartographic inventor, a pioneering mapmaker who was generations ahead of his time. He was not. Snow was not a man out of time, but a man of his times, one who took advantage of the myriad opportunities of his age. His mapping of cholera occurred in the context of both the medical and scientific mapping that had been ongoing for at least a generation, appearing ever-more frequently in general publications, official documents, and scientific studies. Thoroughly single-minded, Snow would use whatever media seemed most capable of advancing the investigations that engaged him.

Cholera 1849

In the midst of Snow's successes—professional and scientific—cholera returned to England in 1849. By the time the epidemic had run its course in London, 14,600 deaths or 6.2 deaths per one thousand people would be recorded (Winterton 1980, 11). The epidemic was especially severe in the Berwick Street area of Soho near Snow's home and practice. The accepted medical and social explanation was that miasmatic, foul, poisonous airs were being generated by urban refuse to the detriment of the health of the city's citizens, especially the poor. It was the general argument advanced by Seaman and Pascalis, one still opposed to the argument of direct disease transmission.

A letter from a Soho Square area resident, published July 3, 1849, in the *Times of London* gives the flavor of the time and the power of the anticontagionist argument. The fever was already entrenched in an environment whose lack of sanitation, good drainage, and secure water was "disgustin." That the letter was published on the eve of a new cholera epidemic makes it the more poignant, and for those who believed in a miasmatic theory of disease, more central. If filth and its noxious airs caused disease, why not believe that this level of uncleanliness and urban abandonment contributed to the new epidemic as well?

John Scott and his fellow residents lived in the general neighborhood in which Snow, too, lived and worked. His home and surgery were near enough to make him both personally and professionally familiar with the residents' complaints. They lived in an overcrowded environment with abysmal sanitation not dissimilar from that of the miners he had cared for in Newcastle on Tyne twenty years before. In the almost twenty years that had elapsed since Snow's apprenticeship during the 1830s epidemic, he had developed his skills as a physician and as a researcher. Over the years, he had, in the midst of his other medical studies, kept abreast of writings and reports on cholera, the research whose maps were briefly reviewed in the previous chapter. Beginning in 1849, Snow focused his considerable energies on cholera and its causes, cutting back on his anesthetic and general medical practices to devote more time to this research. Among the qualities that would distinguish Snow from his contemporaries was the manner in which he folded environmental and social elements into a detailed argument of cholera transmission.

In 1849, Snow published a long two-part paper on cholera in the *Medical Gazette and Times* (Snow 1849a; 1849b) as well as a short monograph, *On the Mode of Transmission of Cholera* (Snow 1849c). A

We print the following remonstrance just as it reached us and trust its publication will assist the unfortunate remonstrants.

The Editor of the Times Paper

Sur, may we beg and besearch your protection and power, we are sur, as it may be living in as wilderness, so far as the rest of London knows anything of us, or as the rich and great people care about. We live in much dirt and filth. We aint got no priviz, no dust bins, no drains, no water splies and no drain or suer in the hole place. The Suer Company of Greet St., Soho Square, all great rich powerful men take no notice Watsomedever of our complaints. The stench of a Gully-hole is disgustin. We, all of us, suffer and numbers are ill, and if Colera comes Lord Help Us.

Some gentlemans comed yesterday, and we thought they were comishoners from the Suer Company, but they was complaining of the noosance and stench our lans and carts was to them in New Oxford Street. They was muched surprised to see the seller in No. 12 Carrier St., in our land, where a child was dying from the fever, and would not believe that sixty persons slept in it every night. This here seller you couldn't swing a cat in and rent is five shilling a week, but there are a grat many sick sellers. Sur, we hope you will let us have our complaint put into your hinfluential paper, and make these landlords of our houses and these commissioners (the friends we spose of the landlords) make our houses decent for Christian to live in.

Praeyr Sur com and see us, for we are living like pigs and it ain't fair we should be ill treted.

We are your respectful servantgs in church land carriers,

John Scott and Residents.

---

more detailed, second edition of the monograph in 1854 eclipsed this work, which until recently was largely forgotten. In his 1936 reprint of the 1854 monograph, for example, Richardson wrote that "it has seemed unnecessary to reproduce the first paper(s) in this volume, since it is included, for the most part in identical or slightly revised language in the second edition" (Richardson 1936, xv).

True, perhaps, but the 1849 edition of *On the Mode of Communication of Cholera* was an impressive document, "a complex blend of epidemiological evidence, pathological observation, and bold analogies" (Vinten-Johansen et al. 2003 22–33). From our perspective it is hard to remember how radical his thesis was: "First, that cholera is a local affection of the alimentary canal; and secondly, that is communicated from one person to another" (Snow 1849a, 746). Thus, while Snow shared a general sanitarian concern with the miasmatists, who sought a cleaner city, his understanding of cholera itself was fundamentally different. They thought foul surroundings created poisonous air. He thought the

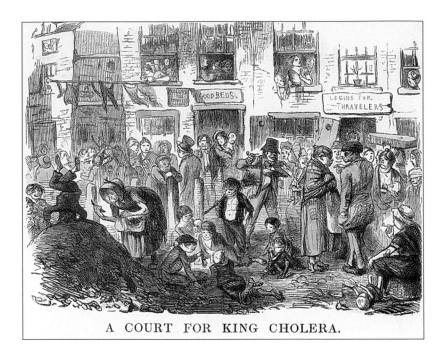

A COURT FOR KING CHOLERA.

Figure 4.5 A magazine illustration, presumably from *Punch,* of the popular view of the relation between cholera and urban waste. The image has been made into a postcard currently available at the John Snow Pub in London.

Source: British Library.

failure to treat waste adequately led to the contamination of water or food as an unseen animalcule was passed from contaminated sites to dense urban populations, and then between them, person to person.

It is important to understand that Snow did not challenge the miasmatic theory of disease but rather the assumption that cholera was a typical disease that could be understood as miasmatic. He did not doubt that some things were transmitted in the air (nor do we today, of course), only that cholera was a different type of condition that did not fit the then-accepted model. Instead of a general theory, Snow offered a narrow argument about cholera. While he argued on the basis of compelling evidence that he did so without the support of a broader general theory of disease was to cause skeptics to question his focused thesis.

Among his arguments was the idea that "the duration of cholera in a place is usually in a direct proportion to the size of a city or towns' population" (Snow 1849b, 942). Based on an analysis of data from the 1832 epidemic published in the *Transactions of the Royal Medical and Chirological Society* in 1844, he published a table of epidemic duration as a function of population. The greater the population of a jurisdiction, the longer the epidemic lasted. The point was that "this difference in the duration of cholera points clearly to its propogation [sic] from patient to patient. If each case were not connected with a previous one, but depended on some unknown atmospheric or telluric state, why should not the twenty cases that happen in a village be distributed over as long a period as the twenty hundred cases which occur in a large town?" (Snow 1849b, 925).[3]

No. of places	Duration in days	Average population
52	0–50	6,624
42	50–100	12,624
33 to 44	100 and upwards	38,123 or 78,823
A table extracted from Snow's work showing the positive correlation of population and duration of cholera.		

Figure 4.6 Table of relation of outbreak duration and population.

Source: Adapted from work of John Snow.

His answer was that cholera, introduced into the area through the water, "supplies a number of scattered cases which diffuse the disease more generally" (Snow 1849a, 749). Epidemics had a longer duration in larger cities because there was greater opportunity there for the disease to be spread to those who came into contact with the excretions of the affected either through recontamination of local water (washings that flowed into the street and a local well) or personal contact. In effect, he had hit upon the idea of a threshold population, a critical community size above which the agent of a specific disease will thrive and an epidemic can spread.[4]

For Snow, only the likelihood of person-to-person transmission explained both uneven patterns of disease occurrence and the greater intensity of outbreaks in the densely settled tenements of the working poor. "The bed linen nearly always becomes wetted by the cholera evacuations, and as these are devoid of the usual colour and odour, the hands of persons waiting on the patients become soiled, and unless these persons are scrupulously clean in their habits, and wash their hands upon taking food, they must accidentally swallow some of the excretion, and leave some on the food they handle or prepare, which has to be eaten by the rest of the family, who amongst the working classes often have to take their meals in the sick room" (Snow 1849a, 746–747).

More generally, he believed cholera spread in the city and across the nation not simply from individual contact in localized epidemics but from water contaminated with the cholera "poison." "There is often a way open for [cholera] to extend itself more widely, and that is by the mixture of the cholera evacuations with the water used for drinking and culinary purposes, either by permeating the ground and getting into wells, or by running along channels and sewers into the rivers" (Snow 1849a, 747). In London, that meant the city's private and competing waterworks, which drew their waters from the polluted Thames River, were somehow complicit.

This was a radical, bold, innovative, controversial argument unique in its detail and its attention to diffusion at various scales and as an outcome of socioeconomic conditions and urban infrastructure limits. Others, however, were arguing similarly, if less completely, that cholera was waterborne not airborne. In the *Medical Times and Gazette,* for example, Charles Coswell published his theories of waterborne contagion, focusing his work on the first points of epidemic outbreak. In "Propagation of cholera by contagion" he suggested "that the disease, in entering an insulated field, has constantly begun its ravages at the seaports, is no new observation; but this peculiarity has not, that I am aware, been so stated as to assume the form of an experimental result . . ." (Coswell 1849, 752).

Reviewing the history of cholera up to 1849, and its constant first appearance in seaports, he wrote that "the malady has at least observed method in its migrations to places insulated by water from those where it previously existed; in other words, has consistently extended itself over this barrier by means of naval intercourse" (Coswell 1849, 752). Snow, too, had noted the frequency of first occurrence in seaside towns—it was a point made again and again in the 1840s maps of the 1831–1834 outbreak—but his theory was not based upon it. In effect, Coswell's argument was concurrent and supportive but independent, one based on the mapped pattern of urban diffusion (and its temporal progression) generally argued in Brigham's map, for example, rather than deductive clinical reasoning. As important, perhaps, Coswell argued independently of Snow that the disease could not be miasmatic because were the cause a "morbific state of the atmosphere," it must necessarily affect all persons who breathed it. But "the effects are only partial; and, if we take the persistent class of agents, why do they not constantly give rise to the disease?" (Coswell 1849, 752). His answer, like Snow's, was both contagion and contact.

Snow was therefore not alone in his argument even if the method of his investigations and the completeness of his argument were, within a few years, to eclipse those of his contemporaries. In 1849, his was one voice among several that argued similarly from a review of the then-available literature. One thing that distinguished Snow from his contemporaries was his clinical background. He was first and foremost a physician. Another factor was his constancy. His research did not end with the 1849 epidemic. In 1851, he presented a paper on his research at the London Epidemiological Society that he had helped organize in 1850 "to one special end—the investigation of epidemic or spreading diseases" (Vinten-Johansen et al. 2003, 238). In it Snow summarized the argument of his 1849 papers and restated his view of epidemic disease as "communicable from one patient to another, this communication being probably the real feature of distinction between epidemic and other diseases" (Snow 1851, 559).

Further, he contended that the evidence suggested that poor sanitation contributed to the spread of the disease through water "vitiated by the contents of sewers and cesspools" (Snow 1851, 610). He thus advanced his two-step theory of cholera contagion and diffusion at two distinct but related scales. At one level, drinking water was polluted by the diarrhea of individuals already infected, or by some other carrier of an unknown, microscopic animalcule or unseen "poison." *Á la* Coswell, the first cases may have come from the sailors and passengers on sailing ships, or the ships themselves when they drained their bilges in the Thames harbor. Second, he argued that individuals so infected might spread the disease in their households or neighborhoods through person-to-person contact, and more generally through the physical materials (bed sheets, clothes, food) they contaminated. Their washing presented a point of interpersonal contagion for family members caring for a patient, and as local waste water improperly disposed of, a potential source for community infection. In effect, miasmatic theories of exhalation and contagion were transposed into a theory of diffusion based on general sanitation, and at the second scale, interpersonal contact.

To maintain the first, the role of the water supply as a vector of diffusion, he drew on an 1849 *Cholera Map of the Metropolis* prepared by Richard Grainger for a report to the Board of Health (Grainger 1850, appendix B). The map attempted to show relative density of occurrence in London by coloring lighter and darker areas of occurrence on a map of city districts. The careful notation of individual cases

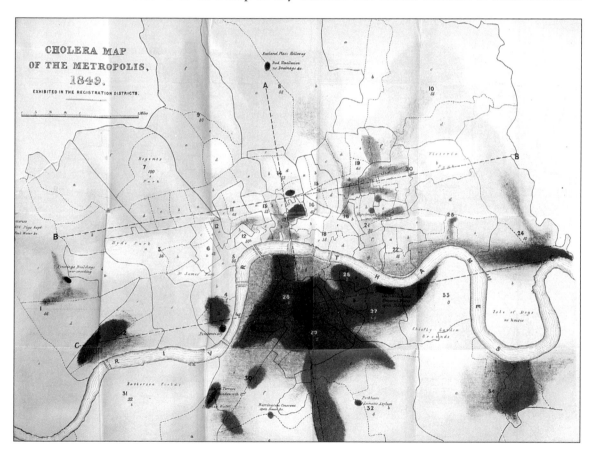

Figure 4.7a Grainger's density map of the 1849 cholera epidemic in London showing occurrence by political district and subdistrict.

Source: Reproduced courtesy of College of Physicians of Philadelphia.

(Seaman and Pascalis), or the careful coloring of specific districts (like Rothenberg's 1836 map), was rejected in favor of a boldly general aggregation of occurrence, a range laid over the physical domain of the city and its political districts. Inked by hand on a lithograph of Greater London's parish jurisdictions, the result looks like a schoolboy's botched copybook spoiled by ink stains, spills on a map of the urban political and geographic landscapes.

In the end, three different densities can be seen. The heaviest is in areas where the cholera outbreak was most severe. These included the Soho area to the west of district 16, and five districts south of the Thames: St. Savior, Southwark (number 25), St. Olave, Southwark, (number 26), Bermondsey (number 28), St. George, Southwark (number 28) and Neington (number 29). A somewhat less-dense shading can be found to the east of the main outbreak, near Greenwich (number 34), and near the penitentiary to the north of the river. Other lightly shaded areas show either minor outbreaks north of the city near Shoreditch (number 19) and Bethel Green (number 20), in West London, and in the area of Poplar proximate to the Thames.

Small numerals designating elevation above sea level are included on the map in support of the theory that generative, miasmatic airs tended to settle around low-lying riverbanks. And there did seem to be a correspondence. Incidence of cholera appeared to be highest in those areas nearest the Thames where elevation was lowest. Where cholera did occur at higher elevations Grainger carefully mapped local circumstances that might have contributed to the epidemic's severity. Thus, in Islington (number 8) "bad ventilation and no drainage" is written near a darkly colored, localized outbreak. In Westminster, "over-crowding" was noted in the area of Fennings Buildings where a dense outbreak's epicenter is surrounded by a pattern of moderate occurrence. "Open sewers" are mapped near an outbreak at Barrington Crescent in Lambeth (number 30), "putrid water" near Lambeth Church sub-district (number 30).

Grainger's map distilled a range of data pertinent to at least two competing theories of cholera's origin and diffusion. Elevation and water sources are joined in a map of political jurisdiction on which a surface reflecting disease density is laid over. That the splotchy nature of the inking is difficult to read and thus perhaps hard for us to interpret does not diminish the thinking it presented. Those believing the disease to be waterborne would point to its relative density in areas near the Thames, and to outbreaks near otherwise contaminated sites away from the river. Those arguing a miasmatic theory of cholera in which increasing altitude was assumed to provide cleaner air might point to the same data and draw a wholly different set of conclusions. For them, too, the correspondence was clear.

Either way, Grainger's map detailed disease incidence in the city in relation to the city's water sources, especially the Thames. Infamously polluted (Porter, D. H. 1998), the river was at once the city's primary source of water and its principal sewer. If the source of the epidemic was indeed waterborne, Snow maintained that the manner of its general diffusion must be in the water supplied by public companies to the city. "The water works that supply the south of London take water from the

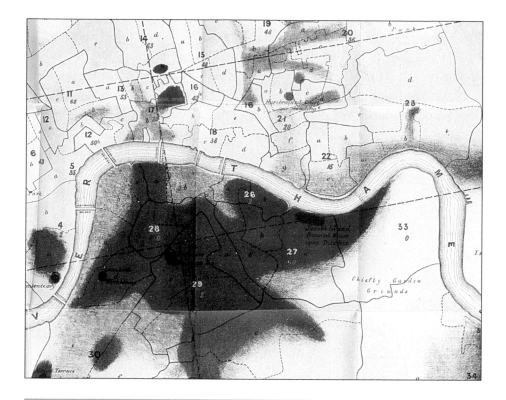

Figure 4.7b Detail of Grainger's density map "Cholera Map of the Metropolis." Small numerals designate altitude above sea level while larger numbers represent urban districts under the then operative Poor Law.

Source: Reproduced courtesy of College of Physicians of Philadelphia.

Thames mostly at places near which the chief sewers run into it. Moreover, the wells in this part of London are very liable to be contaminated by the contents of cesspools . . . these are the chief sources of the high mortality on the south of the Thames, and where they are not in operation there has been comparative immunity from the disease" (Snow 1849a, 749).

For Snow, the epidemic was most severe in urban areas near the river into which the city's sewage flowed and from which much of the city's water was drawn. But those areas were remarkably odiferous, and into the 1860s it was as much the smell as the health problems that might result that argued for the river's rehabilitation through an expensive embankment (Porter, D. H. 1998). To make his case, Snow would need somehow to show a direct correspondence between cholera and the urban water supply. If he could not demonstrate the existence of invisible, waterborne creatures that transmitted the disease, a fantastical idea in the 1850s, he would need to prove their existence in another way.

Ideally, the proof he presented would also have to explain the apparent congruence between epidemic occurrence and altitude. The proposition he wished to argue was that cholera was related to water (irrespective of altitude or local odors), and that some water sources were contaminated while others were not. To make his case, Snow had to show both how a water source was contaminated and then how that contamination was transmitted through the population by means that were not airborne. To do this, he first needed a database of cholera patients and the source of their water. As Snow himself had admitted, "as we are never informed in works on cholera what water the people drink, I have scarcely been able to collect any information on this point" (Snow 1849b).

The South London study

In 1853, cholera returned to England with scattered outbreaks through the winter, erupting in the summer of 1854 in a sustained epidemic that lasted approximately fourteen weeks. William Farr's staff at the General Register Office (GRO) compiled the *Weekly Return of Births and Deaths in London* whose records included the reported cause of death of London citizens. While favoring an airborne argument based on altitude rather than on individual transmission, Farr was sympathetic to Snow's thesis. Alas, he wrote, data that might prove Snow's theory was almost certainly unobtainable. "To measure the effects of good and bad water supply, it is prerequisite to find two classes of inhabitants living at the same level [elevation], moving in equal space, enjoying an equal share of the means of subsistence, engaged in the same pursuits, but differing in this respect, that one drinks water from Battersea [water supply], and the other from Kew . . .." (Vinten-Johansen et al. 2003, 278; General Register Office 1853).

What Farr did not perceive was that the weekly mortality returns his office published would provide the raw data Snow required to test his theories. In one study, Snow used data from Farr's Weekly Returns to compare the incidence of cholera in South London's populous districts and subdistricts as they occurred in the 1854 epidemic, and retrospectively, as they had occurred in previous epidemics. In this work he correlated the incidence of death by population with the one feature that he believed distinguished areas of greater and lower incidence: water supply (Snow 1854b). The Southwark and Vauxhall Water Company, whose waters were drawn from the Thames near Battersea, supplied some districts. The Lambeth Water Company, whose waters came from other less obviously polluted sections of the Thames, supplied others. Snow's assumption was that the Battersea area intake drew from water polluted by the city's waste while those farther from the city did not. In some areas, the waters of both companies were commingled, and in still others, smaller companies were the principal water suppliers. The general population affected was three hundred thousand people "of both sex, and of every age and occupation, and of every rank and station" (Snow 1855, 75). This was, as Snow insisted, experimentation "on the grandest scale."

"As there is no difference whatever, either in the houses or the people receiving the supply of the two Water Companies [Southwark-Vauxhall and the Lambeth water companies], or in any of the physical conditions with which they are surrounded, it is obvious that no experiment could have been devised which would more thoroughly test the effect of water supply on the progress of cholera than this, which circumstances placed ready made before the observer" (Snow 1855c).

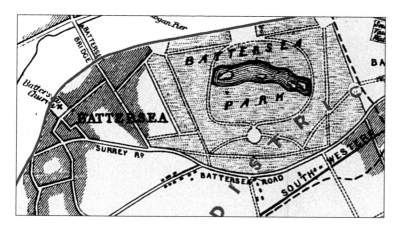

Figure 4.8 Detail of Snow's South London cholera map showing deaths along Battersea Road on the south of the Thames. Parish boundaries are shown with a dotted line running diagonal to the park.

Source: Reproduced courtesy of College of Physicians of Philadelphia.

Using as a starting point the data provided by the weekly mortality returns published by William Farr's office, Snow and "a medical man, John Joseph Whiting, L.A.C." personally investigated 336 cholera deaths, inquiring into the sources of household water of the decedents (Vinten-Johansen et al. 2003, 269). That data, published in an appendix to Snow's 1854 *On the Mode of Communication of Cholera*, fleshed out the registrar's broad statistics recording at least three thousand deaths collected by William Farr's registrars. Snow's grand experiment, one encompassing the epidemic in the whole of South London, was too big for an individual investigator. The General Registrar, Farr directed his registrars to investigate the water sources for at least three thousand deaths in the South London jurisdictions. While these local registrars "could not be expected to seek out the landlord or his agent, or to apply chemical tests to the water as I had done," Snow wrote (1855c, 86), they did yeoman work. While critical data for 2,877 houses was unrecorded, that limit occurred within a population area of more than 439,000 dwellings. For Snow, the sheer size of the sample overwhelmed its limits (Snow 1856, table V).

The results were extraordinarily rigorous for their time, with multiple tables calculating cholera deaths per ten thousand inhabitants for every parish, for aggregated urban areas, and deaths by source of urban water provided. He considered death, in a partial list, by age, occupation (house butlers versus charwomen versus sailors), and sex. The central finding, presented in table IX, was the complicity of water supplied by the Southwark and Vauxhall Company compared to that from either the Lambeth or other sources.[5]

Cholera deaths by water company			
	Number of deaths	Deaths from cholera	Deaths in each 10,000 houses
Southwark and Vauxhall Company	40,046	1,263	315
Lambeth Company	26,107	98	37
Rest of London	256,423	1,422	59

Figure 4.9 Summary of cholera deaths by water company for each of the three primary water sources in South London.

Source: Reproduced courtesy of College of Physicians of Philadelphia.

Snow attempted to distill his argument in a single, comprehensive, four-color graphic foldout map that was attached to the publication (Snow 1855c). It shows the city by administrative district (parish and subparish borders) with its parks, important buildings, streets, and of course, the Thames. Marked as well are the water intakes of its principal water sources and, with small dots, the homes of those whose deaths he and Whiting investigated. The map attempts to create a surface of water jurisdiction with three distinct colors used to show the service areas of the Lambeth and Southwark-Vauxhall water companies as well as those areas where their service was commingled.

The result was a glorious failure, the mapmaking insufficient to do what Snow intended. It was not simply that the colors were muddied, the "purple" of the intermingled areas difficult to distinguish from the "blue" of those supplied by Southwark Vauxhall Water Company, the "red" of the Lambeth Water Company districts a pinkish orange. District and subdistrict names are hard to read beneath the choropleth coloration and deaths, dots inked by hand on the map are too small to be easily read, their relation to the different districts lost. Modern cartographers would say the map was overloaded; its inclusion of everything meant nothing in the map would clearly stand out.

More importantly, the topographic approach to mapping that served Snow so well in the Broad Street study failed him in this study. This map sought not simply to define a relation between "this" (cholera) and "that" (different water sources), but to do so in a way that was statistical and graphic at once. Alas, the relation between deaths and water sources in the individual districts is hopelessly obscured. The map is of areas supplied by different water sources, not the data he recorded on deaths per ten thousand people in each district. Snow's text tables detailed districts (table V) and subdistricts (table VI) on the basis of population, deaths, and water source.[6] In table VI, for example, mortality per district population is derived, and water supplier noted, to arrive at a general comparison (Snow 1855c, 71–73). It was this that Snow had hoped to map (and calculate) not at the coarse scale of the water company but at the finer scale of the subdistricts themselves. It was this that he failed to accomplish in either map or table, at least in part because all the data he needed on individual subdistricts was not available. As a result, the map stands not as a distillation of Snow's *crucial experiment*, as he called it, but

Cartographies of Disease

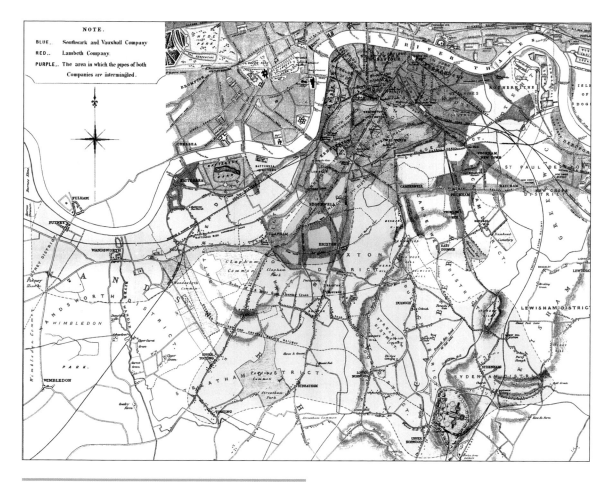

Figure 4.10 Snow's map of the relation between public water supply and cholera in London. Color variations distinguish between Southwark-Vauxhall, Lambeth, and conjoined water jurisdictions.

Source: Reproduced courtesy of College of Physicians of Philadelphia.

as a statement of the problem he faced: cartographically, statistically, and conceptually (Snow 1856) in attempting to analyze the effect of water on deaths in South London's subdistricts.

If the map did not serve Snow's hope of a fine-scaled analysis, it remains important for its ambition. Looking back, it is easy to show how a different system of symbolization or a different scale of abstraction would have improved the result. That is hindsight, however, pure and simple. These were the days in which the procedures of medical mapping and medical statistics were developing, an era before an aesthetics of mapping or a rigorous sense of statistics were developed. The attempt Snow's map presented perhaps is best understood today as both ambitious and laudable even if the results

TABLE VI.

Sub-Districts.	Population in 1851.	Deaths from Cholera in 1853.	Deaths by Cholera in each 100,000 living.	Water Supply.
St. Saviour, Southwark	19,709	45	227	
St. Olave	8,015	19	237	
St. John, Horsleydown	11,360	7	61	
St. James, Bermondsey	18,899	21	111	
St. Mary Magdalen	13,934	27	193	
Leather Market	15,295	23	153	Southwark and Vauxhall Water Company only.
Rotherhithe*	17,805	20	112	
Wandsworth	9,611	3	31	
Battersea	10,560	11	104	
Putney	5,280	—	—	
Camberwell	17,742	9	50	
Peckham	19,444	7	36	
Christchurch, Southwk.	16,022	7	43	
Kent Road	18,126	37	204	
Borough Road	15,862	26	163	
London Road	17,836	9	50	
Trinity, Newington	20,922	11	52	
St. Peter, Walworth	29,861	23	77	
St. Mary, Newington	14,033	5	35	Lambeth Water Company, and Southwark and Vauxhall Company.
Waterloo (1st part)	14,088	1	7	
Waterloo (2nd part)	18,348	7	38	
Lambeth Church (1st part)	18,409	9	48	
Lambeth Church (2nd part)	26,784	11	41	
Kennington (1st part)	24,261	12	49	
Kennington (2nd part)	18,848	6	31	
Brixton	14,610	2	13	
Clapham	16,290	10	61	
St. George, Camberwell	15,849	6	37	
Norwood	3,977	—	—	
Streatham	9,023	—	—	Lambeth Water Company only.
Dulwich	1,632	—	—	
First 12 sub-districts	167,654	192	114	Southwk. & Vaux.
Next 16 sub-districts	301,149	182	60	Both Companies.
Last 3 sub-districts	14,632	—	—	Lambeth Comp.

* A part of Rotherhithe was supplied by the Kent Water Company ; but there was no cholera in this part.

Figure 4.11 Snow's 1855 table of cholera in London subdistricts in 1853. This was the heart of his "grand experiment" investigating deaths in South London on the basis of water supply. Deaths are assigned by subdistrict on the basis of population. Calculation of the effect of water source is then summarized in the table (Snow 1855c, 73).

Source: Reproduced courtesy of College of Physicians of Philadelphia.

were unsatisfactory. Science, after all, is one of those activities where ambitious failure sometimes leads us further than cautious success.

St. James, Soho

The South London study imposed itself—a research opportunity Snow could not pass up—at the same time that he was investigating a more localized outbreak in Soho's St. James Parish, "the most terrible outbreak of cholera which ever occurred in this kingdom" (Snow 1855c, 38).[7] Within 250 yards of its Broad Street epicenter "there were upwards of five hundred fatal attacks of cholera in ten days. The mortality in this limited area probably equals any that was ever caused in this country, even by the plague; and its was much more sudden, as the greater number of cases terminated in a few hours" (Snow 1855c, 48). This was an area Snow knew intimately. The Firth Street apartment where he had lodged while studying medicine was in the area, and in 1854 so, too, were his office and home and those of many of his patients.

If the South London investigation was an opportunity to consider the thesis that cholera was spread in large urban areas through the water supply, the St. James Parish outbreak permitted a detailed study at the scale of an urban neighborhood. In his writings up to 1854, Snow had framed a fundamentally ecological hypothesis based on clinical insights into the nature of the disease he was investigating. With the Soho outbreak he was able to map that thesis at the neighborhood level, one that permitted a type of detail prohibited by the grand scale of the South London study.

In his Soho study, Snow attempted to relate three distinct elements to the incidence of cholera: disease occurrence (individual cases), density of occurrence (aggregated cases), and proximity of water sources. In the Soho area, the water sources were wells from which residents drew their water. Neighborhood travel to and from the well sites was largely pedestrian, and the assumption was that people would drink from wells closest to their homes and shops. The proposition was that the well nearest the center of the outbreak would be the one complicit in its generation, especially if cases were clustered densely in the immediate area of that well.

To turn this thesis into an effective argument required case-by-case consideration; Snow had to prove that those affected drank water drawn from the Broad Street pump. It also required attention to neighborhood traffic patterns and a general sense of distance between the homes of the afflicted and different wells they might draw from. In addition, to understand the disease's progress, Snow had to consider major work sites—breweries, churches, dockyards, schools, workhouses, and so on—destinations where people could be assumed to congregate. Did people working in the area walk by the suspect well, and were they known to drink from it?

The fruits of his investigations were presented in an oversized (18 x 22.75 inches) map that first appeared in the second edition of *On the Mode of Communication of Cholera* in 1854. On a commercial map of the district "all the deaths from cholera which were registered in the six weeks from 19th

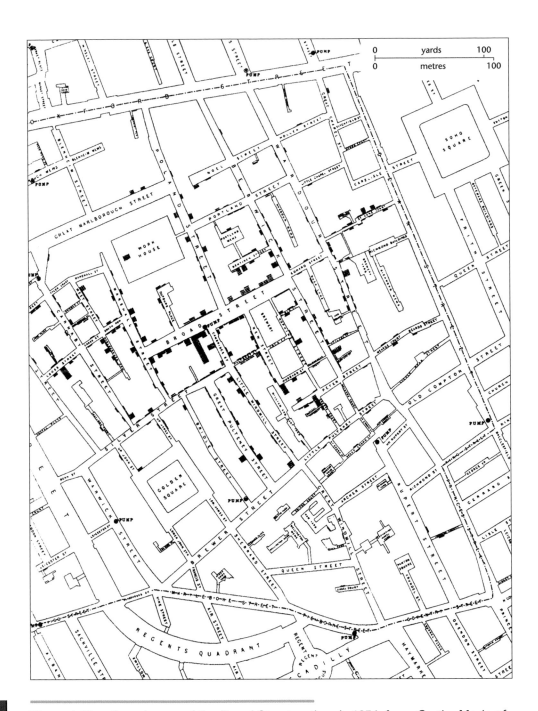

Figure 4.12a Snow's map of the Broad Street outbreak, 1854, from *On the Mode of Communication of Cholera, Second Edition.*

Source: Reproduced courtesy of College of Physicians of Philadelphia.

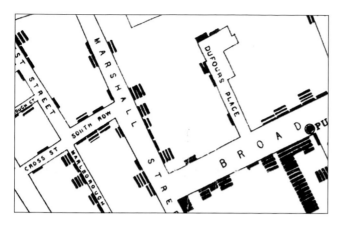

Figure 4.12b Detail of Snow's map of the Broad Street pump area.

Source: Reproduced courtesy of College of Physicians of Philadelphia.

August to 30th September within this locality, as well as those of people removed into Middlesex Hospital, are shown in the map by a black line in the situation of the house in which it occurred, or in which the fatal account was contracted" (Snow 1855c, 46).

Where there were multiple deaths at a single address, he stacked the black line symbols representing individual deaths inward from the street. This permitted both a general assignment by address for each death and a visual measure of intensity from the stacked symbols indicating multiple deaths at a single address. In the end, Snow mapped 574 deaths in a district with thirteen public water pumps, including four north of Oxford Street and technically outside the study district. A dash and dot line (– • –) was used to define the district's jurisdictional limit. In the map the apparent epicenter of the outbreak, and thus its most likely cause, was the Broad Street pump. "It might be noticed," Snow wrote, "that the deaths are most numerous near to the pump in Broad Street" (Snow 1855a, 109). That the intensity of the outbreak was centered upon the Broad Street pump was not a statistical conclusion, one based on the statistical mean, for example, but instead argued visually (and generally) from the map.

Snow was cautious in arguing a simple correspondence between Euclidian distance and real travel time in the neighborhood. He knew that, as the *Punch* map of dead-end and truncated streets had argued, distance was not always easily computed when measured by time traveled in a Byzantine street network. With regard to the Rupert Street pump, for example, Snow cautioned, "that some streets which are nearer to it on the map are in fact a good way removed on account of the circuitous road to it" (Snow 1855c, 45–46). For those who drew and carried well water daily, it was effectively more distant than it appeared on the map, and thus even less likely that its geographic location suggested it as a source of the concentrated outbreak in the Broad Street area.

A crucial function of his map was to orient readers unfamiliar with Soho and its environs. It is this pictorial aspect of the map that has misled some to assume its function was primarily illustrative

(Vinten-Johansen et al. 2003, 332), or at best merely descriptive. Nothing, however, can be farther from the truth. "This 'picture part' is raised only because the map intends to say something about it" (Kaiser, Wood, and Abramms 2005). The city streets, the workhouses, breweries, and dockyards *all* played a part in Snow's analysis. The "picture" distills the complex whole, one in which the range of cholera deaths is joined to that of water sources within an urban environment of homes and shops in streets. The result is what Snow called a "diagram of the topography of the outbreak" (Snow 1855c, 45). In this way the idea of a medical topography advanced a generation before came to bear surprising fruit.

Through its attention to detail of both individual cases and their urban situation, Snow's map also served to critique, at least implicitly, the miasmatic theory of airborne disease which, if correct, he noted, would result in a uniform pattern of incidence rather than the intense variations he had observed street by street and house by house. To make his argument, however, Snow had to explain why some homes and workplaces closest to the Broad Street pump were free of the disease. Despite its proximity to the Broad Street pump, for example, the Poland Street workhouse was relatively free of cholera cases. "The Workhouse in Poland Street is more than three-fourths surrounded by houses in which deaths from cholera occurred, yet out of five hundred and thirty-five inmates only five died of cholera, the other deaths which took place being those of persons admitted after they were attacked" (Snow 1855c, 42).

On visiting the workhouse Snow learned it had its own pump-well on the premises and that "the inmates never sent to Broad Street for water." Had the mortality in the workhouse been equal to that of the houses and shops surrounding it—those whose water was drawn from the Broad Street pump—Snow estimated that more than one hundred inmates would have died.

Similarly, the more than seventy workers employed at Huggins' Brewery at the intersection of Broad and New Streets, near the epicenter of the outbreak, remained free of the disease that affected others living and working in the area. The reason, the manager told Snow, was that when thirsty his employees drank either from the brewery's private well or the malt liquor it produced: "the men were allowed a small quantity of malt liquor" (Snow 1855c, 42). They did not drink water drawn from the Broad Street pump.

Snow also had to consider those who lived nearer to other pumps but who still contracted cholera. These included, for example, the cases of a young girl from Ham Yard (South of Brewer Street) and another from Angel Court off Great Windmill Street. Surviving family members told Snow the children typically drank from the Broad Street pump on their way to or from a school off Broad Street. So, too, he discovered, did another deceased schoolchild from Naylor's Yard, off Silver Street. The seemingly anomalous death of a Noel Street boy, who lived north of Portland and east of Wardour Streets, was explained by his attendance at the National School at the western end of Broad Street.

Not all anomalies involve schoolchildren. Prior to contracting cholera a tailor living at 6 Heddon Court west of Regent Street had spent most of his time on Broad Street; a woman from 10 Heddon

Court who died had been nursing a Broad Street friend who also died of the disease. Snow carefully investigated each case, each line on his map. It was all there in the map, accessible to the reader who could find the home of the deceased child or worker, look for the workplace he or she would travel to, and see the path that might take the deceased past the Broad Street pump. In the text there was the information provided by a mourning parent or fatalistic boss saying, yes indeed, they'd stop for a sip every day. It was in the text and distilled in the map for everyone to see.

In a second map accompanying his report to the 1855 St. James Cholera Inquiry Committee, Snow addressed issues of density of occurrence and proximity to the Broad Street pump in a unique and innovative way. Except for minor corrections and additions, including the addition of the Hanover Square water pump, the map was basically the same as the one included in his 1854 publication. But

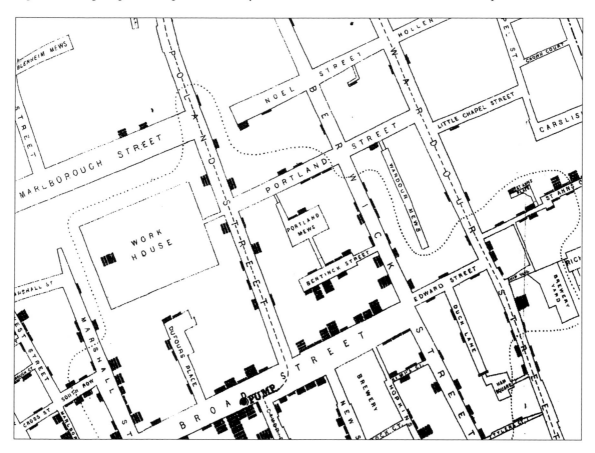

Figure 4.13 Detail of Snow's 1855 map of the Soho outbreak showing the dotted line of equidistance he calculated from the Broad Street pump.

Source: Reproduced courtesy of College of Physicians of Philadelphia.

on this one Snow created an "inner dotted line" defining the area of the outbreak in which incidence of cholera was closer to the Broad Street pump than to any other.

"By the most careful calculation," Snow wrote, he had drawn an eccentric and irregular polygon approximating the median distance by foot between the Broad Street and other local pumps (Snow 1855a). This new domain, a surface polygon based on travel time rather than Euclidian distance, was then used to consider the relation between the dense occurrence of deaths and the pump at their center. "It will be observed that the deaths either very much *diminish*, or *cease* altogether, at every point where it becomes decidedly nearer to send to another pump than to the one in Broad Street" (Snow 1855a, 109). Again, Snow's argument was visual rather than quantitative, a cartographic rather than statistical conclusion. In fact, the boundary defining "nearer" by time contained approximately two-thirds of all deaths included in his database and reported on his map. All but eight of the cases occurring outside this boundary were shown to be related to the Broad Street pump through Snow's interviews with their surviving relatives.

The Broad Street outbreak map was extremely selective and what was left out was important. For example, the map symbolized *only* those cases of cholera mortality reported to the registrar by local physicians through September 9; not those occurring between September 9 and September 30 because, Snow wrote, "I deemed the above inquiry sufficient to establish the cause of the outbreak" (Snow 1855c). Nor, of course, did he map the location of the greater cholera population who in fact survived the disease. Snow also knew of, but did not map, the cases of "work people and others who contracted the cholera in this neighborhood and died in different parts of London." In his text, for example, he reports the case of a West End widower who had a bottle of Broad Street water brought to home each day. Her husband had been a percussion-cap maker in the Broad Street neighborhood and she preferred its taste. Both she and a niece visiting her died of cholera even though there was otherwise "no cholera at the time, either at West End or in the neighborhood where the niece died [Islington]" (Snow 1855c, 44–45).

Finally, Snow mapped only those cases where the diagnosis of "Asiatic cholera," was clear. This meant some cases where physicians insisted the cause was simple "English cholera," a common gastrointestinal complaint we would call food poisoning today, were omitted. In the second edition of *On the Mode of Transmission of Cholera* (1855c), Snow hints at this problem in his appendix of 336 South London cholera deaths. Each death is listed with, among other data, the cause pronounced by the attending physician. These included Asiatic cholera, cholera, cholera Asiatic, cholera biliosa, choleraic diarrhoea, cholera maligna, cholera sero-spasmodica, diarrhea, English cholera, malignant cholera, premonitory diarrhea, and spasmodic cholera.

Diarrhea was a distinguishing clinical symptom for all these variously named conditions. Asiatic cholera was most often diagnosed (as mentioned earlier) by the "rice water" appearance of the diarrhea, the thin, liquid discharge that included white epithelial cells from the lining of the intestine. Others made their diagnosis based on the appearance of the dehydrated patient, the darkened coloring of the advanced patient, and post-mortem on thickness of the blood resulting from dehydration. Still, the confusion was real.

In his writing Snow admitted to these and other exclusions but dismissed their relevance, arguing that, "the deficiencies I have mentioned, however, do not detract from the correctness of the map, as a diagram of the topography of the outbreak; for, if the locality of the additional cases could be ascertained, they would probably be distributed over the district of the outbreak in the same proportion as the large number which are known" (Snow 1855a, 108). And in retrospect, Snow was correct. The cases collected and mapped for the 1854 and 1855 reports were sufficient to establish his argument based on the topography of the outbreak. One suspects that not only did he not see the necessity of adding the cases occurring between September 9 and 30 (his sample was statistically sufficient) but that he did not know how to map the cases of persons living elsewhere whose condition originated in the Broad Street area. Nor was it clear how to map cases of those who survived the cholera: adding a new symbol for the 80 percent of the cholera population that survived literally would have blackened the map with symbols.

Finally, Snow's attention was simultaneously engaged by the ambitious South London study. In thinking about the decisions he made, it is well to remember that he was not a full-time epidemiologist or government scientist but an amateur, a practicing physician in a neighborhood overwhelmed by an epidemic disease. He was as well a specialist whose anesthetic services remained in demand. Like all researchers everywhere, Snow made critical decisions based not only on his sense of the research problem but as well on a range of practical, prosaic limits and constraints. While history absolves him, his contemporaries did not. Others, equally involved in considering cholera presented at least equally rigorous reports whose conclusions were different from Snow's. They, too, mapped their arguments. Unlike him, they did so from within the confines of the general theory of disease then current. It is in the comparison of their work and Snow's that a fuller portion of the medical science of the day can be seen.

Endnotes

1. Given the wealth of materials written about John Snow's work and its contribution to medical science, biographical material is surprisingly limited. One reason for this is that he was not lionized in his own time. His real fame blossomed only decades after his death, and thus decades too late for the type of personal reminiscence that typically accrues around the famous. Equally restricting is the almost total absence of personal data from Snow, a bachelor, who left neither letters nor private journals for the instruction of later biographers. Besides the bare facts of his life, there are his articles, with brief glimpses into his character and history, and the professional work he produced in profusion. That said, knowledge of Snow's life has been enlarged enormously by a recent study of Snow's work and life by an interdisciplinary team from Michigan State University (Vinten-Johansen et al. 2003).

2. This appears to be the first example of a "sketch map" so described. The term took on great importance in the 1960s when geographers, psychologists, and urban planners began to ask citizens to "sketch" their images of the city, to make amateur maps that could be used to understand their relation to the environment and the means by which it was cognitively constructed.

3. In 1855, Snow expanded the argument in a paper "on the comparative mortality of large towns and rural districts, and the causes by which it is influence." Presented at the Epidemiological Society on May 2, 1853, the presentation was eventually published in the inaugural issue of the *Journal of Public Health, and Sanitary Review* in 1855. Here he considered the "popular impression that living in town is itself injurious to people of all ages" and showed that, in fact, London "which is prodigiously larger than any of the great provincial towns, has a much lower mortality than they have" (Snow 1855b, 21).

4. The precise definition of a threshold population, or of a population reservoir, are twentieth-century concepts rigorously developed only after World War II with a serious study of diffusion practices. Measles, for example, requires a threshold of between 250,000 and 300,000 for a disease to take hold (Haggett 2000, 23).

5. A host of lesser water companies supplied water to individual districts in Greater London, including the New River and East London Water companies, Chelsea Water Works, East London Water Works, West Middlesex Water Works, and Hampstead Water Works.

6. While many have discussed the South London study in epidemiology (for example, Rothman 2002, 59–61; 86–89), relatively few have carefully considered Snow's actual data. Among those who have, for example Vinten-Johansen et al. (2003, 273–277), the assumption is that Snow successfully completed his grand experiment at the scale of the London district and subdistrict. New analysis of Snow's 1856

paper suggests, however, that errors in his analysis ultimately preventing anything but a coarse scale of consideration at the level of the water companies despite appearances to the contrary. A new analysis of this work with contemporary cartographic and statistical tools, now nearly completed by my friend and coworker Ken Denike and myself, is tentatively scheduled for publication in 2006.

7. There are several Web sites where Snow's maps are well considered, and as importantly, well displayed. The University of California, Los Angeles, School of Public Health has a particularly useful Web site dedicated to the study of John Snow and his maps. (*www.ph.ucla.edu/epi/snow.html*).

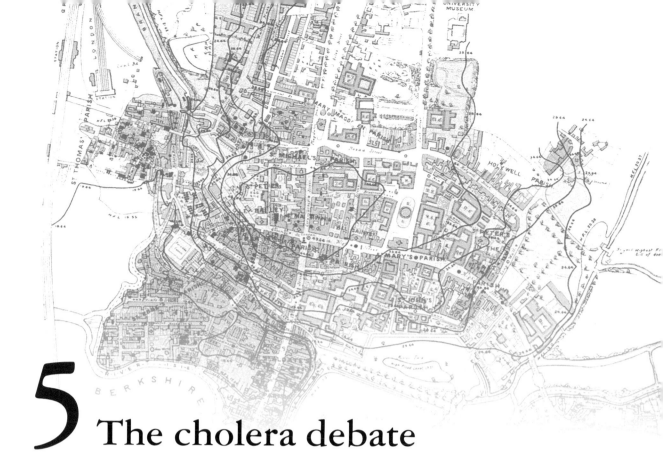

5 The cholera debate

John Snow has become the "patron saint," the progenitor, not only of medical cartography and geography but also of the disciplines of public health and epidemiology (Vinten-Johansen et al. 2003, chapter 16). Everyone teaches Snow and his study of the Broad Street outbreak, his mapping, and his brilliance. His map has become an icon and Snow himself an almost mythic figure (McLeod 2000). Few focus, therefore, on Snow's failure to convince his contemporaries of his argument, the limits of his thesis in the context of his time. It is easy in retrospect to sneer at those who did not perceive what today we understand from the perspective of modern bacteriology and virology. But if we are to do that we must sneer at Snow, too. After all, he did not offer a new theory of disease that would include the issues of airborne vectors of disease (influenza, for example) as well as waterborne diseases. His was instead a limited argument, a "special case" about a disease rather than a general theory of disease. He thus had to fight his battle on two fronts. The first concerned the proposition relating water sources to the incidence of cholera. The second would have required he offer a general understanding of disease including "obviously" miasmatic data while justifying the proposition he sought to prove.

In retrospect, perhaps Snow's greatest failure was tactical. Single-mindedly focused on his limited theory of cholera, he made no real effort to present it within a more general disease theory. As importantly, in his writings he gave short shrift to the propositions of others with contrary viewpoints. He assumed in the 1854 edition of *On the Mode of Communication* that "it is not necessary to oppose any other theories in order to establish the principles I am endeavoring to explain" (Snow 1855c, 113). Mapping neither the sewer lines which "passed within a few yards of the well" (Snow 1855c, 52) nor "the supposed existence of a pit in which persons dying of the plague had been buried about two centuries ago" (Snow 1855c, 54), he left himself open to contrary arguments by others for whom these were at least potentially complicit environmental factors.

Unlike Grainger, Snow mapped only data supportive of his argument, his topography irrespective of that offered by others who also used mapping to distill their theories and test alternative propositions. For example, the London Sewer Commission ordered its engineer, Edmond Cooper (1854), to carry out a sanitary inventory of the area in order to consider the possible complicity of the area's sewer lines, including those built over the burial site of former plague victims. Another, by Reverend Henry Whitehead, published with Snow's in the 1855 Saint James Parish Committee Report, included both Cooper's and Snow's data as part of a more comprehensive map of the outbreak. Perhaps the most

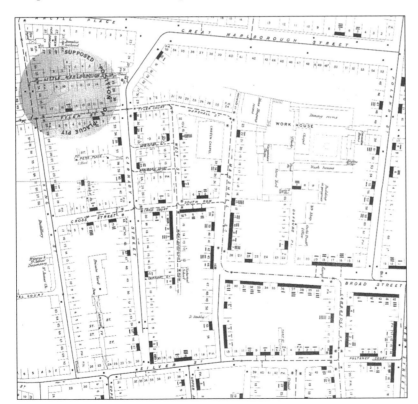

Figure 5.1 Detail of Cooper's map of the null relation between incidence of cholera and the location of existing sewer lines in 1854 in Soho, London. Dotted and solid lines on different streets are sewer lines built in different years.

Source: London Metropolitan Museum.

comprehensive mapping of an urban cholera outbreak was carried out not in the Broad Street area of London, however, but by Henry Acland (1856) in Oxford. His work was at least equally exhaustive and his conclusions, supportive of Farr's thesis inversely relating altitude to incidence, wholly contradicted Snow's conclusions.

Cooper and the Soho sewer system

In 1854, the Metropolitan London Commission of Sewers sent Edmund Cooper to investigate complaints by St. James Parish residents who believed sewer lines (including one running through a seventeenth century plague burial area) vented miasmatic gases that caused the Broad Street area outbreak. If the sewer line was complicit, it might be because it disturbed the noxious gases that resided in this old burial area on which housing and streets had been built. Cooper sought to prove or disprove the belief by seeking a correspondence—or lack of it—between specific sewer lines, the old plague area, and the incidence of disease.

SCHEDULE—*continued.*

NAME OF STREET.	No. of House.	No. of Deaths.	Whether opposite Air Shaft.	Whether opposite untrapped Gully.	Condition of Dust Bin.	Description of Drainage, whether Brick or Pipe, and condition thereof.	Whether any Cesspools, and Number.	REMARKS.
Brought forward...	...	41						
Broad Street—*cont.*......	29	2	Yes	No	Good	... ...	... ...	House shut up.
	31	2	No	ditto	ditto	Not ascertainable	Uncertain	Probably old brick drains; no knowledge of cesspool being destroyed.
	32	3	ditto	ditto	ditto	Pipe drains about 4 months	No	Water-closet defective, and bad smells.
	33	2	ditto	ditto	ditto	Brick drain	Uncertain	Bad smells; brick drains; no knowledge of cesspool being destroyed.
	36	1	ditto	ditto	ditto	Pipe drain	No	Drainage good.
	37	3	ditto	ditto	ditto	Not ascertainable	Uncertain	Probably brick; no knowledge of cesspool being destroyed.
	38	1	ditto	ditto	ditto	ditto	ditto	ditto ditto ditto
	39	3	ditto	ditto	ditto	ditto	ditto	ditto ditto ditto
	40	3	ditto	ditto	ditto	ditto	ditto	ditto ditto ditto
	41	1	ditto	ditto	ditto	Pipe drains good (1 year old)	No	Drainage good, but soil from top of house discharged on paving of yard.
	42	1	ditto	Yes	ditto	Old brick drains defective	Uncertain	No knowledge of cesspool being destroyed.
	43	1	Yes	ditto	ditto	Not ascertainable	ditto	Probably brick; no knowledge of cesspool being destroyed.
	44	2	No	No	ditto	ditto	ditto	ditto ditto ditto
	45	3	ditto	ditto	ditto	ditto	ditto	ditto ditto ditto
	52	1	ditto	ditto	ditto	Old brick drains defective	Yes, 1	Offensive cesspool, and bad drains.
	53	1	ditto	ditto	ditto	Not ascertainable	Uncertain	Probably brick; no knowledge of cesspool being destroyed.
	54	1	ditto	ditto	ditto	ditto	ditto	ditto ditto ditto
Dufour's Place............	1	1	ditto	ditto	ditto	Pipe drains, 1851	No	Drainage efficient.
	7	2	ditto	ditto	ditto	Not ascertainable	Uncertain	Probably old brick drains; no knowledge of cesspool being destroyed; bad smells at times.
Marshall Street	1	1	ditto	ditto	ditto	Brick drain, old and bad	ditto	No knowledge of cesspools being destroyed.
	2	1	ditto	ditto	ditto	Pipe drains	ditto	Drainage effective.
	3	1	ditto	ditto	ditto	Not ascertainable	No	Drainage good.
	5	1	ditto	ditto	ditto	Pipe drains, 6 months	ditto	Drainage effective.
	7	4	ditto	ditto	ditto	Not ascertainable	Yes, 1	An offensive cesspool, and probably old brick drains.
	8	1	ditto	ditto	ditto	Brick drains	Uncertain	No knowledge of cesspool being destroyed.
	9	1	ditto	ditto	ditto	ditto	No	Brick drain appears in good condition.
	10	2	Yes	ditto	ditto	Not ascertainable	Uncertain	Probably brick; no knowledge of cesspool being destroyed; drains said to be good.
	11	2	No	ditto	ditto	Pipe drains to water-closet	ditto	No knowledge of cesspool being destroyed.
	13	4	ditto	ditto	ditto	Not ascertainable; lately repaired	ditto	Most probably brick drain; no knowledge of cesspool being destroyed.
	22	1	ditto	ditto	ditto	Brick drains good	ditto	No knowledge of cesspool being destroyed.
	34	2	ditto	ditto	ditto	Pipe drains	No	Drainage effective.
	39	2	Yes	ditto	ditto	Not ascertainable	Uncertain	Probably old brick drains; no knowledge of cesspools being destroyed.
	42	1	No	ditto	ditto	Brick drains	ditto	ditto ditto ditto

Figure 5.2 Cooper's report on sewers and drains carefully considered a range of potentially relevant environmental factors at homes where people died in the 1854 cholera outbreak (Cooper 1854, 6).

Source: London Metropolitan Archives.

In service of this brief he cataloged 343 cholera deaths reported in the Registrar-General's *Weekly Reports* and then mapped them onto an engineering map of the parish that showed sewer gratings and lines, distinguishing between lines built before 1851 ("a firm dark line _____"), lines added in 1851 (– • – • –) and those whose construction was begun in 1854 and completed before the end of that year (-------). In symbolizing deaths from cholera, he marked a broad, solid line horizontally at every house where a death had occurred and beneath them a series of shorter, thinner horizontal lines to indicate the number of deaths at each location.

Methodically, he investigated the conditions of the sewers and drains at each house in which one or more persons had died, noting their condition on his worksheet. For every house he carefully reported the location of airshafts, gullies, dustbins, and the condition of the drainage system itself. In addition, he noted the presence of cesspools at homes along the sewer line, many of which were in fact unconnected to the sewers. The sewer lines thus served only partially as potential conduits of disease because half the homes disposed of their wastes in the cesspools located beside or behind them, or in the gutters of second- or third-story tenements from which the waste washed down to the street itself.

All in all, Cooper's was an exceedingly thorough report. His conclusion was that "the number of deaths which have occurred seems to be equally divided between that part in which the sewer was built in 1851, and the part in which a sewer has existed ever since the year 1823" (Cooper 1854, 1–2). Intensity of occurrence did not vary between older and newer sewer lines. Nor did he find any reason to indict the ancient plague pit, located incorrectly on his map as a darkened regular oval hovering over Tyler and Little Marlborough Streets just to the east of King Street.

Like Snow's reading of pump complicity, Cooper's reading of the sewer lines was graphic and visual rather than calculated statistically. Unlike Snow, however, Cooper was not investigating the nature of cholera, only the proposition that cholera occurred more frequently nearer to rather than farther away from the sewer lines. Cooper's map was expanded upon by the Reverend Henry Whitehead in his report to the Parish of Saint James committee (Whitehead 1855), formed in November 1854 to consider the epidemic that had recently ended. A 29-year-old assistant curate at the neighborhood's St Luke's Church, Whitehead had ministered throughout the outbreak to affected parishioners. In developing his report he went back to many homes, interviewing the survivors, and uncovered what in retrospect appeared to be the index case of the outbreak at 40 Broad Street.

After four days of violent diarrhea, Sarah Lewis's five-month-old daughter died September 2, 1854. During the child's illness, Mrs. Lewis had emptied pails of water used in washing her daughter's diapers into a cesspool beside the house and near the Broad Street pump it almost certainly contaminated (Whitehead 1855, 159). Hers was the first case chronologically, one whose importance was underscored when Saint James Parish Committee engineer J. York examined the Broad Street well and found seepage from the area between the 40 Broad Street cesspool and the wall of the Broad Street pump (York 1855, 168–172).

On a parish map that included most local schools and shops, including those Snow referred to but did not map, Whitehead included Cooper's sewer lines and grates as well as the "erroneously supposed position of the ancient plague pit shewn in the map of the commission of sewers." A large, darkened, irregular rectangle correctly identified the "extent of Craven Estate corresponding with site of pest-field," the "ancient plague pit" on which homes and sewers had later been built, as well as Cooper's incorrectly situated and too small oval. Were miasmatic airs to rise from the dead, the map said, they would be from this area, now correctly located. Were specific sewer lines complicit, they would be those that ran beneath the old Craven Estate onto which homes had been built.

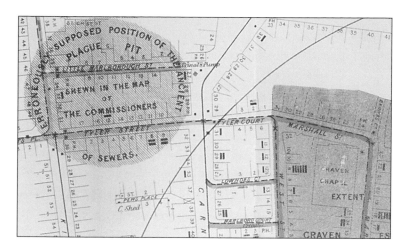

Figure 5.3a Detail of Rev. Whitehead's map of the Broad Street cholera outbreak, including recent 1854 sewer lines (in red), and those laid earlier, shown with a dotted or straight line. Whitehead's circle of greatest incidence sits between the erroneously located "Plague Pit" in Cooper's map and the edge of the correctly located area.

Source: British Library.

To this surface Whitehead joined a full set of 697 cholera-related deaths, including those occurring after September 9, the cut-off date for Snow's data. Whitehead's dataset also included those who had contracted the disease in Saint James Parish but died elsewhere in the city. These deaths were symbolized using a thick horizontal line, á la Cooper, at the home they had visited, with not horizontal but thin, vertical lines beneath the bar to show the number of deaths.

Most important cartographically was the circle drawn by the Reverend Whitehead to encompass the vast majority of cholera deaths in the area. With it he attempted to define the extent of the outbreak through the imposition of a regular analytic field—called today a "buffer"—whose sole characteristic is its relation to one or more sets of mapped data. The buffer is an abstraction fused to the surface of the map, an element of the analytic landscape distilling elements of the dataset itself. In this case, the circle described the boundaries of the outbreak through location of deaths within the parish landscape. Fitted by hand to the map with a compass, the circle, whose radius indicated 630 feet, was centered near the Broad Street pump intersection, also the center of Snow's irregular, polygonal walking path. In Whitehead's map both Cooper's oval "plague pit" and the Craven Estate lands were notably distant from the epicenter of the outbreak, the center of choleric mortality.

Whitehead also proposed a second method of aerial definition; a districting that was almost equally interesting. "It has been shown by Mr. Whitehead that the limits of the Cholera District are also very accurately defined within an irregular 4-sided figures, the north and south angles of which are placed respectively near the middle of Poland Street and at the South End of Little Windmill Street" (Whitehead 1856, 9). This unmapped irregular rectangle defined the area of the outbreak rather than the area of greatest intensity defined by Snow's irregular polygon. Whitehead's goal was to define the epidemic's boundaries rather than to determine its center of activity. His circle (and rectangle) thus complements Snow's polygon, serving an administrative rather than a clinical purpose.

Whitehead's was an impressive piece of work, one that expanded upon Snow's more limited topography, showing the schools and churches of the district that Snow discussed but did not map. The mapped argument that Whitehead presented included both the deaths Snow mapped and those occurring later in the epidemic. Furthermore, Whitehead struck upon an imaginative symbolization permitting the inclusion of those who could be shown to have contracted the disease in the Broad Street area but died elsewhere. The database was exhaustive, the theories considered in the mapped argument broad, and the mapped result innovative.

Whitehead's report and its mapped argument did not support Snow's focused argument for contagion even if it did concede the centrality of the Broad Street pump and its importance in the outbreak. In an ecumenical fashion, Whitehead included data pertinent to each of the three theories of diffusion then extant. For the majority insisting upon a miasmatic posture there was the corrected location of the former pest field in relation to the deaths that occurred in the district. If nothing else, this mapping gave credence to the miasmatic theory of cholera. The map lacked only a system of lines and isolines showing the direction of the wind during the outbreak to be a complete contributor to a thesis of airborne cholera; isolines of altitude would have satisfied Farr's approach.[1] For the Sewer Commission there were the lines that ran through the area, each line dated by the year of its construction. Their apparent lack of complicity laid to rest the fears of many in the neighborhood. And for Snow there were the water pumps with the Broad Street pump central to the deaths that Whitehead had mapped.

Critical concerns

The Saint James Parish Committee Report authors did not endorse either Snow's general conclusions or those of the miasmatists. They left open a statement on the nature of cholera, opting instead for a more limited declaration implicating the pump without endorsing Snow's argument about its importance. The problem was that this small-scale study was, while clearly suggestive, not definitive. True, Snow's theory of the pump's culpability afforded, in his words, "an exact explanation of the fearful outbreak of cholera in Saint James parish." But it was not the explanation, one all would be compelled to accept upon the weight of its evidence. Clearly, he believed his mapped argument permitted "no other

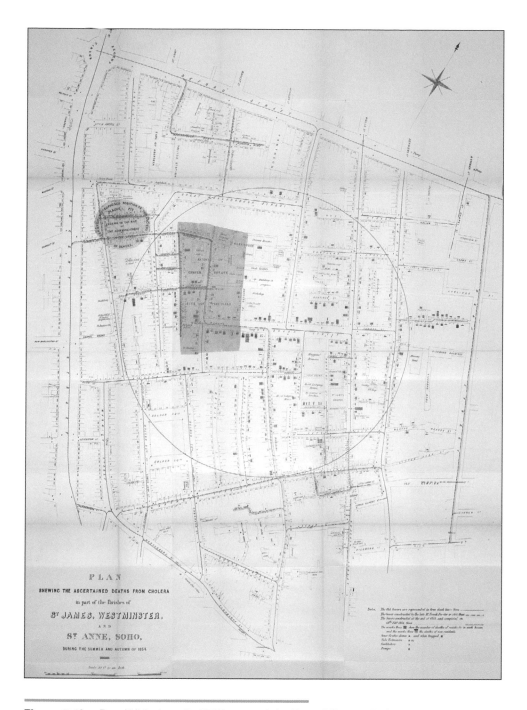

Figure 5.3b Rev. Whitehead's 1855 map of the Broad Street cholera outbreak in 1854, prepared for the Saint James Parish committee.

Source: College of Physicians of Philadelphia.

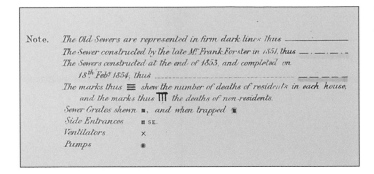

Figure 5.3c Legend from Rev. Whitehead's Broad Street outbreak map, showing his method of symbolizing location of sewer lines by year, house-by-house data (sewer grates, etc.), the pumps and different categories of deaths.

Source: British Library.

circumstance which offers any explanation at all, whatever hypothesis of the nature and cause of the malady be adopted" (Snow 1855c, 54). Cooper's sewer map showed that "there is nothing peculiar in the sewer or drainage of the limited spot in which this outbreak occurred" (Snow 1855c, 54), removing the new lines as an explanatory factor. Finally, the old plague pit was, Snow noted, "just out of the area in which the chief mortality occurred." All this was insufficient to convince his contemporaries of the waterborne nature of cholera, however.

Famously, Snow had argued the Broad Street pump's handle should be removed. When that occurred, the outbreak's intensity decreased. A pin of the modern John Snow society immortalizes the moment. "In consequence of what I said," it reads, "the handle of the pump was removed . . ." *(figure 5.4)* In fact, Snow himself admitted that "the attacks had so far diminished before the use of the water was stopped, that it is impossible to decide whether the well still contained the cholera poison in an active state [when the handle was removed], or whether, from some other cause, the water had become free from it" (Snow 1855c, 51–52). And, he continued, "Whether the impurities of the water were derived from the sewers, the drains, or the cesspools, of which there are a number in the neighborhood, I cannot tell." Without knowing that, there was room enough for doubters.

Critics of Snow's theory used the maps of Snow and Whitehead to argue for a continued miasmatic interpretation of the disease. Edmund Parks, for example, observed that the centralized pattern of the outbreak, centered upon the Broad Street pump, was exactly what one might expect if a localized, noxious miasma was in fact the cause of the disease. Parks did not say why the outbreak was centered there—he didn't have to, only that it was possible. Furthermore, he pointed out, there were so many pumps in the area that no matter where the epidemic had its center one would surely be close by (Parks 1855).

As important, not *every* case Snow and Whitehead investigated could be assigned to the Broad Street pump and its water. Snow believed this was likely the result of the difficulty of collecting data postmortem. What was important, he insisted, was that the preponderance of cases could be shown to be pump-related. "As regards the eight cases in which I could trace no connection with the water of the

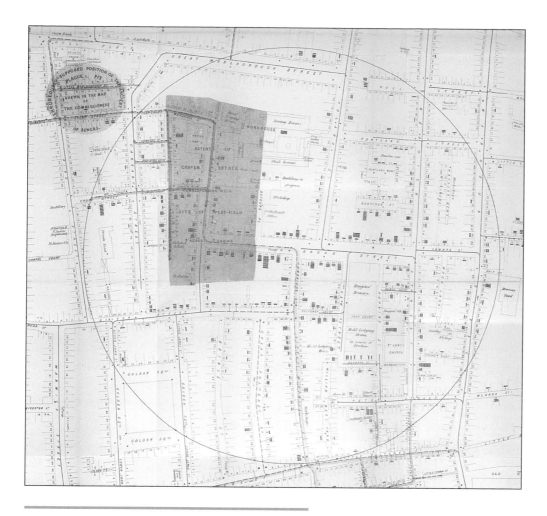

Figure 5.3d Detail of Rev. Whitehead's cholera outbreak map with a circle defining the epidemic's boundaries, the irregular rectangle of the old "pestilence pit," and Cooper's erroneously located "plague pit" included.

Source: College of Physicians of Philadelphia.

pump in Broad Street," Snow wrote, "it may be observed that they form but a slight mortality for the large area in which they occurred; a mortality not greater than was occurring in surrounding parishes, and probably not greater than would have taken place in this district if the greater outbreak had not occurred" (Snow 1855a, 116).

In retrospect we, too, assume these were likely fatalities resulting from other causes, probably the dehydrating diarrhea of "English cholera," or severe salmonella. We, however, have the advantage of knowing about the bacterium that causes cholera and its precise mode of transmission. For doubters

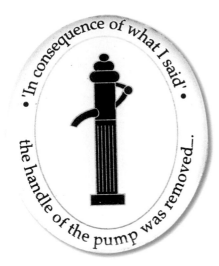

Figure 5.4 Pin of the Broad Street pump from the John Snow Society, London. The myth states that the removal of the pump resulted in the end of the Broad Street outbreak. Snow himself did not believe this to be true. Still, the quote is famous and presented proudly on a pin available at the John Snow pub in London.

Source: John Snow Pub, London.

like Parks in the mid-1800s, the anomalous cases were sufficient to cast doubt upon Snow's conclusions. So, too, was the undeniable fact that not everyone who drank from the Broad Street pump got sick. If it was the water, they said, then anyone drinking from the pump should be affected. Had that been the case, the deaths would have been far greater. Snow's explanation was an unsatisfactory analogy: "The eggs of the tape-worm must undoubtedly pass down the sewers into the Thames, but it by no means follows that everyone who drinks a glass of the water should swallow one of the eggs" (Snow 1855c, 113). In other words, whatever it was that got into the water did not seem to get into every glass of water that was drawn from the pump.

For skeptics, this was a giant hole in the center of Snow's argument and would remain a sticking point for some even after Robert Koch identified the bacillus *Vibrio cholerae* as the one responsible for the disease. In 1892, for example, the German scientist Max von Pettenkofer drank a glass of diluted *Vibrio cholerae* during an outbreak of the disease in Hamburg in an attempt to disprove Koch's work advancing the bacterium as the cause of the disease. Von Pettenkofer did not become deathly ill but neither did he turn back the then overwhelming tide of sentiment admitting bacteriology as the principal mode by which disease like cholera could be defined and explained (Dimenstein 2003).

In 1854, the limits of Snow's argument were too great to be ignored by contemporaries who weighed his data with that presented by others, his non-theory of disease with one developed over centuries. Simply, his critics argued, Snow had erred by permitting his beliefs to get ahead of his science. "Is this evidence scientific?" the *Lancet* asked in an 1855 editorial (Wakley 1855; Vinten-Johansen et al. 2003, 344), "Is it in accordance with the experience of men who have studied the question without being blinded by theories?" The answer, the author Thomas Wakley insisted, was no. "The truth is, that the well whence Dr. Snow draws all sanitary truth is the main sewer. His *specus*, or den, is a drain.

In riding his hobby very hard, he has fallen down a gully-hole and has never been able to get out again" (Wakley 1855). Wakley did not have to distinguish between unproven theory and established knowledge, between the unseen poisons Snow posited and the foul miasma everyone could smell. The evidence seemed incontrovertible, and on balance little of it was interpreted as favorable to Snow's point of view.

Miasmatic researchers

To understand Snow's inability to convince his contemporaries, it is useful to consider the detailed, often exemplary work of others, like Farr, whose research was as rigorous and whose conclusions were distinct. Remember that Snow was the innovator and radical whose argument was based upon an unproven theory of invisible poisons born nobody knew where and then somehow passed from person to person. Its acceptance demanded a leap of faith. Those whose views differed from Snow's favored a posture that built upon the Hippocratic tradition whose general perspective of good and bad airs and environments carried the weight of a millennium of medical writing, thinking, and research. Where the data seemed to be supported by long-accepted theory, it gained in importance as a result.

One of those whose work stood in opposition to Snow's was Farr, an able statistician whose analyses were frequently published in the *Lancet*. He quantified the relation between altitude and deaths per ten thousand people resulting from cholera and choleric diarrhea in London in 1849, 1853, and 1854. In general, he found, deaths were greater at sea level along the Thames River than inland. The fit was not exact, but the general pattern was sufficient for Farr who believed that in the absence of other equally rigorous correlations, the relationship between altitude and incidence of cholera was explained by his zymotic theory of disease, a variation on the miasmatic. Disease fermented where foul airs congregated at lower levels where waste washed down to the riverbank from the city. Cholera was less frequently found at higher levels where the air smelled cleaner and waste was less evident.

Nor was Farr alone in his assumptions. Augustus Petermann, a German cartographer elected a fellow of the Royal Geographical Society in 1846, mapped the 1831–1833 cholera epidemic and saw a similar relationship. "He also discussed the relation of the disease to relief and observed that a cursory glance at his map apparently corroborated the belief that cholera rarely penetrated mountainous countries and never reached the tops of hills. The cholera districts in the British Isles 'seemed to lie all in the lower grounds and valleys'" (Gilbert 1958, 178).

While Farr and Petermann argued the proposition that increasing altitude resulted in a decreased incidence of cholera, other researchers were at pains to determine the elements that might explain that relationship. In its report to Parliament, the General Board of Health included a complex and detailed chart based upon readings from twenty-four meteorological stations in Greater London (General Board of Health 1855). On a daily basis, a range of data was recorded, including air pressure, air temperature, barometric pressure, cloud cover, humidity, precipitation, Thames river temperature, and wind velocity.

Farr: Altitude and cholera

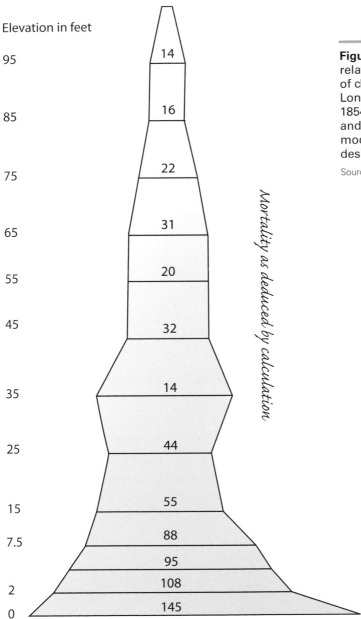

Mortality from cholera

Elevation in feet

95 — 14

85 — 16

75 — 22

65 — 31

55 — 20

45 — 32

35 — 14

25 — 44

15 — 55

7.5 — 88

— 95

2 — 108

0 — 145

Mortality as deduced by calculation

Figure 5.5 A graph showing the relation between altitude and incidence of cholera or diarrhea per ten thousand London inhabitants in 1849, 1853, and 1854. Farr's original graph was traced and reproduced, albeit with more modern fonts and simpler textual design.

Source: Adapted from Farr (1855).

An attempt was made to correlate any (or all) of these to the incidence of cholera historically (using data from 1848 and 1832 epidemics) as well as to the cholera epidemic of 1853–1854.

The chart joined the incidence of cholera (blue) and diarrhea (yellow), the former fatal while the latter was not, with a daily record of climatic variables. Together, both diseases present the now-common bell-shaped wave of an epidemic against a background of endemic disease. Along the yellow base line at the bottom of the chart, representing cases of endemic diarrhea, the incidence of both cholera and diarrhea explode at the end of June, with the epidemic peaking at the end of August and then subsiding through October. A combination of climatic variables peaked around the time the epidemic began and then slowly declined as the epidemic eventually waned. The effect of these variables on the odiferous, miasmatic airs along the river served to explain, at least for Hippocratic-minded anticontagionists, the generation of choleric airs.

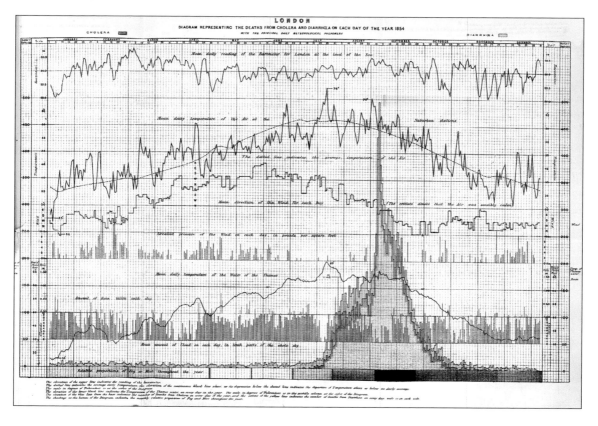

Figure 5.6 A graph of climatic variables joined to incidence of cholera (blue) and chronic diarrhea (yellow) in London, 1854. The map was based on readings from twenty-four urban recording stations in London and prepared by the General Board of Health for a report to both houses of Parliament.

Source: College of Physicians of Philadelphia.

The beginning of the epidemic in late July coincides with a period of fog or mist represented by the progressively darker colors in the bar at the bottom of the graph. The epidemic's peak occurs in the period of greatest fog or mist in early September, as if the clouds themselves held the potent cholera before the city's eyes. The relation to temperature is also obvious, with the epidemic beginning during the days when daily mean temperature was at its peak (75 degrees), and the temperature of Thames River water was 69 degrees. As water and air temperature declined into autumn, so, too, did the incidence of disease. And except for perhaps three days of rain in late July, the epidemic took place during a relative drought with little wind.

It was presumably obvious to everyone. High temperatures and low winds were the conditions that generated cholera in the odiferous wastes that sat in the heat along the banks of the Thames. The smell would have been strongest where the riverbank dried and the sun beat most strongly on the urban effluvia that washed onto it. Winds were insufficient to blow away the poisonous, choleric air. At higher altitudes the temperature would be cooler and winds possibly more fulsome. The evidence was in the nose, of course, because at those altitudes one did not smell the stench so evident at the riverbanks and the people therefore were healthier.

Acland: Oxford

Further evidence was presented by H. W. Acland in his extraordinarily comprehensive *Memoir on the Cholera at Oxford,* an examination of cholera outbreaks in that city between 1830 and 1854. In this study, perhaps the most comprehensive of its day, Acland used charts and maps to create a topography that was at once geographic and topographic. The incontrovertible conclusion, he argued, was, *á la* Farr, that altitude was "a more constant relation with mortality from cholera than any other human element" (Gilbert 1958, 181–182).

A physician, Acland carefully considered 290 cases of cholera occurring in 1854 in Oxford. His database, published in the book-length memoir, included both cases of cholera and "choleraic diarrhoea," distinguishing between those that were mortal (n=128) and those that were not (n=162). For each case occurring in 1854 he included in his published tables the age, date of onset, diagnosis and outcome (death or recovery), occupation, residence by street, and the sex of the patient.

On a map of the city, Acland symbolized the 1854 outbreak cases of diarrheic cholera (a single brown dot) and cholera (double dots placed horizontally) above the location of a patient's house.[2] In the streets themselves, he marked cholera cases from the 1849 records with a blue, horizontal bar, and for the 1832 cases, a blue dot. His map thus included data from all three epidemic outbreaks, imaginatively changing symbol shape, color, and placement relative to the homes of persons affected for each range of cases categorized by year.

The map's domain was simultaneously geographic and sanitarian. On a detailed plan of the city, he included large brown dots to identify "unhealthy" sites based upon the research of previous sanitarian

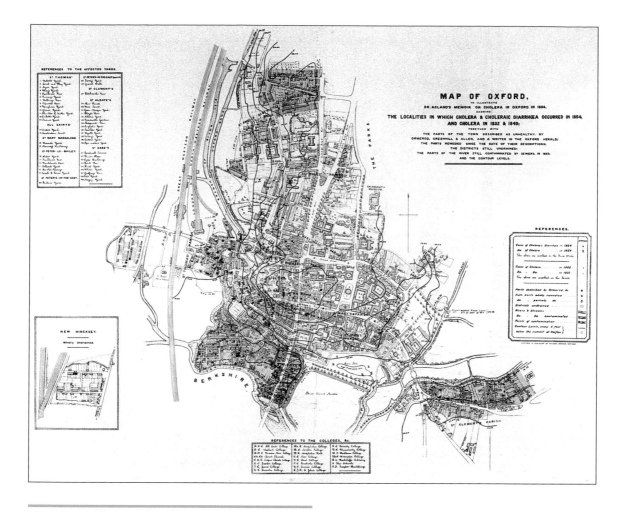

Figure 5.7a Map by H. W. Acland showing the relation of altitude to disease incidence in three separate cholera epidemics in Oxford.

Source: Rare Books and Special Collections, University of British Columbia Library.

investigators. He also distinguished between contaminated (parallel blue line with dots inside it) and unpolluted rivers (a blue river line). Finally, to this he added contour lines marking altitude in five-foot gradients below the town's highest point, the "summit of Carfax." The result was, Acland believed, conclusive. Deaths occurring in all three epidemic outbreaks were clustered in areas of lower as opposed to higher elevation. In every outbreak, the disease attacked persons in lowlands more strongly than persons who lived at higher elevations within the city. This was true even where previously documented unhealthy sites could be found at significant altitude (for example, near the Carfax summit). The only logical conclusion was that cholera was a miasmatic disease fostered in lowland airs that did not rise to greater altitudes.

Here was Farr's inverse correlation of altitude and disease incidence expanded upon and mapped to glorious, expensive, multicolored perfection. Not only did it include data from three epidemic outbreaks, it also argued that the correlation between disease and altitude held despite evidence of known sites of ill health and of contamination in areas of relative altitude. In this manner, it

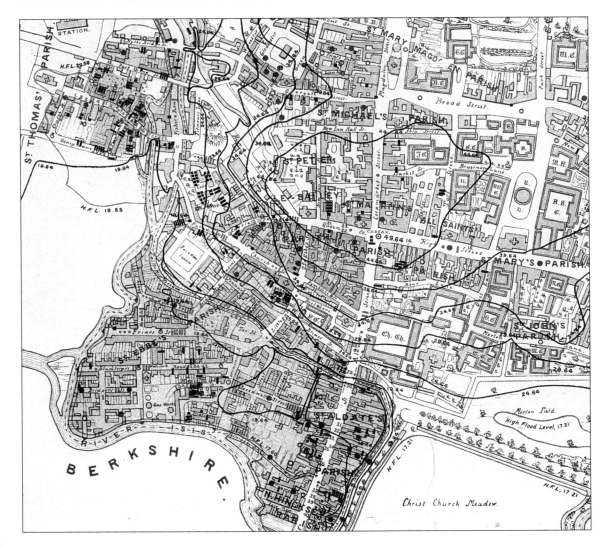

Figure 5.7b Detail of Acland's map of cholera incidence in 1832, 1849, and 1854 in an environment whose areas of pollution are noted with five-foot altitude gradients.

Source: Rare Books and Special Collections, University of British Columbia Library.

Cartographies of Disease

advanced previous studies like Grainger's in a substantive fashion. To hammer home the point, Acland included an extraordinary chart of the incidence of cholera (black), choleraic diarrhoea (yellow), *and* diarrhea (red) reported in Oxford before, during, and after the epidemic of 1854. Similar to the board of health's climatic chart of London, this one's power was the greater for the fineness of its scale. If altitude was inversely related, the chart said, the effect can be explained by the temperature, sunlight, wind, and rainfall that promote choleraic airs (and horrid smells) in the lower altitudes. In his text the effect was considerable: See the relation in the map, understand it through the charted data.

On the horizontal axis is a range of climatic conditions, including ozone levels, minimum and maximum daily temperature, rainfall and humidity, barometric pressure, wind speed and direction, and cloud cover. Each of these is charted against the incidence of the diseases over the time of the outbreak. Every attribute was considered in relation to the data distilled in the map and the theory the whole advanced. The chart expanded the argument of the map, its relation of disease incidence over more than thirty years to local geographic conditions. Map and chart together used an analysis of climatic and physical determinants to explain variations in disease incidence.

Acland's careful work was state of the art but not cutting edge. Others were using similar techniques in their attempt to understand the biogeographic nature of other diseases. In an 1859 report for the British Parliament on a yellow fever epidemic in Lisbon, for example, Robert Lyons published an extremely legible if oversized multicolored foldout chart of the daily state of the atmosphere in Lisbon during the prevalence of the cholera in the summer of 1856. With four months of data on barometric pressure, temperature, wind speed and direction, etc., the chart distilled pages of tables from the Royal Observatory in the same way the maps of this period distilled spatial arguments.

Among the things that distinguished Acland's efforts was that, like Snow's Broad Street study, he chose a scale of analysis that permitted an almost encyclopedic mapping of a single disease outbreak. Acland then fleshed out his thesis by changing scales and considering the effect of the Oxford outbreak on surrounding towns. In an enterprising fashion, he found a way to represent different intensities of relation between town and hinterland. In this way, he was among the first to map the dynamic exurban spread of an epidemic disease.

The problem was how to categorize the towns on his map. His simple answer was that towns in which no cholera was reported (Headington, for example) were simply named on the map. Those where the disease was reported (Abingden, Brill, Oakley, etc.) were enclosed in an oval. Towns with a small number of cases that could be traced to Oxford were linked to that city by a simple double line. Those linked with a double line ending in a star indicated towns in which a more general outbreak resulted from an individual case that could be traced to Oxford. The mapping linked topography—"valley incidence and relative relief with poor drainage" (Learmonth 1988, 148) to the relative intensity of cholera's diffusion from Oxford to the surrounding towns with which Oxonians interacted.

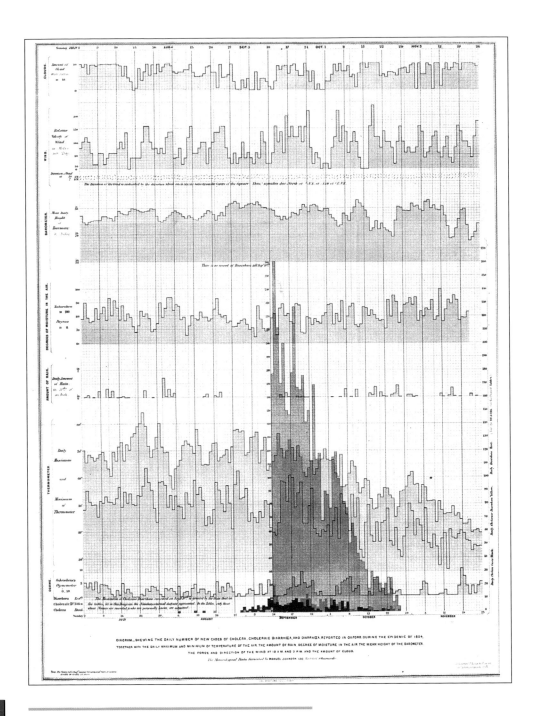

Figure 5.8 Acland's chart of cholera, diarrhetic cholera, and dysentery, relating disease incidence to climatic conditions in Oxford.

Source: Rare Books and Special Collection, University of British Columbia Library.

It also distinguished an urban hierarchy of town to hamlet that one hundred years later would take on extreme importance.

In the late twentieth century researchers would begin to understand not only environmental determinants of health and disease but also the manner of their diffusion and the demography of the effect of epidemics on populations. Here, however, is an early attempt remarkable for its completeness and rigor. Like much of the science of every era, it missed an intervening vector. It missed as well the fact that water sources at higher elevations typically relied on well water draw from aquifers or highland streams rather than the polluted Thames. But the mapping—and here, the mapmaking—were clear, consistent, and, if ultimately incorrect, still rigorous.

Snow was unconvincing within the greater context of his day. In science, the value of any study is decided not against an abstract rule of "truth" or a yardstick of objective "reality" but instead by the acceptance of an argument by a jury of one's peers. It is not enough to be right; one has to be right in the context of one's times (Nuland 1989, 239). That is what science has been about at least since Robert Boyle first insisted that, "matters of fact be established by the aggregation of individual beliefs" (Shapin and Schaffer 1985, 25). The science that results is what the majority of scientists together believe. Snow was not sufficiently convincing to build that aggregation in the face of a medical tradition whose theories were both entrenched and strongly supported by the work of investigators, like Acland and Farr, which was as rigorous, and as rigorously mapped, as Snow's own.

This is not to say Snow failed, simply that in the context of his day his work was insufficient. What Nuland says of another adventurous researcher serves equally well here: "When the cultural milieu is just right, when the technological tools have been invented, and when enough restless minds have begun to chafe under the status quo, some one spunky spirit comes forward to deliver the enlightening goods" (Nuland 1989, 239). Snow was enlightening. That others rejected his ideas based on seemingly firm evidence and very strong theory is a sneer neither at Snow nor his critics. Science was just making its way, applying available technologies in the context of theories that encouraged ever-more rigorous analysis of the data at hand.

Cholera and mapping

Snow understood the limits of his Broad Street investigations. It was in part because of them that he was simultaneously engaged in the more ambitious and potentially definitive project, the South London study. Because the Soho study was not conclusive does not mean the work was unimpressive, however, or unsuccessful; it only means it was incomplete and its conclusions unacceptable to the majority of his contemporaries. Today some assert that maps and mapping were peripheral to Snow's (or Whitehead's or Cooper's) thinking. They were at best an afterthought, simple graphics almost inexplicably added to the official reports (see, for example, Vinten-Johansen et al. 2003, 332).[3] But the maps Snow and his contemporaries produced were neither simple graphics nor casual addendums

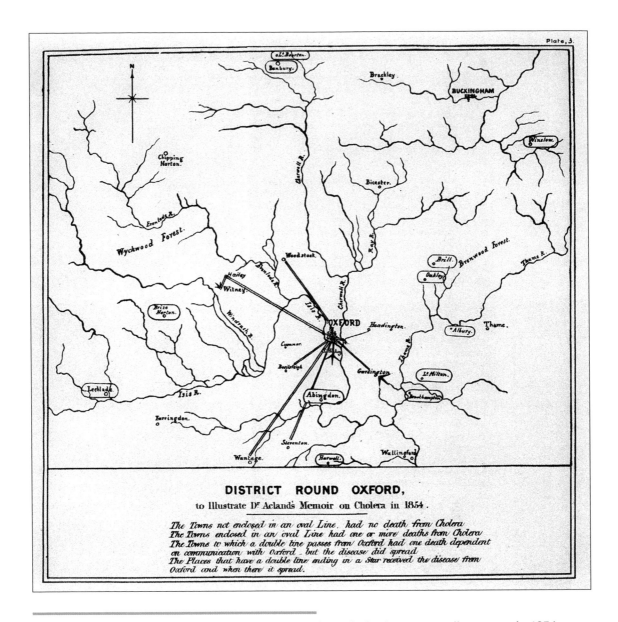

Figure 5.9 Acland's map of the spread of cholera from Oxford to surrounding towns in 1854.

Source: Rare Books and Special Collections, University of British Columbia Library.

used to spice up a report. Rather, they were the inevitable consequence of the thinking they presented powered by the technologies of their day. They were necessary elements of their respective reports, as important as the datasets on which each was based. The propositions the researchers were arguing were spatial. Maps were, by the 1830s, an accepted tool for the analysis of spatial propositions and the distillation of spatial arguments. They were integral to the thinking of the era, the work of the researchers and the understanding of the readers then debating differing theories of the nature of cholera as an example of a pandemic disease.

It is perhaps more accurate to insist that the debate in the 1850s and 1860s over the nature of cholera was *all* about mapping, about the ability to link incidence to topography in a way that made sense. Acland's contour lines, Cooper's sewers, Snow's irregular polygon and Whitehead's circle were evidence of the way mapping was being used not only to transform datasets grown too large to easily manipulate in tables alone but more importantly to relate disease incidence to a relevant and concrete topography. The mapping naturally resulted in maps (and charts and tables) because, from Acland to Whitehead, the real problem was to frame propositions that would reveal the relations that promoted or inhibited interaction between agent and host within a single population and between varying population centers.

In this effort to understand those relations, the medical and statistical were joined in the map. Snow mapped the incidence of cholera and the location of the water sources in Saint James, Soho. He calculated both death as a percentage of the population and projected deaths if the brewer workers or persons in the Poland Street poorhouse had only drunk Broad Street water. For the South London study he mapped not only cholera by district population but also by water supplier, calculating deaths per district to make his point. Farr was a statistician *par excellence*; Acland mapped both disease incidence and contours showing altitude to make his case. All had the examples of Chadwick and his contemporaries to build upon. Here were reams of cold, hard data that together could be used both to identify a relationship and the conditions that explained their effect. Altitude was at fault in periods of low rain and high heat when, with little wind to dispel it, the foul miasmatic odors generated the bad air that resulted in the epidemic.

At stake in this debate was not simply the origin of cholera but, more generally, the way in which epidemic (and perhaps chronic) disease was to be understood. Every age has its critical illness (Sontag 1978)—plague, cancer, cholera, tuberculosis, and more recently AIDS have all served the role—the study of which becomes the focal point of medicine's struggle to identify the broader determinants of disease, and thus, perhaps, the constituents of health. In the 1850s, that disease was cholera, and the lessons learned in its study would power medical science forward in the coming years.

Maps were a logical, almost inevitable medium to report the work that resulted. It was in the mapping that the importance of both the absence of cholera at the Poland Street Workhouse, and the nearby brewery, is best seen. And it was in the maps that the relative density of occurrence in the area of the Broad Street pump (defined by Whitehead's circle or Snow's irregular polygon) was demonstrated. Acland's maps made clear the inverse relation between altitude and disease incidence over three epidemics that Farr had argued in his more abstract chart. The climatic charts of Acland and the

General Health office can only be read today as a part of the mapped argument in an emerging science that was graphic and numerical at once.

And while the miasmatic, contagionist conclusion was wrong, the inverse relationship that was used to argue it was accurate. That Acland and Farr missed the meaning of the relation is a fault neither of the researchers nor the mapping they did. In contention were different theories of disease, different perceptions of the city, and different assumptions about the data required for a disease study. One cannot blame a scientist for being limited by the science and knowledge of the time.

In retrospect, the arguments of Acland and Farr, Whitehead and Snow present a pristine example of the best of science struggling in the face of ignorance and uncertainty. The remarkable thing is not that Snow perceived what others did not but that these researchers together were able to advance the science of a man they admired. The proof was to be seen in the next several decades as different researchers built upon the work of all these men, seeking better explanations for the diffusion of cholera and the reasons for its spread. That this work was heavily mapped and carefully graphed as the propositions became more rigorous, the studies more ambitious, is not surprising because, at least in this period, mapping and charting were integral to the evolving sciences—medical, physical, and social—that were together advancing.

Endnotes

1. While scientists had mapped wind direction and deviations in barometric air pressure as early as the 1820s, it was not until somewhat later in the nineteenth century that these symbols were combined in a substantive manner. Indeed, it would not be until the early twentieth century that climatic mapping would be sufficiently advanced to permit relatively precise weather mapping (Monmonier 1999).

2. Gilbert (1958, 179–182) includes four black-and-white maps of Acland's map, separating the physical contours, the incidence of disease (choleraic diarrhoea and cholera), and areas of ill drainage into separate plates. As he did with the work of others, his modifications to the original work were accompanied without comment as if the black-and-white plates—and modifications to them—were the original author's work. Learmonth (1988, 148) describes field trips Gilbert would lead through Oxford to give students and visitors a sense of the nineteenth-century city and the environment Acland described.

3. In writing about Snow's 1854 map of the Soho outbreak, Vinten-Johansen and his colleagues make the map an inexplicable afterthought. "For some reason [Snow] decided at that point to prepare an illustrative map of the Golden Square Outbreak and made brief references to it in the manuscript" (Vinten-Johansen et al. 2003, 332).

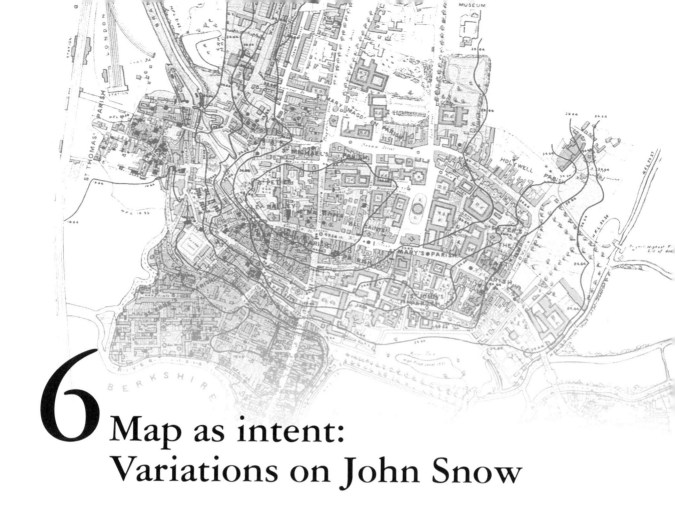

6 Map as intent: Variations on John Snow

The work of Acland, Cooper, Farr, Whitehead, and the other nineteenth-century researchers is forgotten today by all but a few medical historians. What we remember is John Snow and his maps. In the twentieth century, the myth grew of the Promethean researcher who single handedly proved cholera was caused by waterborne bacteria. He was considered the lone pioneer who created medical cartography (McLeod 2000), and not coincidentally, the disciplines of epidemiology and public health. The myth obscures the more interesting, and certainly more complex, reality. Snow was not a loner but a collegial fellow who thrived in his attendance at the weekly meetings of his peers. He was a familiar of Farr, Whitehead, and scores of other researchers, a man of his time who read widely and published extensively in the journals of the day.

Snow's work built upon that of others and appeared as one example—and not necessarily the best—of mapping as an analytic tool in medical research. The definitive map of the Broad Street outbreak was Whitehead's *(figure 5.3a-d)*. It was his dataset that was the most inclusive, including the deaths of those who contracted the disease in the Broad Street area but who died in other parts of the city. It was he, not Snow, who corrected and incorporated Cooper's mapping of the sewer lines and the old plague pit as alternative hypotheses to be investigated graphically. Whitehead created the circular zone that described the extent of the epidemic, the forerunner of the buffers medical mappers use today.

Snow's preeminence grew not from his mapping but the thinking his maps sought to present. Cooper asked a smaller question, seeking only to know whether or not local sewer lines were complicit in the outbreak. Whitehead was interested primarily in describing the outbreak that affected his parishioners, not understanding the nature of the disease itself. Snow's great legacy is his consideration of the Soho outbreak as an example of a more general problem, the environmental elements that promoted a disease within a specific host population. His maps reflected his thinking, excluding data that was extraneous while focusing on the topography of an outbreak as a way to understand the nature and diffusion of cholera, the relation between disease agent, host population, and the environment that promoted that relationship.

It is useful to think of Snow as an early ecologist seeking to describe a range of elements contributing to the understanding of a specific phenomenon. All the elements of his stated concern were focused in his charts, maps, and texts on the discussion of the diffusion of the waterborne cholera that affected his community. As it had been for Pascalis and Seaman before him, a vertically structured investigation of the specific outbreak occurred within a more general, horizontal sanitarian concern for the contextual determinants of public health.

Snow's real genius lay not in the maps he made but in the questions he asked and his ability to combine clinical and ecological perspectives in his search for relevant data. He was not a medical cartographer making maps as a way to uncover the epicenter of a disease outbreak or the vector of a specific pathogen. Indeed, he was not a mapmaker at all. He was instead a mapper who worked upon a commercial map sufficiently detailed to include the work places—a brewery on Broad Street and a workhouse on Poland Street, for example—to which he referred in his text. The result was a "diagram of the topography of the outbreak" (Snow 1855c, 45), the essence of the ecology he considered textually.

The mapping that resulted was an outgrowth of his hard thinking (Brody et al. 2000) about a collection of cases in an environment he believed complicit in their propagation. In this he reminds us "what the map's about—what is really at stake—is whatever the discourse facilitated by this pointing [mapping] is about" (Wood 2002). Snow's discourse was well in advance of that of his contemporaries even if the maps that were a part of his work, and the statistics they employed, were wholly in step with that of other researchers of his day.

Perceiving the degree to which authorial intention is a defining characteristic of all scientific work is often difficult. The results seem so "real," so impersonal and obvious that the centrality of the researcher in their construction is easy to forget. Like statistics, maps confer a sense of authority. They seem to be independent of the author, a distillation of facts that by the nature of their graphing or mapping appear to be firm, undisputed. Because maps have been long assumed to be a representation of reality rather than first and foremost a reflection of the author's intention, the idea that maps, like statistics, are authorial tools has been largely overlooked. Instead, the mapping literature typically has concerned itself with how best to prepare a map so that it will reflect the supposedly objective data it seeks to present. Thus, mapping theory has largely concerned itself with issues of symbolization and design rather than more substantive concerns (Crampton 2002, 638). That is, for most general cartographers the maps serve a fundamentally communicative rather than substantially investigative function.

The central issue of medical mapping is not the clarity of the representation, important as that is, but the definition and method of consideration of a phenomenon and its causes. In medicine as in all things, objectivity and the science that supposedly presents it "exists only as a product of human activity" (Turner 1991). The data we collect, the manner in which it is considered, and the thinking that results (graphic, mapped, statistical, and textual) reflect the researcher and his point of view as much as the phenomenon he or she seeks to consider. "Each map [or chart or graph] is made from a particular perspective and for a particular purpose" (Heersink 2001, 136–37).

Purpose defines the subjectively grounded result. The question, therefore, is rarely "how to lie with maps" (Monmonier 1996) or statistics (Huff 1993) or charts (Jones 1995). Most of the "damned lies and statistics" (Best 2001) contained in reports—graphic and textual—are offered in the best of faith. Cooper told the truth to the best of his ability. So, too, did Whitehead. Farr's proof of the inverse relation of altitude to incidence of cholera was no more mendacious than Pascalis's or Seaman's of the relation of furry miasmata to yellow fever. The critical question is not what is "true," or "real," but what truth or reality do we seek to express and how do we present it within the context of our interests.

That is the lesson not simply of Snow but of the myriad researchers who have used Snow's data and maps for their own purposes. Vinten-Johansen and his colleagues (2003, 297–299) count twenty-seven instances where Snow's maps have been appropriated by later researchers. Hundreds of others (including myself, see Koch and Denike 2004) have used Snow's map—or maps based upon his work—as icons that speak to the importance of spatial analysis, fine-scaled studies, and medical mapping. What is most interesting about the myriad redrawings of Snow's maps is how different they are from Snow's own work.

Every author since Snow has had access to the maps and reports that he and his colleagues produced. And yet, in almost every case not only does the interpretation of Snow's map and work change in the retelling, but in most the map itself is twisted, turned, and truncated—violated, for want of a better word—by this or that mapmaker's mindset and point of view. Even in its most "scientific" mode—a GIS version by the U.S. Centers for Disease Control (CDC) designed for teaching purposes—the context of its making redefines its appearance and its content in ways that are at once demonstrably false and inaccurate. A review of the history of Snow's map says a great deal about mapping as an analytic technique, and more important, about the role of authorial intention in research generally.

W. T. Sedgwick

William T. Sedgwick (1911) was not a practicing physician lecturing in a school of medicine but a professor of sanitary science and public health in Boston. His interest, and that of his fledgling discipline, was, as the title page of his book made clear, the *Principles of Sanitary Science and the Public Health with Special Reference to the Causation and Prevention of Infectious Diseases.* His text was a casebook in which, chapter by chapter, issues of sanitation, and especially clean water, were the villains of the story, the causes of the infectious diseases that students of sanitary science and public health were being trained to fight at the end of the nineteenth century. Here the horizontal issues of health and wellness were constructed within an academic context that used vertically researched disease outbreaks as principle examples.

Sedgwick's evolving discipline was a modern incarnation of the sanitarianism earlier argued by Pascalis and Seaman, one that built upon a general view of public health as a function of local conditions of sanitation. That sanitary science and public health deserved to be recognized as a unique and systematic discipline was the not overly subtle subtext to Sedgwick's work. The quote on the title page of the book gave the sentiment of the age: "The triumphs of sanitary reform as well as of medical science are perhaps the brightest page in the history of our century." Public health was to be perceived as, if not an equal, then at least a junior partner in the best advances of medicine's late-nineteenth-century technical revolution.[1]

At the time of Sedgwick's writing, "sanitary science" and "public health" were relatively new disciplines struggling for their place in academe. They tended to be intellectual domains allied with, perhaps, but distinct from medicine, studies whose legitimacy was based on nonclinical investigations of the incidence of disease in specific environments. Here the model was less Dr. Snow than Rev. Henry Whitehead, a nonmedically trained but still gifted researcher. The Broad Street outbreak served Sedgwick as an iconic example of public health thinking and reasoning. "As a monument of sanitary research, of medical and engineering interest and of penetrating inductive reasoning, it deserves the most careful study. No apology, therefore, need be made for giving of it here a somewhat extended account" (Sedgwick 1911, 170). His retelling of the Broad Street outbreak was the most extensive case study in Sedgwick's book. The whole presented, he told readers, "one of the earliest, one of the most famous, and one of the most instructive cases of the conveyance of disease by polluted water" (Sedgwick 1911, 170).

Sedgwick summarized Snow's work in loving detail. Over 50 percent of the chapter consisted of quotes taken directly from Snow's 1855 report to the St. James Cholera Inquiry Committee. He paid special attention to Snow's fieldwork, considering the null cases, the lack of cholera at the brewery and the minimal number of cases at the Poland Street Workhouse, as well as Snow's description of cases occurring elsewhere in the district. Also commended in Sedgwick's text was Snow's careful description of how direct, person-to-person transmission occurred in densely habited dwellings. Here, after all, were examples of the networks of occurrence and transmission over time that Sedgwick's students presumably would pursue when confronted with a disease outbreak.

In this telling, Rev. Whitehead's discovery of the index case of the outbreak at 40 Broad Street was presented as confirmation of Snow's theory. The *pièce de résistance* of the story was a physical examination of the well itself. In a report to the St. James committee, its engineer secretary, Jeremiah York (1855), found that the main drain of 40 Broad Street, the house of the outbreak's index case, was less than three feet from the side of the well. Around the drain, used solely to carry sink waters, was a badly constructed cesspool into which the effluvia of a privy in the home drained. The cesspool was clogged and overflowing into the surrounding soil that abutted the Broad Street well where York found the bricking to be substandard. "No doubt remains upon my mind that constant percolation, and for a considerable period, had been conveying fluid matter from the drains into the well," Sedgwick wrote, quoting York (Sedgwick 1911, 180).

For Sedgwick, York's examination of the well for the parish committee was the final step in a seamless investigation that began with Snow's generative thesis and mapped analysis. It was then advanced through Whitehead's discovery of the index case and ended with the confirmation bestowed by York's evidence. Snow's neighborhood study—one neither he nor his contemporaries thought definitive—was presented by Sedgwick as authoritative. Implicitly, the whole became, in Sedgwick's telling, proof of the importance of sanitary science as a discipline seeking to promote health by preventing disease through a close examination of the environment in which it might breed. York's report was so important to Sedgwick that he reprinted much of the engineer's report verbatim, reducing the font to eight-point size to fit it to the textbook page.

In addition, Sedgwick (1911, 181) redrew York's original diagrams. With his report York submitted two detailed diagrams of the house at 40 Broad Street. The first included the relation of its rooms, drains, water closet[2], and underground cellars to the nearby well and the city's sewer line. Each element in his map was carefully named to help readers to follow his argument. His second drawing focused upon the subsurface bricking separating the well from the house's cellars and drain. Unlike its predecessor, this drawing included a scale permitting readers to see for themselves the proximity of the well to the drainpipes and the cesspool.

York's text provided a careful assessment of the drain, cesspool, water table, and well structures in an attempt to describe as completely as possible the manner in which the wastes from 40 Broad Street flowed through this drain and its cesspool, and from there into the proximate bricking of the well. He needed detail that Sedgwick did not. In his retelling of the Broad Street story, Sedgwick had only to show through his illustration the general framework of the engineering details. Nobody needed to be

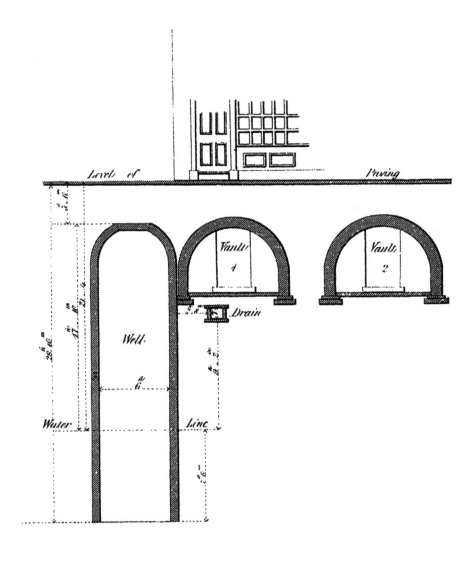

Level of   Paving

Vault
1

Vault
2

Drain

Well.

Water   Line

Scale of ⏉ 10 9 8 7 6 5 4 3 2 1 0   10   20 Feet

T. Brandt, lith 25 Rupert St

a

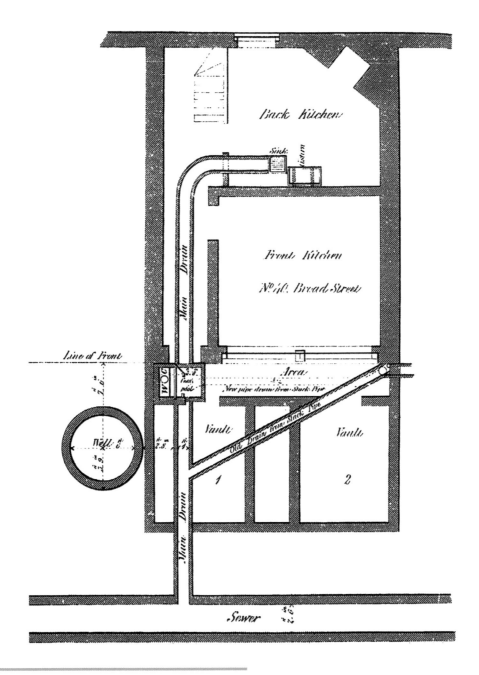

Back Kitchen

Sink

Cistern

Front Kitchen

No. 40. Broad Street

Main Drain

Line of Front

WC

Cess pool

Area

New pipe drain from Stack Pipe

Well 4'

Old Drain from Stack Pipe

Vault

1

Vault

2

Main Drain

Sewer

b

Figure 6.1a and b   Jeremiah York's 1855 illustrations of the relation between 40 Broad Street and the Broad Street pump. (Left: elevation or section view) the relation between the house at 40 Broad Street's substructure and the Broad Street well and (right: plan view) the house plan in relation to the sewer, well, and drainage infrastructure.

Source: Rare Books and Special Collections, University of British Columbia Library.

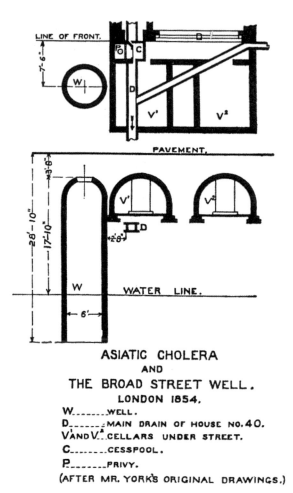

Within the figure:

LINE OF FRONT.

7'-6"

W

P O C

D

V' V²

PAVEMENT.

3'-6"

28'-10"

17'-10"

V' V²

D

2'8"

W

WATER LINE.

6'

ASIATIC CHOLERA
AND
THE BROAD STREET WELL.
LONDON 1854.

W........WELL.
D........MAIN DRAIN OF HOUSE NO. 40.
V'AND V²..CELLARS UNDER STREET.
C........CESSPOOL.
P........PRIVY.
(AFTER MR. YORK'S ORIGINAL DRAWINGS.)

Figure 6.2 Sedgwick's simplification of York's illustration of the house and sewer at 40 Broad Street.

Source: Reproduction courtesy of University of Toronto Library.

convinced in 1911 of the theory in dispute in 1855. York's two diagrams were therefore conflated into a single, simplified graphic that served to give the sense of the solidity of York's original work. In it, legibility was increased at the expense of detail critical to the original.

In precisely the same way, and for the same reasons, Sedgwick simplified Snow's 1855 map of the Broad Street epidemic. The result appears curiously denuded. Only those streets most critical to the story (Broad and Dean Streets, for example), or those most likely to be familiar to the reader (Oxford and Regent Streets), are named in this version. Otherwise, streets are anonymous and shorn of their character. On Snow's maps, the Broad Street brewery is identified generically, while on Whitehead's it is given its proper name, "Huggins' Brewery." In Sedgwick's map, however, it is just empty space without symbol or sign. The bold bars used by Snow to symbolize deaths have been transformed into dots, each still representing a single death. Nor does Sedgwick's version include the locations of those who contracted cholera in the Broad Street area but later died elsewhere, deaths included in Whitehead's but not Snow's mapped analysis.

The reasons for the changes result from the very different goals of Snow and Whitehead, the original investigators, and fifty years later, Sedgwick, the lecturer in sanitary science. The former were interested in the topography of a disease within a specific environment whose elements he believed complicit. To relate the individual cases, especially those somewhat distant, to the Broad Street pump, they needed to not only identify the young girls from Ham Yard and Angel Court, but also to name the streets they walked. The original maps suggest the synchronicity, spatial and temporal, that Snow and Whitehead unpack in their texts to show that geographically distant persons did in fact walk to and then drink from the Broad Street pump. Their readers needed to see in the map the individual routes that carried the deceased by the pump on their daily trips from home to school or work. Sedgwick required only the apparent density of cases surrounding the Broad Street pump to prove the correctness of Snow's hypothesis.

Snow's 1855 map carefully considered time as an element defining the relation of local residents to their water system. The irregular, shortest-distance polygon he drew around the Broad Street pump distilled data on proximity, measuring Snow's walking time between the pumps. In this way he sought to relate the pump's centrality in relation to cholera deaths in time within a map pertinent to the lives of those who died from cholera. His districting by time insisted upon not just "nearer and farther" but "sooner rather than later" as an element critical to his investigation.

Sedgwick's map included the irregular polygon but ignored the idea behind its creation. It is simply a "boundary of equal distances between Broad Street Pump and Other Pumps," nothing more. In his map, "all parts of the surface coexist at the same time" (Beck and Wood 1976, 215). Snow's careful measure of temporality, walking time, had become Sedgwick's of metric distance, drawing the reader to the clustered density of aggregated cholera cases clustered around a central point within a single omnipresent time frame. But then, Sedgwick did not need Snow's complex consideration because by the early twentieth century everybody knew what cholera was. What he needed was to make the case for a "sanitary science" whose focus was "public health." Sedgwick did not deal with the messy casework of epidemiology, the unraveling of the elements of people in context whose daily life patterns might affect their relation to a disease.

The question is not simply communicability, good and bad graphic presentation. Snow's and Whitehead's maps both communicated very well indeed. Nor is it simple legibility, emphasizing the data in a way that is more easily accessed by the reader. The purpose of the maps had changed in the intervening years. The 1855 maps sought to distill the range of individual deaths in relation to the domain of the pumps in a manner that considered the time and space of the lives of those who died in a consideration of their relation to local sources. The dominance of the Broad Street pump was a conclusion that only took on meaning in this context. To be a useful summation of Snow's argument, or

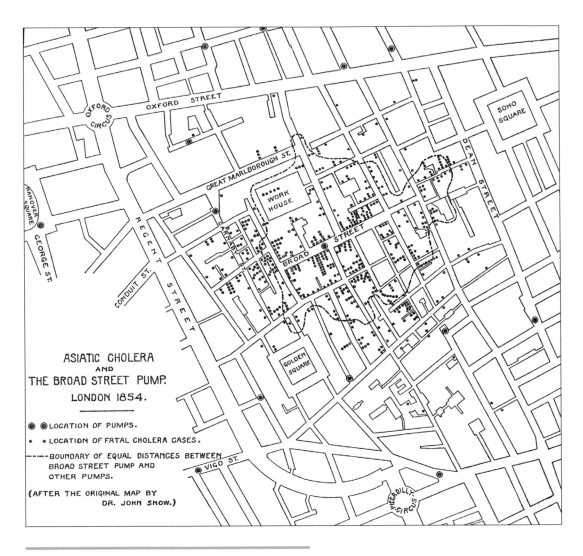

Figure 6.3 Sedgwick's 1911 adaptation of Snow's 1855 map of the Broad Street epidemic for Sedgwick's textbook on public health and sanitary science.

Source: Reproduction courtesy of University of Toronto Library.

Whitehead's, the aggregation of the cholera cases had to be done in a manner that permitted the sum of individual relations, the lives of those affected, not simply their deaths, be perceived within their maps. The complicity of the Broad Street pump was then to be deduced on the basis of not simply density of occurrence and proximity to source. As importantly, it was deduced from a deep knowledge of the life habits patterns of the people who lived and died in the study area, the children who walked to school and the men who worked at the brewer or in the workhouse.

By 1911 (and indeed by the text's first edition in 1901), however, the waterborne reality of the bacterium *Vibrio cholerae* was a given. Sedgwick, therefore, did not require Snow's complex argument but instead a symbol of Snow's sanitarian argument to serve as a teaching example in his book. The power of his appropriation lies in the now-obvious centrality of the Broad Street pump in mapped relation to a large number of deaths. It is "after the original map by Dr. John Snow" not simply historically but also both conceptually and in purpose. Unpacking its synchronicities and acknowledging its dense ecology would have detracted from the "obvious" complicity of the Broad Street pump that Sedgwick sought to argue. By eliminating street names and local landmarks, Sedgwick enforced an anonymity upon the resulting landscape that permitted his readers to see the Broad Street pump as a generic case, one whose general lesson could be anywhere applied. Snow's real triumph, Sedgwick argued, was the "boundary of equal distances" whose means of calculation Sedgwick left unstated.

Thiessen polygons—Voronoi network

Snow's cholera area defined by walking time is the source of the erroneous but entrenched myth of Snow as the originator of Thiessen polygon analysis, creating interlocking, regular polygons in a Voronoi network based on a "nearest neighbor" analysis using simple Euclidian distance (McLeod 2000). But Snow neither drew a polygon network nor used one to calculate relative rates of death for the thirteen pumps in his study area. He drew a single irregular polygon based on the time required to walk in the area from a pump to adjacent homes.

What Snow contributed was, perhaps, the idea of districts based on a calculation of proximity. Whitehead suggested another innovative solution by imposing a single compass-drawn circle around all cases in an attempt to define a general cholera area. His goal was very different from Snow's effort to identify the densest cluster of deaths based on proximity to one or more pumps. That the epicenter of Whitehead's circle was near the Broad Street pump would later provide medical cartographers with an example of centrality as a critical measure (spatial mean, for example) of spatial phenomenon, and of a simple buffer analysis, too.

The myth that Snow discovered polygon analysis likely began with Sedgwick's map. In the denuded landscape it is easy to assume that Snow may in fact have continued the exercise, measuring deaths across the mapped environment for all the pumps, quantifying on his map deaths by distance for every pump and well. The potential of polygon analysis promised in Sedgwick's map was later advanced in, for example, the 1980s when Cliff and Haggett (1988, 53–55) used Snow's data to demonstrate how a Voronoi network of Thiessen polygons might be created (figure 2a).

The modern result was a series of regular polygons based on Euclidian distance, not walking time, within which a sum of "nearest neighbor" deaths were easily calculated. Every death was assigned to the single pump to which it is nearest. The result is an analytic procedure in which the relation between range and domain is assumed to be based on a single variable, in this case Euclidian distance.

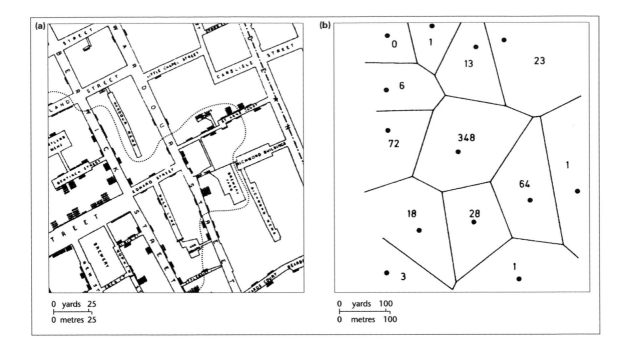

Figure 6.4a and b Two views of polygons: Cliff and Haggett (1988, 54) used Snow's cholera map (a) as a tool to describe districting using a Voronoi network of Thiessen polygons (b). Numbers in individual polygons represent deaths occurring within each (b). In his 1855 map, (a) Snow used an irregular distance measure to create a single boundary around the Broad Street pump.

Source: 6.4a. Snow, 1855. 6.4b. Cliff and Haggett, 1988.

No other distinction between members of either class is permitted by this approach. Lost is the eccentricity of the street network that might make this or that location practically more proximate to one pump than another. Nor can the approach capture the real-life eccentricities that Snow's map and text carefully considered: the brewery worker or workhouse employee whose occupation or residence removes them from the neighborhood set despite proximity or the spatially distant person whose school or work brings them closer.

The modern turn

The next appropriation of the 1855 maps and their data occurred in the 1950s during a period of extraordinary medical advance. During World War II, the introduction of penicillin and sulfa drugs had led to a general acceptance of antibiotics that promised treatment for a host of common and previously serious infectious diseases. After the poliomyelitis pandemic of 1951–1953 a vaccine was introduced that promised an end to one of the more terrifying diseases then known. A host of new

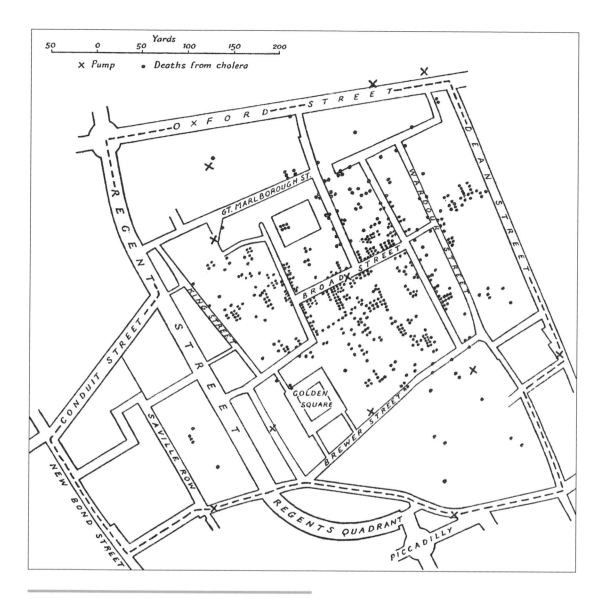

Figure 6.5 Gilbert's appropriation of Snow's 1855 map of cholera, *Geographical Journal,* 1958. Later, many mistakenly assumed it was Snow's original and not Gilbert's appropriation.

Source: Blackwell Publishing.

surgical approaches were announced, and new diagnostics were being introduced on what seemed like a monthly basis. It was a "medical age" in which, by the end of the 1960s, officials would proudly, if erroneously, proclaim that infectious, epidemic diseases had been conquered by western science.

It was in this context that in 1958 E.W. Gilbert published an influential review of "pioneers maps of health and disease." Its explicit goal was to inform the then "lively interest in medical geography," (discussed here more fully in chapter 9) through consideration of its modern antecedents. Gilbert's article presented a small set of nineteenth-century maps purporting to describe the incidence or diffusion of various diseases in England. Not surprisingly, perhaps, the first was "Dr. John Snow's map (1855) of deaths from cholera in the Broad Street area of London in September 1854." Gilbert described Snow as the man "largely responsible for demonstrating the waterborne origin of cholera" and offered Snow's map as a model of its kind. The map Gilbert presented as Dr. John Snow's bore little resemblance to the original, however. It was not even Sedgwick's.

In this version, two pumps located above Oxford Street in both Snow's and Sedgwick's maps are eliminated. So, too, is the Hanover Square pump Snow included in the 1855 but not the 1854 map. Similarly absent is the 1855 map's irregular polygon, its signal contribution. The street system is not only largely anonymous but severely restricted. Over half the streets named by Snow and mapped anonymously by Sedgwick are in this version wholly absent, off the map entirely. Of those retained, only a few are named, including, this time, the famous clothier's street, Seville Row. Cholera deaths are again presented with dots rather than bars, but in this version the pumps are presented as small x's rather than larger dots within circles. All in all, the ecology is denuded of myriad elements that made the original richly useful and informative.

Following Sedgwick, Gilbert "up-dated" Snow by converting the latter's idiosyncratic Victorian argument into a standard 1950s-style dot map. It continued the process of simplification begun by Sedgwick. By removing all secondary streets within the cholera area identified by Snow and Whitehead, and by symbolizing the pumps as less distinct x's, everything is focused on Broad Street and the swarm of cholera deaths that now seem to be attracted to it. Where the originals maps were dense and complex, artifacts of detailed studies, Gilbert's self-consciously assigns a single, very legible correlation to Snow: many deaths, one pump, and therefore one source for the outbreak. Everything in the original maps that did not contribute to this goal was removed.

Clearly, Gilbert was not interested in the complex ecological portrait that John Snow crafted in his effort to make sense of the 1854 outbreak. Nor was he involved in the details by which a localized disease outbreak could be investigated, something that had captured Sedgwick. By the mid-1950s, these had become as generally accepted, as taken for granted as the bacteriology that in 1883 identified *Vibrio cholerae*. Nor was Gilbert interested in issues of public health, sanitation, or epidemiology. He appropriated Snow's map to serve the then-evolving myth of Snow the mapmaker, the man who "discovered" the cause of cholera through mapping a simple covariance. In this he followed Sedgwick's lead but without the latter's interest in public health or sanitation. In Gilbert's hands, the focus becomes John Snow as a self-conscious and analytic mapmaker, not a mapper graphically distilling data to present a specific argument.

In 1964, Gilbert's map became the basis for a new Dr. John Snow map. Created by L. D. Stamp for a text on medical geography, the book briefly described Snow's "major breakthrough in the battle against cholera" in 1848. Alas, Stamp got the year wrong. In his map, Stamp changed the symbol for the pumps from x's to parking lot symbols, black circles around a white capital P to emphasize their prominence. "Notice the affected pump in Broad Street," Stamp's caption says. "The handle of this pump was removed at Snow's request and incidence of new cases ceased almost miraculously" (Stamp 1964, 16), his text insists, a myth as much as the map Stamp creates after Gilbert. Snow himself wrote

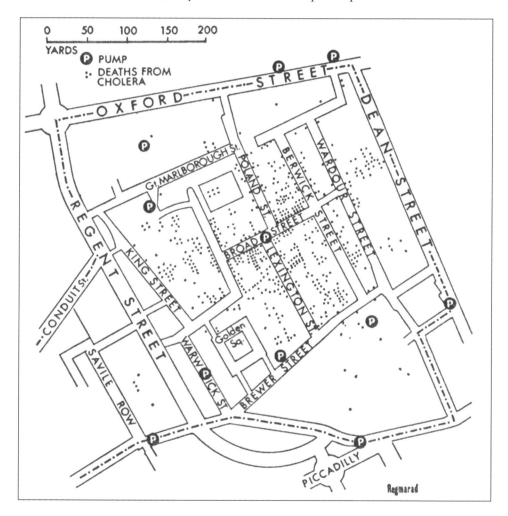

Figure 6.6 Stamp's version of "Snow's map of cholera deaths in the Soho district of London, 1848. Notice the affected pump in Broad Street" (Stamp 1964, 16).

Source: By permission of Oxford University Press.

that the decrease in deaths after the pump handle was locked was likely a result of the natural waning of the epidemic rather than solely the closure of the pump itself.

It is at this point that the distinction between "mapping" and "mapmaking" (Wood 1993b) becomes critical. John Snow mapped elements pertinent to the cholera outbreak in Soho in an attempt to advance an argument about the nature of the disease through an investigation of the Soho outbreak. The map was not a stand-alone analytic tool but one simultaneously locating and distilling a wealth of data discussed in his monograph, papers, and report. Gilbert the mapmaker created a graphic, a map designed to show a clear correspondence between the incidence of a disease outbreak and a single source of contagion. He eliminated the elements of Snow's map that did not contribute to this goal, in the process transforming Snow's complex investigation into what Roland Barthes (1983) called a "simple signification."

The progressive abstraction of Snow's and Whitehead's working maps results in an impoverished domain (fewer streets without identifying landmarks like the brewery) that makes of the original a generic statement. The result is a "signification," an abstraction that transforms the map's signified elements. The general process, one in which the supposedly simple, iconic representation is shown to be a general symbolic argument, is summarized in the accompanying illustration.

The level 1 signifier is the set of individual marks by which the topography of the outbreak is signified, the deaths and the pumps located within the named street environment that are the "Broad Street map." At level 2 this becomes the sign, a true representation of x, that at level 3 is transformed into a new signified (Snow's argument) at another level as the raw material by which objects or words (the topography) are further transformed into a general statement (it's the water pump!). The end result is a general myth at level 4. In this way, the mapping of deaths and pumps in the Broad Street area becomes a representation of the topography of a cholera outbreak (level 2) and then a general statement of the relation between deaths and water source in disease (level 3). Here it becomes both a general statement of the relation between disease source and incidence (signifier) and of the way that relationship is revealed (signified). The resulting "myth" at level 4 is that the map itself was the

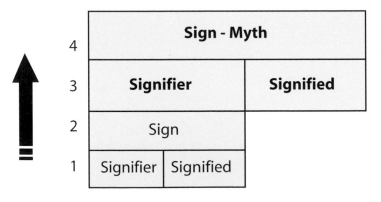

Figure 6.7 The process by which signs are generated and myth created, based on the work of Roland Barthes (1983), based on the work of Roland Barthes (1983) and applied by T. Koch (1990).

Cartographies of Disease

critical problem solver and that mapmakers ("pioneers of medical geography") were the heroes of this breakthrough in medical science.

In the progression from the specific to the general, the map's synchronicity becomes assumed; the potential for individual case consideration is replaced by the anonymity and conformity of all cases. This process, begun in Sedgwick's map and text, is continued in Gilbert's through the truncation of the street network to emphasize the density of the "cluster" of deaths now "obviously" centered on the Broad Street pump. Removed in the process is the very specificity the level 1 signifiers gave the original maps. Gone with them is the map's real utility to the original researchers.

The myth that evolves at level 4 is that, "maps reveal disease sources," and more generally, that "maps serve medicine;" or more precisely, "medical science." Gilbert crafted a myth precisely as Roland Barthes defines it, a "kind of speech better defined by its intention than its literal sense" (Barthes 1972, 105). The resulting image exemplifies the "naturalization of the cultural" (Barthes 1972, 104) in support of a system of values that, in this case, revolves around the potential of medical mapping both practically, at level 2, and generally at level 4. The whole represents not a lie but an "inflection," (Barthes 1982, 116), an emphasis in service of a view of maps as scientific tools. In the process, the myth becomes not Sedgwick's view of Snow as the prototypic sanitarian and public health researcher but instead Gilbert's creation of Snow as the man who single handedly introduced analytic mapping to nineteenth-century medical research while solving the problem of cholera. How do we know this? We have Snow's iconic map *à la* Gilbert as evidence.

The Tufte contribution

Gilbert's map took on a life of its own. In the 1970s, it was reproduced as "the famous dot map of Dr. John Snow" in Edward R. Tufte's influential *The Visual Display of Quantitative Information.* Tufte presented Gilbert's version as Snow's work, praising it as "an early and most worthy use of a map to chart patterns of disease" (Tufte 1983, 24). Snow did not "chart" the patterns of disease in his map. That implies a rigor and completeness Snow's map did not present and Snow did not claim. Because there were pockets of cholera distant from the pump and areas near Broad Street that were cholera-free (the brewery and the workhouse), Snow was careful not to assert that his map offered conclusive proof of his theory or a complete description of the generative elements of disease on which conclusions resulting from a simple relation or equivalence be drawn. Indeed, for Snow himself the Broad Street area study was not definitive. The apparent complicity of the Broad Street pump was sufficient, he believed, only to argue its centrality in this outbreak and to suggest the relation between water source and cholera generally. That was one reason why Snow undertook the larger, more complex South London study.

The niceties of Snow's cautions were lost on Tufte, however, who argued that Gilbert's 1958 map (he apparently did not see the original) was Snow's, and that it represented an extraordinary technical advance in analytic mapping, a historically unique presentation and consideration of epidemiological data on a two-dimensional plane. Tufte's interest and expertise lay neither in medicine nor medical history but in the "visual display of quantitative information."

From that perspective, Gilbert's simplification based on Sedgwick's appropriation served better than did Snow's original. It permitted Tufte to talk about Snow not as a mapper but as a map*maker* who created a dot map to "chart" the disease to reveal a simple correlation between cholera and water, and between the cholera deaths in Soho and the Broad Street pump. Lost in this process was Snow the "map thinker" (Brody et al. 2000) considering a problem—the nature of cholera and its means of diffusion—whose solution was, at the time of mapping, hotly contested. What Tufte gained was a simple argument represented by a simple icon. Lost were the complicated reality Snow considered, and, ironically, the means by which he sought to consider it. Communicability came at the cost of the very elements of mapping that made the original maps so useful.

In 1997, Tufte returned to Snow's work in a new book, *Visual Explanations.* There he included Snow's 1854 map rather than simply Gilbert's appropriation of it. Unlike his earlier text, in the more recent work Tufte quoted extensively from Snow's own writing, especially the St. James Parish Committee report. In this newer analysis, he gives Snow's thinking about the Broad Street outbreak far fuller consideration. Unfortunately, Tufte does not consider the concerns of Snow's contemporary critics, nor Cooper's and Whitehead's maps. Nor does he consider Snow's own cautions about conclusions drawn from the Broad Street map or, alas, the South London map published in 1855. The myth is intact and he can safely discuss the "saintly" Dr. Snow as pioneer forefather of epidemiology and medical cartography. Tufte does not, of course, mention the limits of his own, earlier work. Nor does he consider the broader historical context of Snow's work, thus missing the reasons why Snow's contemporaries saw Snow's work not as groundbreaking but, more commonly, as cranky and unscientific.

The Monmonier contribution

Tufte's 1983 book, *Visual Display of Communication,* became a standard, and his appropriation of Gilbert's simplification of Sedgwick's interpretation of Snow's work became the standard referent. Indeed, the default assumption among many researchers, especially medical geographers, became that the Gilbert-Tufte appropriation was Snow's map. Since Tufte, other authors have felt free to modify the Gilbert-Tufte icon for their own purpose and call it "Dr. Snow's." In *How to Lie with Maps*, for example, Mark Monmonier (1996) uses the Tufte-Gilbert-Sedgwick map to create his own "reconstruction" of "Snow's Dot Map."

In this map, symbols, especially for the pumps, are once again modified. Monmonier's new symbols are based on Gilbert's map and yet another appropriation (Monmonier 2005), a version of the Broad Street map published in 1964 by Lawrence Dudley Stamp (1964, 15). The vastly enlarged circles become the significant range upon a now-uniform, attenuated street network. Variation in width between primary and secondary streets, pronounced in Snow's map and Sedgwick's appropriation, here virtually dissappears. The deaths from cholera become the general domain that is joined to the diminished set of eleven pumps (compared to the 1855 map's fourteen pumps) represented by grossly oversized symbols. What is signified becomes "Snow discovered the pump that caused the outbreak," not Gilbert's "Snow mapped a correlation between deaths and water sources" or Sedgwick's "Snow discovered through mapping that cholera is waterborne."

The result is no longer that maps serve medicine, but that maps reveal disease sources. The enlarged circles representing the smaller set of pumps makes this clear. All one needed, the Monmonier map

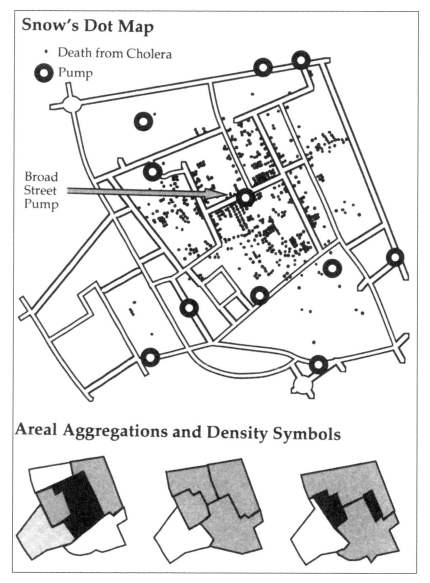

Figure 6.8 Monmonier's version of the Tufte-Gilbert map version of Snow's. From *How to Lie with Maps,* 2nd ed. (1996, 158).

Source: University of Chicago Press.

says, is data relevant to a simple proposition equating water source to deaths, a proposition that necessarily returns a single pump as the obvious culprit. With the message secured (maps serve medicine) and the potential of mapping for epidemiology encoded (maps reveal disease sources) not only the original map but also the Snow myth and the map icon itself could be dispensed with.[3]

Indeed, from the start, for Monmonier (1996, 158–159), Snow's map was a vehicle to introduce issues of data aggregation and the various results different approaches to aggregation achieve. To that end he added a second illustration below "Snow's Dot Map" in which the whole becomes an example of the dangers of aggregation. But Snow neither aggregated his data nor collected data from an outbreak where aggregation would serve the analysis. Monmonier's point is irrelevant to Snow's argument about the single-source neighborhood outbreak he considered using a topographic approach to analyze graphically the data he collected. For Monmonier, the map, however, is just propaganda, "and copycat propaganda at that," (Monmonier 2002, 155).

Thus in 1997, Monmonier dismissed Snow as largely irrelevant to contemporary epidemiology and public health. "Real epidemiology isn't like that, at least not in late-twentieth-century America. Cholera is rare, if not extinct, and contagious diseases like pneumonia and influenza are less troublesome than heart disease, cancer, stroke, and numerous degenerative ailments once ascribed to old age" (Monmonier 1997, 263). But heart disease, cancer, influenza, and stroke are mapped today by epidemiologists attempting to define clusters and to determine causal patterns in a manner similar to the one Snow pioneered (U.S. Department of Health and Human Resources 1997). Nor is cholera any more extinct or benign than pneumonia and influenza. At the time of Monmonier's writing in the 1990s, the world was in the midst of yet another international cholera pandemic that began in 1961 and by the early-to-mid 1990s was spreading through the Americas (CDC 2000a). The Pan American Health Organization (PAHO) reported 391,751 cases in the Americas in 1991, and in 1995, 85,805 cases (Arbona and Crum 1996). As the CDC wrote in an editorial note on a 2003–2004 cholera outbreak in Zambia attributed to raw vegetables "Cholera, which is still propogated by many of the same vehicles described by John Snow in the mid-1800s, remains a public health threat in sub-Saharan African and certain Asian countries" (CDC 2004, 2077–2078).

As importantly, through the 1990s the U.S. Centers for Disease Control (CDC), the World Health Organization (WHO), and PAHO *all* presented data, often in map form, on epidemics and pandemics of AIDS, cholera, flu (influenza), hepatitis, and the West Nile virus, to name only several diseases. Data for these and more localized outbreaks of specific diseases (meningitis and salmonella, for example) were and are frequently mapped by international, national, regional, and local health organizations concerned with precisely the type of disease investigation that John Snow pioneered in the 1850s.

U.S. Centers for Disease Control

It is because mapping remains a critical tool in modern epidemiology that in 2000 the U.S. CDC began distributing a mapping program, Epi Map, with its epidemiology software, Epi Info™ 2000 (CDC 2000b). First distributed in 1985, Epi Info is a series of freely distributed programs "for use by public health professionals in conducting outbreak investigating, managing databases for public health surveillance and other tasks, and general database and statistics" (CDC 2000b, 7). Originally DOS-based, in 2000 the program switched to a Microsoft® Windows® format that facilitated the inclusion of its mapping program as one more aide to statistical visualization and analysis. "Thus one can produce a map similar to John Snow's original map of cholera cases and pump locations in London" (CDC 2000b, 18). Data based on Snow's 1854 study of the Soho outbreak is included as an example of mapping as a tool for epidemiology and the statistical analysis of health events.

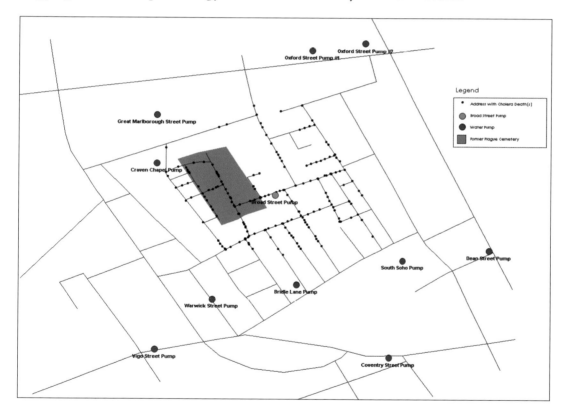

Figure 6.9 Map based on CDC's Epi Info data for the Soho cholera outbreak. A limited set of deaths are aggregated by location rather than individually displayed.

Source: Koch, based the CDC's Epi Map 2000 program settings.[4]

While touted by some (Lang 2000), the map that results from the projection of the Epi Info database bears very little resemblance to Snow's. As in Monmonier and Tufte (after Gilbert), the number of pumps is reduced to eleven. Except the location of the plague pit, which was included in Whitehead's but not Snow's map, all significant elements of the environment (brewery, workhouses, schools, etc.) are excluded. Cholera deaths are represented not individually but instead georeferenced by house location (street number and name assigned) on a severely truncated network of undifferentiated streets of uniform width.

No symbolization is employed to distinguish sites of multiple deaths at a specific street address from those where only a single death occurred. Nor does the program's manual suggest that this would be a smart thing to do. Thus, the map that results appears to present an outbreak with a total of 206 cases rather than the 456 deaths included its database. Egregiously, 122 deaths are wholly excluded from the total 578 deaths that Snow himself mapped. Those so excised occurred west of Carnaby Street, east of Berwick Street, or south of Brewer Street: deaths whose location outside the Broad Street epicenter required Snow's careful, onsite investigations to determine the relation between the deceased (students and workers) and the Broad Street pump they traveled past in their daily lives.

What results is a clear, visually precise cartographic product that fails by any standard of epidemiological accuracy. This version is all about the visual display of electronically stored health data, not the investigation of the cause of the deaths in St. James, Soho, in 1854. After Monmonier, the size of the pumps in the default settings for the CDC map is exaggerated to emphasize the range's importance and the now obvious centrality of the Broad Street pump. That centrality is further emphasized by the excision of deaths at locations nearer South Soho, Bridle Lane, and the Marlboro Street pump. Because this version advocates implicitly for mapmaking using GIS, the message changes. It is now not simply that "maps reveal disease sources" or that "maps serve medicine," but that "GIS mapping reveals disease sources" and, at another level, "GIS serves medicine." Outliers (deaths nearest to other pumps) are excluded to avoid the necessity of a case-by-case analysis that, while practically critical, is not easily persuasive graphically.

This is not an inevitable consequence of the digitization of data. Nor does it reflect any inherent limit in mapping with GIS as an analytic approach. Rather, CDC personnel involved in the project made of Snow's complex topography a simple, explicit teaching case that argued a mapped approach in the same way that Sedgwick earlier altered Snow's work to argue his sanitarian perspective. By way of contrast, consider the computer-generated map based on a version of Snow's mapped data obtained in 1998 from ESRI. Internal evidence strongly suggests the dataset was digitized from maps that appear originally prepared by Cliff and Haggett (1988).[5] Here the number of pumps is returned to the original fourteen considered by Snow, and the registry of deaths (N=578) is undiminished in a street network that includes those presented in Snow's and Whitehead's mapping.

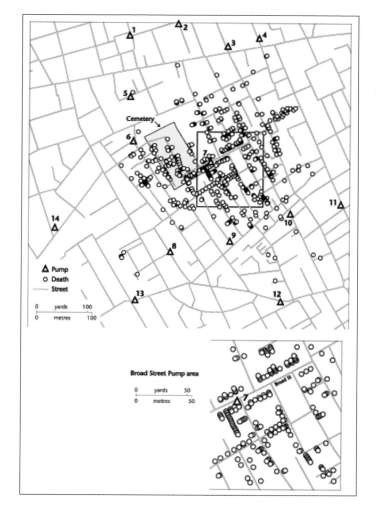

Figure 6.10 A GIS-generated map with data provided by ESRI, apparently based on Cliff and Haggett (1988).

Source: Cliff and Haggett 1988, *Atlas of Disease Distribution*, Blackwell.

Historians have in recent years found GIS technologies useful in recreating historical maps and building analytic approaches to historical events based upon those electronic recreations (Knowles 2002). It may thus seem surprising that the workplaces Snow and Whitehead investigated and mapped (brewery, schools, work house, etc.) are excluded in this dataset. In their work, Cliff and Haggett were careful to make clear they were using Snow's basic dataset to teach specific analytic techniques useful in epidemiology and the study of disease. Their selection from Snow's dataset was consistent and transparent. It self consciously adapted for pedagogic purposes elements of the Snow map and made the fact of that adaptation clear. The same is true of the ESRI adaptation of their datasets and its use both here and elsewhere by the author (Koch and Denike 2004).[6]

Discussion

Sedgwick, Gilbert, Tufte, Monmonier, Cliff and Haggett, researchers at the CDC, and cartographers at ESRI all had access to the original Snow map and the dataset that included (a) deaths from cholera occurring in the Soho area in 1854, (b) the location of public water pumps in that district in that year, and (c) the Soho-area street network. From these, all chose the data to be included in their maps and then manipulated it for their own purposes.

Each mapmaker was engaged in a different discourse; each discourse resulted in a very different map. These maps were not objective and "value-free" but reflections of the individual mapmaker's intentions. But then, data is always a matter of selection and choice. Snow chose not to include the sewer lines or plague pit thought by some to be complicit in the St. James, Soho, outbreak. Nor did he map the latter deaths included in Whitehead's map, or those of people living elsewhere who contracted the disease in the St. James, Soho, neighborhood. Cooper mapped a limited set of cholera deaths good enough to make his case to the Sewer Commission. This is, after all, what researchers do: they select from potentially important facts that material that seems to them germane. They call it data and manipulate it in the way that best seems to address a problem. When they do it right, their choices are made clearly and are transparent, available for all to consider.

In this case, the very different maps based on Snow's reflect not a limit inherent in the mapping process but instead the process by which data was defined and selected to serve this or that author's goal. For his part, Snow was interested in creating a "topography of cholera" to summarize a wealth of data potentially pertinent to an understanding of the Soho outbreak. He worked in ignorance of the bacterium that was the specific disease agent. His map was designed both as an analytic tool (the apparent density in the area closest to the Broad Street pump) and as a general distillation of his propositional and ecological arguments. It existed not apart from, but embedded within, a text that paid special attention to the topography of the neighborhood and the socioeconomic realities of its inhabitants.

Sedgwick's interest was the promotion of the then-new discipline of sanitary science within the context of public health, a goal Snow himself presumably would have applauded. He modified Snow's work to fit the needs of his textbook and its greater goal of advancing the sanitary science he taught and believed in. Gilbert's interest was not cholera (or epidemiology) but "pioneers" of medical cartography, the very idea of which served both a growing myth of Snow and of the mapmaker-as-scientist. In service of this interest, his map emphasized the correlation between the incidence of disease and its single source, thus advancing the potential of mapmaking for epidemiology, and more generally, medical science.

Tufte built upon Gilbert's treatment of Snow's work in a book about the visual display of quantitative data, and more specifically, mapped displays of that data. Monmonier furthered the adaptation in his own work, one that made discovery of a single pump a mapped inevitability. The CDC map simplified things even further to transform the myth of mapmaking as medical science into one about GIS,

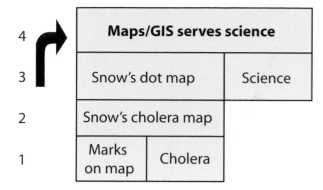

4 ↱	**Maps/GIS serves science**	
3	Snow's dot map	Science
2	Snow's cholera map	
1	Marks on map	Cholera

Figure 6.11 Koch's application of Barthes's signifier-signified sign theory. The transformation of Snow's original map into an icon by later researchers applies Roland Barthes's general perspective to this history.

Source: Koch, based on Barthes's *Myth Today*.

mapmaking, and medical science. The ESRI version did the same thing, although without insisting the result was "Dr. Snow's map," and its manipulation of the dataset was far less egregious. The result is a process of abstraction that can be again represented using Barthes's basic schematic.

The result is that "Dr. Snow's map" in its many modern forms is no longer about the 1854 cholera outbreak, or even about the topography of a disease outbreak, but about the power of GIS, graphic analysis, and the mapmaking that is presumed to result when mapmakers work in service of science. Here the general semiotic process of mythification is focused upon the Snow appropriations. At level 1, the signifier is Snow's map of the Soho outbreak, one whose indictment of the Broad Street pump signified its complicity in the outbreak. At level 2, Snow's basic epidemiology is simplified and then used as a signifier, in Sedgwick's map, to serve as a signifier of the proven methods of sanitary science and the discipline of public health. At level 3, Sedgwick's map is again modified and abstracted in a manner signifying mapping's power as a problem-solving approach to epidemics and medical issues generally. Finally, at level 4, the myth of the map becomes transformed into one that raises GIS mapping to a science in and of itself, a tool that without public health or other approaches may determine the source and cause of an outbreak of illness.

Snow's "the pump is complicit" became Sedgwick's "here is how sanitary science serves." In the hands of Gilbert and then Monmonier the lesson is that "maps serve science or medicine" until, in the CDC iteration, the message is the type of mapping (GIS) that is important: "GIS serves medical science." The whole owes at once everything and nothing to the marks Snow made on his map as part of his consideration of the 1854 cholera outbreak in this district of London.

But these appropriations are based not on Snow the map thinker but on Snow the mapmaker. The appropriations ignore the debate in which Snow was engaged, the degree and manner in which his maps served his argument. Those aspects of Snow's analysis most important to him (look at the map and see the density of deaths around the pump!) disappear with the removal of the streets and local areas in the modern versions. By 2002, Monmonier thus could dismiss the map entirely as mere "propaganda" (Monmonier 2002, 155), an assertion that ignored Snow's own writing and his careful, topographic approach.

The conclusion is unavoidable: Mapmaking is manipulation, a process dependent on authorial background, intent, and perspective. This makes it no different, however, from charting, graphing, or writing. As later chapters demonstrate, the reductionism that came from limited statistical approaches to the incidence of disease would in the 1950s be countered by a more robust ecological approach that used maps as a corrective. In the 1980s, Peter J. Gould would rail against the limits of professional epidemiology, "oblivious to where the epidemic is" in his seminal studies of the diffusion of AIDS (Gould et al. 1991, 82). We are all prisoners not simply of the techniques we use but, more importantly, of the perceptions we bring to the problem at hand.

An advantage of mapping over statistical graphs and charting is that egregious errors, like those in the CDC database, are revealed spectacularly in the map while, in numbered columns or simple charts, such errors are less easy to detect. Most spectacularly, we see in the transformation of the cholera maps based on John Snow's work not simply errors but intellectual trends that are highlighted in the graphics. There is a trend away from the topography of disease and the ecology it sought to present toward a simple correspondence and a simplified perspective. The history of not just medical cartography and geography but of epidemiology and public health reflects a constant tension between the thick ecologic perspective and more narrowly defined propositions relating a suspected disease agent and its host population. This tension easily traced into the twentieth century through the maps of later medical researchers, the arguments they sought to make, and the methods by which they tried to convince others.

Endnotes

An earlier version of this chapter, The map as intent: Variations on the theme of John Snow, was published as an article in *Cartographica* 39:4 (Koch 2004). It was enormously useful to have the opportunity to first develop these ideas in the context of a journal article before enfolding them into the larger texture of this book. The opportunities such smaller canvases provide in the writing of a larger work are not to be minimized. I am, therefore, grateful to the journal's editors as well as both journal and peer reviewers for their comments. This chapter particularly benefited from conversations with Denis Wood on the maps included.

1. That medicine had undergone a revolution, one of which early twentieth-century physicians and writers were justly proud, is clear. Microscopy had become a real tool in both epidemiology and general medicine. It identified a host of bacteria complicit in a range of diseases, including cholera,

and insights into hematology and other now-distinct medical disciplines. Lester's work on sepsis and sterile operating theaters combined with the anesthesiology that had evolved from Snow's day to make of surgery a viable alternative with an ever-declining rate of mortality. Osler had codified diagnostic principles and advanced the teaching of medical science. From our perspective, the medicine was generally ineffective, more diagnostic than curative (Thomas 1983), but from the perspective of the day its advances were touted and its benefits very real.

2. The complicity of water closets in the pollution of the city's water supply was an issue that was to occupy Snow's thinking several years later. The problem was not simply "the fact that water closets cause the pollution of the rivers" (Snow 1858) but that they required "such an inordinate quantity of water" that adequate supplies could not be obtained solely from wells and springs, necessitating the use of polluted river water.

3. Mark Monmonier (2005) took exception to an earlier article, The map as intent (Koch 2004), on which this chapter is based. Those interested can see his comments and my reponse in a 2005 issue of *Cartographica* (Koch in press).

4. Epi Map 2000 was developed by the Epidemiology Program Office of the Centers for Disease Control and Prevention (CDC) using ESRI MapObjects® 2.0 software. ESRI contributed a special, royalty-free license for distribution of Epi Map in conjunction with Epi Info that is free to all researchers (cdc. govepiinfo).

5. I have been unable to track down the mapper who developed the dataset at ESRI. The assumption that this is, in fact, based on Cliff and Haggett (1988) is based on a number of factors. First, the maps that result from this dataset look like those of Cliff and Haggett. More importantly, the street network, the number of pumps, and the number of deaths in the dataset are the same as in the Cliff and Haggett book. As importantly, the deaths are offset from the street in a manner similar to Snow's and reproduced in the Cliff and Haggett version. Also important, of course, is what the map does not include, details of the topography (the churches, workplaces, etc.) that were in Snow's and Whitehead's maps but not in the Cliff and Haggett map. The conclusion is that someone at ESRI digitized this dataset for its mid-1990s demonstration of GIS approaches to medical mapping.

6. It is perhaps appropriate to note in passing that I am currently recreating a complete, digital version of the 1854 cholera maps of Cooper, Snow, and Whitehead. A digital recreation of the South London study is also planned. A brief description of the procedures involved in transforming the original maps to digital versions is included in chapter 11.

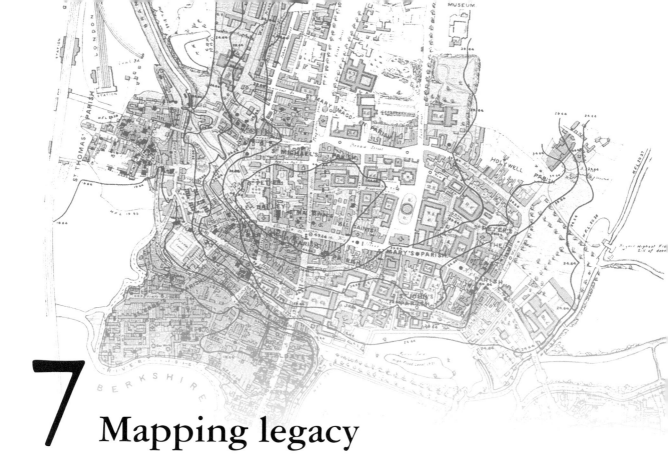

7 Mapping legacy

In retrospect, Snow's Broad Street study and his study of the South London epidemic were the Archimedean point after which nothing was ever the same. They did not convince the majority of his many contemporaries, of course. That would take years, and the clinical lessons of bacteriology. Still, when the next outbreak struck East London, William Farr was "prepared in 1865 to closely scrutinize the water supply" (Morris 1976, 210). He traced the epidemic to the East London Water Company where open ponds of water tainted by sewage were being used as an emergency reserve of water. The company protested, and in letters to newspapers a company officer named Greaves criticized Farr who, he said, had in his analysis used an "obsolete map" whose accuracy was questioned in a way that opened Farr's conclusions to doubt. "The truth about this map question," wrote the *Medical Times and Gazette* on September 8 is that "in the best recently published maps of the two reservoirs and the canal, which Mr. Greaves says are no longer used, are distinctly laid down and described as belonging to the Company; and as their existence in actuality is not denied, it seems to us puerile to quibble about their delineation on a map" (*Medical Times and Gazette* 1866, 254).

Snow showed how to consider the topography of a local outbreak to identify the epicenter. As had Whitehead and Cooper in their maps, Snow described that topography in a way that identified areas of intense disease activity and used mapping to relate that area to its epicenter, the pump, the suspected source of the outbreak. Even for those like Farr who were unconvinced by Snow's general theory of the disease, his basic methodology was, at a practical level, wholly convincing. The question was not about the utility of mapping, but rather about the accuracy of the map that Farr had used, one whose distinctions were sufficiently trivial to be dismissed, in this case, by the prestigious *Medical Times and Gazette.*

Of critical importance was not simply the use of maps but the "shoe-leather," the on-site investigations Snow and Whitehead had pioneered in their studies of the 1854 outbreak. The basic data contained in Farr's weekly *Register*, and Farr's use of it in his argument for the relation between disease and altitude above sea level, was the model for evolving protocols of statistical research based upon official records, an important advance. Snow and Whitehead expanded upon that data through interviews with the relatives of those who died from cholera. The result added depth to the mortality statistics in a way that emphasized the relation between individual case and suspected source. Snow's more general social and sanitarian concerns informed the general context in which those relations were to be understood.

Pascalis and Seaman had looked at the location of disease during outbreaks in New York City, each death an individual event related by proximity to possible sources of an outbreak. Snow collected detailed data on those afflicted in a way that permitted the mapping to detail more defined relations between the individual, the environment (schools, workplaces, water sources, etc.), and the disease itself. This led in turn to an understanding of interpersonal transmission between cohabitants of a house, and especially caregivers and the ill they nursed. In cases of multiple infections within a house, Snow was careful to note who had the disease first and who had it later, which brother or husband cared for an afflicted sister or wife and then became ill himself.

To call this the Archimedean point is to say not only that after Snow people approached the investigation of disease differently than they did before but also that, as *both* researcher and as symbol of the evolving focus of his age, Snow became the intellectual and practical standard for what, by Sedgwick's day, was the accepted process of investigation. Snow was not alone in this, however. Others also mapped the data of cholera's incidence and diffusion at local, regional, national, and international scales. In history's shorthand, Snow has come to symbolize the movement whose spirit was anticontagionist but whose most significant contribution was a way of looking at health and disease.

Seaman's and Pascalis's mapping and thinking were innovative, but their conclusions were incorrect. Snow's thinking and research was radical and spot on, defining an approach first proven experientially and later confirmed by an evolving science. No wonder Sedgwick gave it pride of place in his book. It was the model on which other maps and mapping were based.

Cholera: 1870s

The growing influence of the work of Snow and his contemporaries can be seen in the consideration of the next cholera epidemic, one that began in the 1860s and spread around the world, reaching England in the middle of the decade and the United States on February 8, 1873, when Peter Thomson, a New Orleans sailor, died of "sporadic cholera." By April 1 there had been 109 cases of cholera in the city. Soon after, cholera began to travel north along the Mississippi River. The disease rapidly diffused by steamboat and riverboat until, by June 15, it reached Cairo, Illinois, where the Mississippi and Ohio Rivers meet. From there it traveled along existing waterways and rail lines to Chicago, Indianapolis, and, in an easterly direction, Cincinnati and Pittsburgh. By that winter, when the epidemic subsided, it had affected eighteen states.

In 1874, the U. S. Congress directed the Secretary of War to assign an army medical officer to investigate and report upon the epidemic under the general supervision of the surgeon general of the U.S. Army. The resulting 1,061-page report, *The Cholera Epidemic of 1873 in the United States,* was replete with a series of maps that considered both the history of cholera's repeated international diffusion in various epidemics beginning in the 1830s, and in another set, its then-current spread in the United States. Technically its author was Dr. John M. Woodworth, the U.S. Surgeon General, who contributed a twenty-eight-page introduction.[1] The real author, however, the one who did the work,

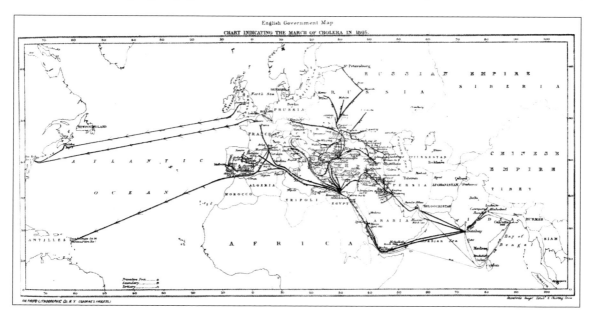

Figure 7.1 A British map of the international diffusion of cholera beginning in 1865 included in the U.S. Congressional report by J. M. Woodworth, 1875.

Source: Rare Books and Special Collections, University of British Columbia Library. Woodworth (1875).

was army physician Ely McClellan. It is his name that is attached to many of the report's maps, which were drawn to his specification. It was McClellan, with his colleague, Dr. John C. Peters, who wrote to medical personnel in every town and state visited by the epidemic to ask for information on its local effect. He then correlated and annotated these reports in a 705-page narrative that remains today one of the most complete studies of a single epidemic, its incidence and pattern of diffusion, ever produced.

In a detailed introductory chapter McClellan made clear the driving intellectual perspective of his report, the manner in which he would understand the reports of local medical personnel in affected U.S. cities that made up the body of his research. He began with the assertion "that cholera is a portable disease is at the present day denied but by few observers; even among those who reject the contagiousness of the disease this fact is recognized" (Woodworth 1875, 54). McClellan based his statement on the authority of "the meeting of the International Sanitary Conference of 1874" where it was "unanimous affirmed [sic.] 'that the Asiatic cholera, susceptible of epidemic extension, is not developed spontaneously, except in India, and when it appears in other countries it is invariably by introduction from without" (Woodworth 1875, 54). Furthermore, he argued, cholera's "pestilential march" in the United States "has invariably been preceded by the arrival of a vessel infected with cholera-sick or laden with emigrants and their property from infected districts."

To support this conclusion, McClellan included maps collected at the Vienna conference. These detailed the diffusion of cholera internationally, including one of "the progress of the Asiatic cholera during the years 1845, 1846, and 1847" prepared for the conference by a French physician. Other maps McClellan used to develop his thesis described the regional progress of the disease in the Middle East, and in India where the disease was endemic. The British "chart indicating the march of cholera in 1865" actually maps the pandemic's diffusion from 1865 into the 1870s.[2] From the pandemic's origin in India, it moves first by sea trade routes and then over land into Africa, the Middle East, Europe, and finally to Britain, from which it travels to Canada and the United States.

The map is not as simply descriptive as it appears at first glance. In fact, it is relatively dense, joining the range of cholera incidence, country by country, to the domain of established international travel routes—overland and by sea. The assumption of its Indian origin and the coincidence of diffusion routes with the more general map of maritime trade routes surely familiar to every educated person of that time are clear. It thus emphasized the international conference's conclusion that cholera originated in India and in every epidemic wave—including the one that struck the United States in 1873—was carried by sailing ship or land-based caravan country to country and, in those afflicted, city to city.

The authority of the conference cannot be overestimated. In 1874, a conference bringing together the world's leading authorities on a medical topic was not a commonplace event. Transatlantic travel was still a major undertaking, time consuming and expensive, and for a medical officer of the United

States Army it must have been a heady affair. The conference permitted McClellan to argue from the start an international consensus on certain "propositions," for example that "it was unanimously affirmed" by delegates that "cholera can be transmitted by personal effects coming from an infected place, especially such as have served for the sick from cholera; and certain facts show that the disease can be carried to a distance by these effects" (Woodworth 1875, 47).

"In this manner a sure transmissibility of the cholera infection is effected, and that a distinct outbreak of the disease may occur by such means at great distances from the seat of original infection" (Woodworth 1875, 47). The proposition that persons contracting cholera "have been exposed to excremental pollution, excremental sodden earth, excrement-reeking air, or excrement-tainted water" was one advanced, McClellan said, at the international conference by the Registrar—General of Great Britain himself. In short, McClellan argued that whether cholera was in the air, the earth, or the water (or all three) it was a "poison," precise nature unknown, whose progress could be traced by considering the traces of disease over time.

Having established an international and expert consensus that a global pattern of diffusion was operative at every scale, McClellan identified two principal vectors in the United States, the railroads and the steamboats. In this manner he argued not simply a method of diffusion but also of cholera's introduction. It entered the United States at the ports and then traveled with other foreign goods across the nation. In the case of the 1873 epidemic, the first cases reported were in New Orleans, from which, McClellan argued, it traveled north on railcars and riverboats.

"During the month of May, in that year, the disease was first brought northward along the line of the Mississippi River by infected boats, and during the ensuing months their agency was felt upon the Arkansas and Ohio Rivers as well as streams of lesser magnitude. Nor was it in conveying the disease from the seat of original infection that their agency was evinced, for we find that the line of infection was turned, and that they conveyed the disease upon return trips to re-enforce the epidemic at the original point of departure" (Woodworth 1875, 52). Importantly, he argued this was not only true of the then-recent epidemic but was also true in the first cholera epidemic, which occurred in the 1830s.

This argument was informed by McClellan's map of the Eastern United States, including the Mississippi, on which the "cholera route, epidemic of 1832" was mapped. On the east coast, cholera entered the ports of New York City and Charleston on English sailing ships. From New York it traveled up the Hudson River and then over land by rail through the Great Lakes as far as Lake Michigan. From Charleston it traveled down the coast to New Orleans—another line of diffusion is from the Caribbean—and from there traveled northward by riverboat and by rail into the minimally developed hinterland of 1830s America. This same pattern of diffusion was repeated in the 1870s, McClellan would insist. But between the 1830s and 1860s, both rail and river transportation systems had matured, providing a more robust vector for the transportation of disease.

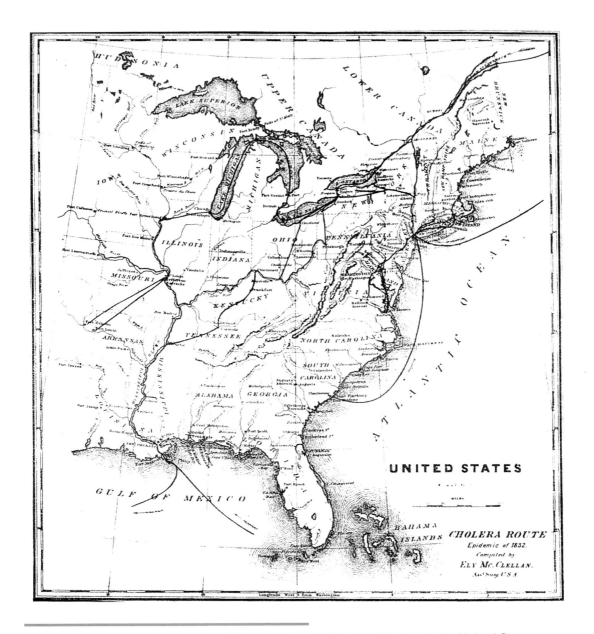

Figure 7.2 McClellan's 1875 map of the route of the cholera epidemic in the United States in 1832.

Source: Rare Books and Special Collections, University of British Columbia Library.

Sanitarian concerns

The argument that cholera traveled between countries along trade routes, or that wells were often complicit in local outbreaks, was not an endorsement of a modern, germ-theory explanation of this pandemic. Indeed, the general theory of cholera generation remained principally contagionist, one Pascalis and Seaman would have understood. The International Conference on cholera accepted the general proposition that "the surrounding air is the principal vehicle of the generative agent of cholera; but the transmission of the malady by the atmosphere, in the immense majority of cases, is restricted to the close vicinity of the focus of emission. As to facts asserted of transportation to a distance of one or many miles, they are not conclusive" (Christie 1876, 476).

The assumption was that "in free air the generative principle of cholera rapidly loses its morbific activity, but that in certain conditions of confinement this action may be preserved during an undetermined time." Miasmatic cholera traveled the world, in other words, but it did so through close contact within the stuffy confines of close quarters. These were precisely the conditions that could be found on railcars and in riverboats. In the first, the "fetid air" trapped in an enclosed space that promoted disease was most notable in the cars of second-class passengers in which open toilets, the "commode de salon," that opened directly onto the train tracks from which the "poisonous dejection falls below the car" (Woodworth 1875, 50).

Here the old distinction between "exhalation" and "contagion" was returned in a new model that owed much to the evolving botany of the day. In the 1850s, Mühry (1856) had argued a theory in which disease-generating miasmas were to be understood as "microscopically small, germinating organisms, most likely fungi and dust-like fungal spores, each with its own toxic properties" (Rupke 2000, 92). Like most plants, these were distributed in the air and the soil. Contagia, a related form of plant-like life, lived in the human body and could be passed between bodies irrespective of local climatic conditions. Science was coming together, miasmatic theories edging toward what would become, with Pasteur and Koch, bacteriology.

These ideas were implicit in McClellan's work where he distinguished in a more practical fashion between the sanitary conditions of the poorer passengers traveling in cramped riverboat quarters who had only the use of a "close and wet closet" from which most necessarily returned "with soiled clothing to the pile of freight" whose space they shared onboard. That soiling, McClellan believed, carried minute elements of excrement that attached to the freight on which passengers rested, and when they vomited, their "involuntary dejections" increased the potential contamination among fellow travelers by infecting cargo bundles that would later be handled by dock hands in individual ports (Woodworth 1875). McClellan thus grafted onto the generally miasmatic, contagionist argument, another based on individual contact with the contaminated discharges of the afflicted.

The point was sufficiently important to McClellan to be emphasized by a pen-and-ink drawing of second-class passengers lying among the cargo bales and bundles that, with them, were also conveyed up and down the river. The people appear if not generally ill then at least enervated, lying dead or asleep with only a woman and a sleeping child in a full sitting position. Walking past them toward the animal pens at the back of the picture is a man with a bucket, probably water, a man whose hat and coat and upright posture suggest a deckhand. The impression is one of malaise, the purpose clearly editorial. This is what it is like for the poorer passengers, the illustration says; this is where the disease is transmitted, not just in the air but also from person to person, person to cargo, and cargo to us all.

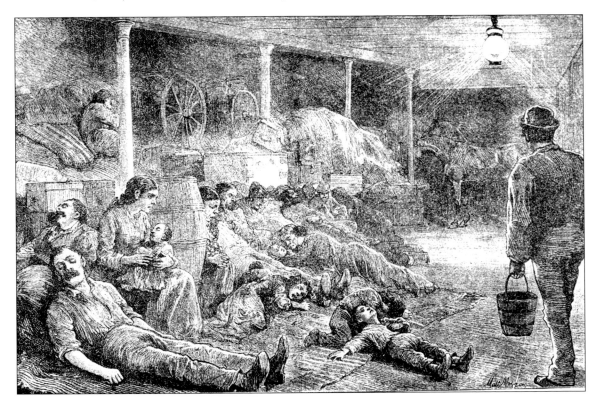

Figure 7.3 An illustration of second-class passengers on Mississippi riverboats used by McClellan in his report on the cholera epidemic of the 1870s to show the inferior conditions.

Source: Rare Books and Special Collections, University of British Columbia Library.

In this way, McClellan transposed the broader sanitary arguments of the city, and the conditions of the poor, to the microcosm of the riverboat and, by extension, to railcars. His introduction foreshadowed a more general urban argument advanced by his coauthors in their reports on epidemic outbreaks in various Mississippi River cities. Time and again, medical officers in cities like Memphis and Nashville noted the disease's greater incidence among the poor than the rich, the early and fierce incidence of cholera occurring among prisoners working on the railroad. In each case various investigators pointed to a lack of urban sanitary infrastructure as a contributor to the severity of local outbreaks.

McClellan: Case studies

McClellan's mapping of the international pandemic in its varying years, and his general analysis of its modes of diffusion in the United States historically, were the context within which he framed the reports of local health officers in cities where cholera struck. The task required diplomacy. His was a federal study in a nation that distrusted federal intrusion, especially in areas such as those dealing with health where responsibility was assumed to rest at the scale of state and local governments. McClellan's respondents were local physicians and members of local or regional health boards who were sometimes chary of admitting to the deficits of the cities that were their charge. And, of course, there were many who did not yet buy the conclusions of the international conference, who wished to believe cholera was local and solely miasmatic, not international and interpersonally communicable.

New Orleans

The New Orleans report by Dr. C. R. White, president of the Louisiana Board of Health, for example, insisted that most physicians in his area "warrant the belief that it was not Asiatic cholera" that struck their state but only an unusually severe occurrence of endemic diarrhea, also called cholera. "The prevalence of cholera at the same period of 1873 may be viewed as the natural tendency of that portion of the year, exaggerated into serious, and deadly, and somewhat general disease, by the presence of local poison, engendered by filth and magnified by unusual meteorological conditions" (Woodworth 1875, 101). In short, summer heat and rains combined with local filth to create the "furry miasmata" of endemic summer diarrhea that, in 1874, was unusual in its intensity but normal in its occurrence.

Within the miasmatic theory of the day, a kind of regional chauvinism pervaded in medicine. It stood to reason that if local airs were important to disease, then local practitioners would be the ones who would know what affected their patients. There was, as well, a southern defensiveness against northern intrusion in this assumption, one that seems to pervade Dr. White's report. "'As surely as there is a distinction between foreign and American medicine,' declared a New Orleans practitioner in the mid-1850s, 'so surely is there a distinction between Northern and Southern medicine'" (Numbers 2000, 219). In as political a manner as possible, McClellan complimented the "admirable and exhaustive report of Dr. White," and then rejected out of hand "the theory that the cholera epidemic of 1873 originated *de novo* at New Orleans." He made his case on the back of White's own data, detailing a two-step process that remains today a model of basic epidemiological thinking.

He first located on a map of the city the cases that White identified, numbering them sequentially on the basis of chronology. McClellan then identified a relation between each case and the harbor itself.

The index case was Peter Thompson, who "died of cholera upon the 9th day of February, after unloading a Liverpool ship" while case five, Edward Nelson, "the husband of case 4, died of a disease similar to that of the wife the previous day; and that at the time of his attack he was working on the steamboat levee" (Woodworth 1875, 105). In several cases McClellan found links to the levee that White and his colleagues had ignored or overlooked. For example, White's study reported that Robert Banks, the sixth case, was "not connected with the shipping" but in fact, McClellan noted, "at the time of his report he was working on the steamboat levee" (Woodworth 1875, 105).

After plotting the location of the homes of these first deaths, McClellan then drew lines connecting the homes of the deceased to the steamboat levee where they worked, numbering the vectors based on the date of diagnosis. The result was what today are sometimes called "spiders," lines of incidence that,

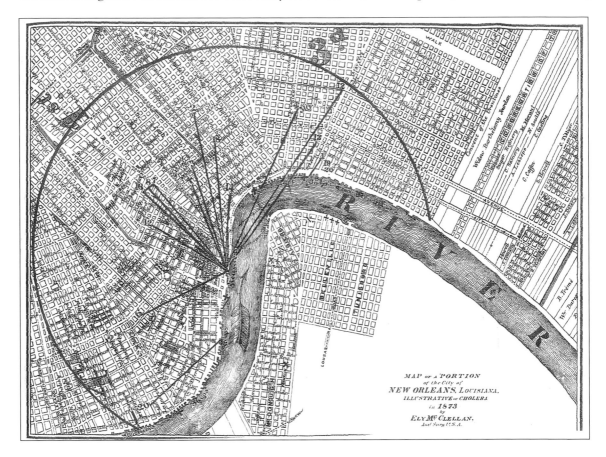

Figure 7.4a   McClellan's map of the New Orleans cholera outbreak in 1873.

Source: Rare Books and Special Collections, University of British Columbia Library.

in this case, all converge at or near the steamship levee or, in one case, the docks at which international sailing ships berthed. In this way, McClellan politely rebutted White's argument for the *de novo* nature of the epidemic. They may live here, and here, and here, McClellan's map said, but they all worked on the levee where the disease was introduced by ship. In this way, he unpacked the map's synchronicity (Beck and Wood 1976) by emphasizing the home-work axis that exposed those affected to the cholera they then carried, at the end of the work day, home to their loved ones and their neighbors.

On the map, McClellan darkened the city blocks on which the homes of cholera victims were located. Some are buried under the spiders, others stand beside them. Where cholera victims lived elsewhere, places where either another line would be illegible or a blackened city square would be hard to read, he marked the house with an x. That most of these homes were on or near the river, or clearly vectored from it (see the x vector from Rampart Street to the levee) added weight to the map's argument.

McClellan then drew a semicircle centered on the steamship levee to define a "cholera area" of greatest incidence. The semicircle served three functions. First, it defined an area of greatest intensity to refute Dr. White's insistence upon a generalized, diffuse diarrhea outbreak of miasmatic origin. Secondly, it localized disease occurrence within the area centered on the steamship levee. Finally, the semicircle served as a signature technique, one common to the work of German geographer Alexander von Humboldt, McClellan would introduce into other maps of cholera in other cities, creating a graphic consistency that argued implicitly that this was the model, one drawn at the epicenter not only of cholera in New Orleans, but across the U.S. epidemic itself.

"Upon the accompanying map a circle has been described, the center of which rests upon the riverfront of Canal streets. The diameter of this circle is long enough to include the locality at which case No. 15 died. It will be observed that the circle embraces but the heart of the city of New Orleans, and that a large portion of the city is without its limits . . . it will be found that the vast majority of the cholera deaths in 1873 occurred within the area of this circle" (Woodworth 1875, 106). Like John Snow with his map of the dense cluster of cholera cases occurring nearest to the Broad Street pump, McClellan argued that were the epidemic local and miasmatic, another more diffuse pattern would be expected.

The conclusion was clear: "The doctrine of 'non-importation' will not stand." He makes the point with a semicircle centered on the levee whose implications Whitehead would have understood. The variation in disease incidence between dock area residents who worked near the levee and those who did not, and were not among the first ill, was important to McClellan. The whole exercise was designed to emphasize that "the unfortunate individuals who contracted cholera upon or near the steamboat levee came in contact with the poison which had been imported in the effects of emigrants from the cholera-infected districts of Europe" (Woodworth 1875, 111).

To drive home the point, McClellan included in his report a table of the number of vessels—with the number of passengers and crew—arriving in New Orleans on a monthly basis from December

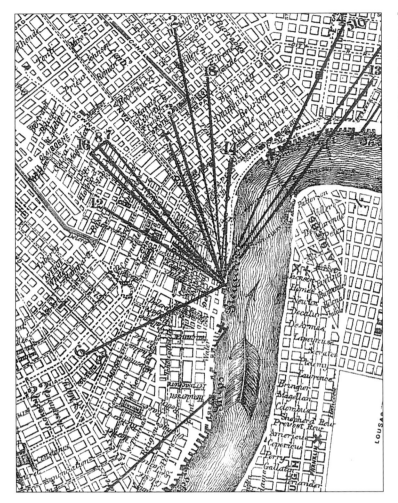

Figure 7.4b Detail of McClellan's map of cholera in New Orleans, in 1873 showing spiders radiating from the docklands to the homes of the earliest cases.

Source: Rare Books and Special Collections, University of British Columbia Library.

1872 to June 1873. He included, too, the basic demographics of emigrants by age and port of origin. To this data he added information on outbreaks among emigrant ships from Europe arriving elsewhere in North America, for example, in Halifax, Canada, where "the most efficient sanitary precautions were at once adopted" when cholera was discovered in contrast to New Orleans, where they were not. The implication was that the epidemic of 1873 in the United States occurred in part because rigorous precautions were not taken in New Orleans that were enacted in, for example, Halifax. Had they been, had attention been paid to arriving vessels and their passengers, the epidemic might have been contained. The message was that the failure of containment and sanitarian measures at the New Orleans port, and presumably in New Orleans itself, permitted the epidemic to spread through the United States.

Memphis

Methodically, city-by-city, McClellan used local medical officials' reports to make the case that "from New Orleans cholera was distributed to the interior of the continent by water transportation" (Woodworth 1875, 111). In Memphis, Tennessee, for example, McClellan's respondent was Dr. H. H. Erskin, "late president, Board of Health," assisted by Dr. J. C. Peters who "came South under the auspices of the New York Board of Health to investigate [the epidemic's] origins" (Woodworth 1875, 137). Unlike White in New Orleans, Erskin and Peters had no doubts of the nature of the disease they faced, the method of its introduction, nor the mode of its diffusion.

The index case in Memphis was diagnosed on April 15 by two local physicians with the death of "an Irishman by the name of Kelly, who had but a few days before come up the river, on what boat is not known, and was lodging at 136 Front Street, between Market and Exchange, in an Irish boarding-house, the surroundings of which were filth" (Woodworth 1875, 137). The next cases were a man named Cunco "who kept an eating house immediately on the river" and then a railroad conductor who, though he died twenty miles from the city, "lived in the square on which Kelly died." These cases are marked and numbered on the Memphis cholera map, as are houses where cholera was later rampant in the city.

On May 4, at least three-quarters of a mile from the river, a woman who lived near the corner of Orleans Street and Marshall Avenue died. Erskin defined her residence as "in a locality highly favorable to the development of the disease. She lived in a small, neat cottage upon the edge of a large pond of stagnant water filled with the filth of the lots whose rear sloped from the adjacent, more elevated streets. It was under the declivity, and near it was the offensive water, whose surface was covered with a green vegetable mold of rank and noxious growth. The atmosphere was full of miasma and supplied the *nidus* for the development of any malignant disease whose germs might be wafted to it" (Woodworth 1875, 138).

McClellan was more than willing to permit Erskin and Peters their contagionist beliefs as long as the essential argument for the mode of transmission was made. "The place was rife with the elements of a great plague, and only needed the specific germ to diffuse it widely and fatal [sic.]," they wrote. What was important, for McClellan, was that a "specific germ" found a hospitable environment for growth in humanity's crowded and unsanitary corners. Erskin and Peters were eloquent on the problem. The city's "sanitary condition was shameful and a disgrace . . .. When cholera was announced the streets were unclean, the alleys reeking with filth, the back yards even in the case of our prominent citizens, who blushed to be made the subjects of public exposure, were full of slops and garbage . . . privies had remained unemptied for years and were in many places running over with the foul accumulations" (Woodworth 1875, 139). Furthermore, the unseasonably cool and extremely damp weather—with near constant rains—contributed to the fetid airs the reporting physicians believed invited cholera into the city.

In considering specific clusters of the disease, Erskin and his colleagues (he names several other local physicians who contributed to his report) paid special attention to the local wells, rating their water by its appearance, assuming their potential as carriers of contagion. Not surprisingly, the poorest citizens—convicts working on a local road gang and members of the "Negro quarter"—suffered most from the epidemic and had the least favorable water sources. In the area of the epidemic's greatest intensity "about fifty [Negro] families lived, thickly crowded in small, ill-ventilated cabins; filthy, careless in habit and diet, purchasing cheap vegetables, stale and unsound, and using water from an alkaline well which, apparently pure, disordered the bowels" (Woodworth 1875, 139).

Nor was the epidemic a single event. That summer there were two distinct cholera epidemics, "waves" we would call them today, and a third of yellow fever. The first began with Kelly's death and the deaths of a group of railroad workers at a camp seven miles out of the city. In May, a group of penitentiary inmates laying track for the Memphis and Ohio Railroad were stricken as well. By the summer, "when the outbreak occurred at Lucy Depot," a railway depot outside the city, a new wave began with outbreaks occurring and recurring throughout Shelby County. As that wave began to subside in early August, "yellow fever followed like an invading army. While its vanguard was busy in Nashville and the interior towns of Middle Tennessee and North Alabama, its rear was still at work [in Memphis], and its effect still visible upon the stragglers who were doomed to fall victims along the line of travel upon which it made its desolating march" (Woodworth 1875, 140).

It is thus understandable, perhaps, that Erskin would say that "the poison was blown to every point of the compass" that summer. For him and his colleagues it must have seemed as if epidemic disease *was* everywhere, a terror as omnipresent as the air itself. Erskin distilled the summer's cholera experience with a map later modified by McClellan.³ "By reference to the map it will be seen that [cholera] had developed in localities distant and separate, dependent upon surroundings more or less favorable to its spread . . . . It left the community enfeebled and alarmed, the more ready victims for yellow fever, which so soon followed" (Woodworth 1875, 141).

The map's concentric circles are almost certainly McClellan's modification of one originally submitted by Erskin. They are a feature of most of the report's maps documenting cholera's progress up the Mississippi, a thematic signature not of individual mapmakers but of the report's principal author. And in each, the center of the circles, or semicircles, is at the docklands on the river. In this map, the assumption of broad, general disease incidence is refocused to an outbreak that begins at the river and is spread from it to the town itself. The earliest cases occur at riverside and the epidemic's greatest toll—each case marked by a darkened city block—occurs within a quarter mile of the rail and docklands on the river. Erskin's insistence upon an outbreak occurring "distant and separate" becomes, in McClellan's mapping, something different (Woodworth 1875). The likelihood that railroad work gangs in fact represented a second, independent point of introduction is suggested in Erskin's report and explained by McClellan's insistence on the vector of interpersonal contamination.

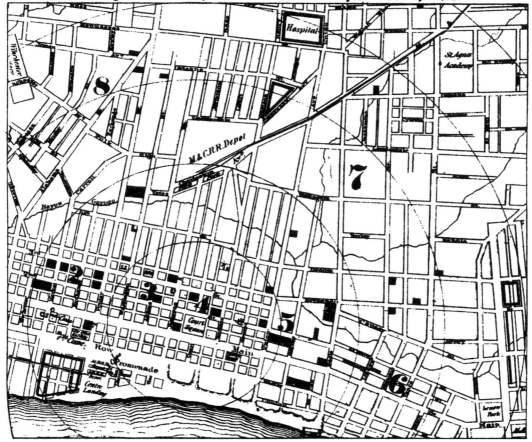

Figure 7.5 Map of cholera outbreak in Memphis, Tennessee, 1873, showing centrality of the riverside docklands to the disease's spread.

Source: Rare Books and Special Collections, University of British Columbia Library.

Bi-directional diffusion

Impressively, McClellan and his Memphis correspondents were perhaps the first to detail a dynamic pattern of infection and re-infection along specific vectors of transmission, the railroads and steamships, which "conveyed the disease upon return trips to re-enforce the epidemic at the original point of departure" (Woodworth 1875). If travel was generally *bi*-directional—with ships going and coming—then it made sense that the disease would be introduced and later *re*introduced along those same vectors. The second epidemic in Memphis was thus, in McClellan's hands, a demonstration of how a contagious disease might first be diffused *away* from its point of initial introduction but then be *returned* at a later date by second-generation persons who first contracted the disease at a secondary or tertiary site of infection up river or down the rail lines.

To understand how important this point is, it is worth noting that the bi-directionality of epidemic infection was a major point relearned during the AIDS pandemic of the late twentieth century, the most mapped pandemic since cholera. In the 1990s, researchers would bring together a similar argument demonstrating that "the U.S. urban hierarchy is a two-way street" in which, "what ever enters the system anywhere flows rapidly into the largest [and then next largest] cities" (Wallace et al. 1997, 940). It was left to modern researchers to rediscover and advance McClellan's understanding of the "complex, dynamic, ecological process in which historically defined socioeconomic and political structures" (systemic poverty, for example) promote reinfection in an urban environment from which a disease earlier diffused (Wallace and Wallace 1995, 341).

Nashville

One more map and city report will serve to complete this review of McClellan's opus. Included with the report to McClellan by three Nashville physicians was a report by the local board of health, "The Water We Drink." Published in 1866, it provided a general description of the city's natural drainage system and the state of Nashville's fresh-water supply. Three-fourths of a mile above the river was the mouth of Brown's Creek. "The topography of the southern slopes from the city shows that a large basin of country emptied its drainage into this stream. The northern boundary of this basin is a ridge starting from the river at the city reservoir, running south of west through the university ground, north of the city, to Fort Negley, thence across a country in a line with the outer defenses of the city. All of that portion of the city south of this line is naturally drained into Brown's Creek" (Woodworth 1875, 143).

The creek itself was polluted by "the immense amount of garbage and filth of every description which accumulates about tenements, and with every rain finds its way into this creek." Added to this the "cleanings of the privy vaults of the city were deposited, not only along the banks, but actually in the channel of this stream." More important to the 1874 report's authors were the hilltop cemeteries, however, "the escapage which drains from these resting places of the dead." These hillside cemeteries were, the 1866 authors had argued, miasmatic reservoirs (like the Craven Hill Estate in Soho) and therefore at least potentially health hazards (Woodworth 1875, 143). More generally, the authors noted that public springs were in generally bad condition. These included Wilson's Spring, which ran beside the U.S. Army barracks (Sixteenth United States Regulars). It was from these polluted water sources that the city's afflicted poor generally drew their water.

McClellan's respondents used the 1866 report to explain the 1873 epidemic. They noted that the army's large privy was daily disinfected, rendered fluid by water, and its discharge then pumped into a cesspool blasted into the area's rock surface. "After each rain-fall the contents of all privies in the city are fluid, and are rapidly drained off; where [they are drained] is a question of undoubted interest to the drinkers of water from the wells and public springs" (Woodworth 1875, 145). Indeed, all the city's creeks drained through areas of relatively dense habitation to the river itself. What the authors said of Lick Branch might serve to describe the general state of the sources of area's well water: "On each side of the creek, and between the fills, (each serving as a dam to keep back from the river the accumulating filth above,) exists a common deposit of every imaginable abomination, which lies rotting, seething, and weltering in the unobstructed sun" (Woodworth 1875, 146).

Nashville suffered from an unfortunate congruence of events. First, there was the Exposition in May 1873, in which "the city was full to overflowing with strangers from all portions of the state . . .. Into this dense mass of humanity, on the 12th of May . . . came a gang of convicts from a cholera-infected camp upon the line of the Memphis and Paducah Railroad. Every one of these convicts, every one of their guards, was suffering from choleraic diarrhea" (Woodworth 1875, 146). While those so afflicted were confined to the penitentiary, "whose walls should have formed a *cordon de santé* to the doomed city," its privies, cesspools, and wash-houses drained into Lick Branch, "whose waters run through almost the heart of the city, and in close proximity to the springs from which so many of the inhabitants obtain their drinking water" (Woodworth 1875, 146).

As important, "the sanitary history of this city shows a most lamentable negligence on the part of her authorities." Simply, local officials had refused to invest in sewage infrastructure or protected water. Finally, fierce public opposition to federal involvement added to the lamentable state of local affairs. "Why should it be necessary to have a national board for the exercise of such control?" some locals asked. "Is it possible that the large cities are so destitute of sanitary learning and experience that they must be remanded to the guardianship of a board commissioned by the general government?" (Woodworth 1875, 146).

The answer for McClellan's correspondents was yes. "Whenever cholera has been upon the North American continent, Nashville has been decimated. Her noblest citizens, as well as the most degraded, have been counted victims by the score, simply because 'doing their own thinking' has been productive of no sanitary reforms, and has resulted in the utter ignoring of the wise and prudent suggestions of her own sanitarians, and the local deficits that were present to add to the epidemic of 1833, were present to augment the severity of the same disease in 1873, and still exist at the close of 1874" (Woodworth 1875, 146–147.)

McClellan mapped this brilliantly. He blacked in the houses of early cholera cases in the epidemic period that most clearly came up river, numbering the cases sequentially. From their epicenter he drew his, by now, familiar concentric rings radiating from the epidemic's dockland epicenter. The point is made once again that the outbreak seems to be centered at the river and to radiate out from the core area peopled by river workers and visitors. To this he adds, however, darkened areas at higher elevations—the barracks and the penitentiary, for example—where cholera occurred in May. These

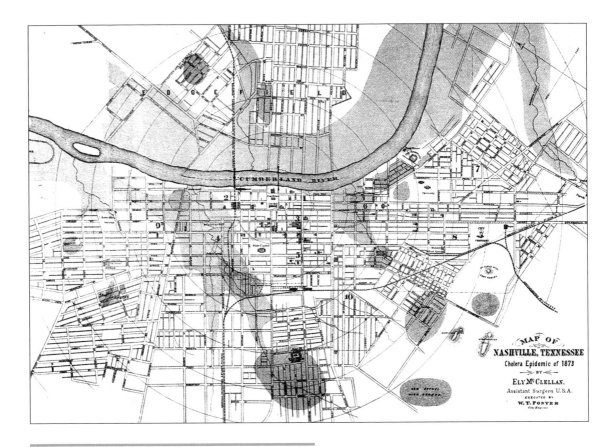

Figure 7.6a Map of the incidence of cholera in Nashville, Tennessee, in 1873. In the federal report the map was notable for its inclusion of detail on local water sources and the incidence of disease, marked by darkened areas in this map.

Source: Rare Books and Special Collections, University of British Columbia Library.

anchor, and in some cases encompass, the creeks that the official report says were polluted. These areas of incidence and elevation also serve as buffers of the river drainage system along which cholera presumably traveled. Smaller circles appear as well to mark areas of outbreak centered on local wells fed by the rivers that flowed downhill from the barracks, the penitentiary, and other outbreak sources like New Bethel.

Here was Snow's topography of an outbreak writ large. The map incorporated Farr's preoccupation with altitude with Snow's concern for water and infrastructure. Incidents of local outbreak at upland areas like the penitentiary and the barracks are joined to lowland cases by local topography. Added to this were the central index cases McClellan needed to continue his greater argument about the course of the epidemic and its vectors along the Mississippi and its tributaries. The whole is set within a political environment of indifference to sanitary concerns and distrust of federal intervention. Also, that political environment contributed to a condition of recurring epidemics (first cholera, then yellow fever) whose pattern could be traced repeatedly first to the river and its commercial traffic but secondly to the water system that flowed down from the hills above the city, picking up urban refuse in its wake.

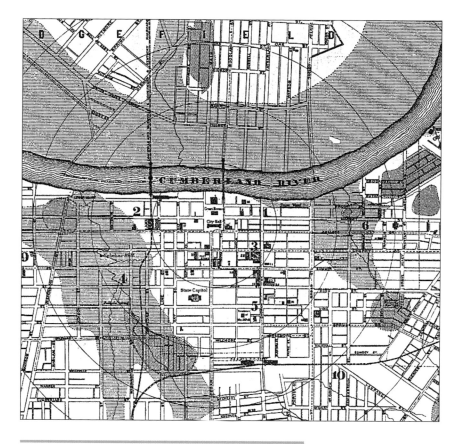

Figure 7.6b   Detail of map of cholera incidence in Nashville, Tennesee, showing areas of drainage and disease intensity.

Source: Rare Books and Special Collections, University of British Columbia Library.

In the absence of a clinically precise, microscopically verifiable germ-theory of disease, miasmatic medicine continued to rule. Within that context, however, the practical utility of considering water supply, one demonstrated in Snow's studies and later others, was accepted. In essence, a special theory of waterborne cholera had come by this time to exist within the greater theory of disease that remained for many Hippocratic and Galenic. Nor should this be surprising. Time and again in the history of science old theory accommodates new data, albeit with progressive difficulty, until new technologies and new theories permit the old to be enfolded in a more comprehensive and verifiable thesis.

Public boards of health

McClellan's study brilliantly organized data provided by local health boards, then a relatively new phenomenon, most of whose members assumed that disease was in the air, a miasmatic result of foul odors. It made sense both experientially and in the context of the evolving science of the day. In the next decade Koch's bacteriology would begin to put to rest the assumption of foul airs as uniquely generative of a class of diseases, reducing olfactory evidence to a secondary and suggestive indicator of areas where disease might breed. But at this time and for several decades public health was about odor, the smell of disease and its causes, just as it had been for Seaman and Pascalis.

This can be inferred from the statements of the public health officials from New Orleans to Nashville. It is clearer, however, in a map created by the Board of Health in Boston in 1878. Organized in 1869 to address the effects of pollution of a local river, the Board of Health published in 1878 a "map showing the sources of some of the offensive odors perceived in Boston," (Board of Health 1878) in which "large areas have been at once, and frequently, enveloped in an atmosphere of stench so strong as to arouse the sleeping, terrify the weak, and nauseate and exasperate nearly everybody . . .. It travels in a belt half way across the city, and at that distance seems to have lost none of its potency, and although its source is miles away, you feel it is directly at your feet" (also quoted in Haglund 2002).[4]

In the map mud flats and marshes along the Charles River, the site of a number of residential and commercial structures that used the river as a sewer, were marked with a red hatching. Three different arrows—each feathered to indicate intensity—showed the direction of prevailing local winds that carried the stench of the mud flats across the city. The outlets of sewers into the river—another locus of foul smells—were marked and numbered as well. The result would have satisfied Seaman had he had access to a printing technology capable of fusing the atmospheric pathways with the locus of urban waste odors to create a map of the environmental pathway of disease carrying foul odors across the urban plane. The Boston map was not disease specific, however. Rather, it mapped a dynamic disease hazard, the local airs that carried the stench that generated disease from this or that locus across the greater city.[5]

The report

Cartographic historian F. J. Spencer (1969, 4) dismissed the maps in McClellan's report because, he wrote, they "have nothing of the clarity of disease dispersion which [Snow's] map portrays." The judgment was too harsh by half. Snow's Broad Street map was of a single subdistrict on which he could mark individual cases without concern for greater, regional influences. McClellan was working with reports submitted by local officials from a host of cities, all of which he had to integrate into a single

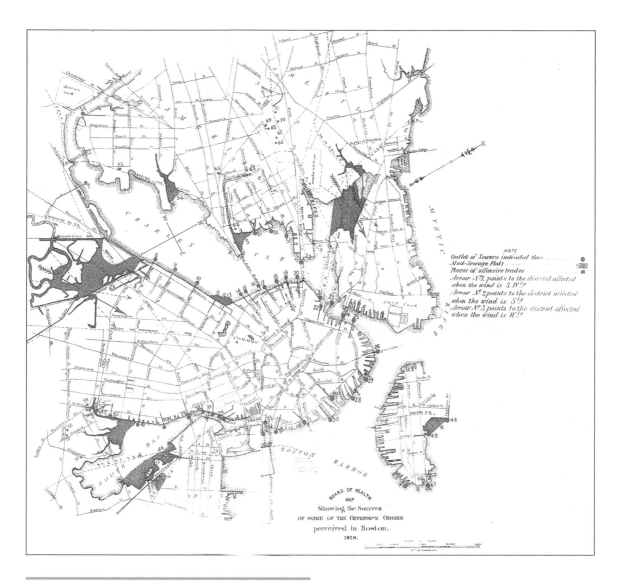

Figure 7.7 Boston map of odors by the Board of Public Health, 1878. Red hatching shows the location of mud flats and marshes, large dots of sewer gratings, from which foul odors were carried across the city by prevailing winds marked with separate arrows. Boston Board of Health, 1878.

Source: Courtesy of the City of Boston.

comprehensive report of his own. Some submitted maps he would modify, both for consistency and to advance his argument; in other cases, he drew the maps himself.

As important, Snow sought only to show the relative density of occurrence in the St. James, Soho, outbreak and its relation to the Broad Street pump that was near its epicenter. McClellan sought in his maps and text to prove the general course of the 1873 epidemic in the United States, its relation to previous epidemics, and to argue the complicity of river and train networks as vectors of transmission. The goals of the two were distinct. The resources they had differed, as did the scale of their arguments. The comparison is simply unfair.

Unlike Snow, McClellan was not his own man. He was a military physician working under a military superior on a project that served a congressional mandate. He was dependent on data from local public health and medical officials who had not attended the 1874 conference in Vienna and whose understanding of cholera was in some cases a generation out of date. Woodworth and McClellan were not at liberty to criticize local informants and officials in a nation that, as the Nashville report made clear, was predisposed to distrust federal involvement in areas of local and state sanitation and health.

It is useful to think of McClellan's report as an atlas for which a series of maps was collected, annotated, regularized, and systematized in a report whose real goal was to add the U.S. experience to an expanding, international body of medical knowledge. To be sure, there is not always the mapped consistency expected of an atlas even in McClellan's day. This is especially true in the historical maps collected from British and French authorities at the international conference. Certainly, the quality of McClellan's maps varies from one to another, in part because of their necessary reliance on material submitted by local medical officials resident along the Mississippi River, many of whom had little if any mapping experience. But taken together the argument was thematically consistent and intellectually ambitious. The maps included by McClellan together argued at a range of scales a commonality of experience that extended from the local event to fifty years of international experience with a dreaded pandemic disease.

From our perspective, McClellan's study suffers from a failure to standardize reportage of the incidence of the disease. But that was not McClellan's brief, and in the 1870s standardized national (or international) reportage of disease incidence was still decades in the future, a dream yet to be dreamt. Instead, McClellan accepted the difficulties of his assignment and the limits of the data provided by local officials whose perspective was typically contagionist and limited. From their reports he created a work whose reading presented the broadest possible portrait of the dynamic ecology of the epidemic that came to the southern United States by ship, diffusing from New Orleans by railway, steamship, and riverboat across a good portion of the nation.

The result did not dispute the contagionist perspective directly. Rather, in his report, it existed simultaneously with the anticontagionist theory of direct transmission. That was the evolving science of the day. Within that theoretical context McClellan argued a systematic pattern of individual and interpersonal contagion that acknowledged sanitarian concerns but insisted upon a process of transmission that in the end was thoroughly modern. Even more impressively, he did this within a broad framework of historical epidemics and global disease transmission.

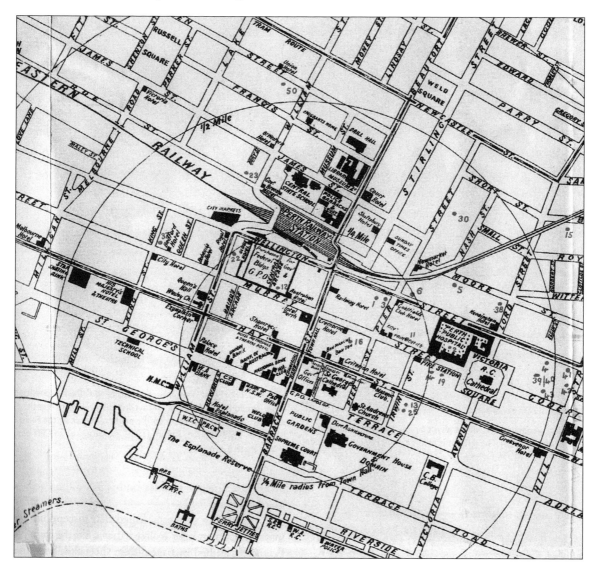

Figure 7.8 Map of an 1893 smallpox epidemic in western Australia shows the degree to which McClellan's mapping served as a general model of disease investigation elsewhere (Cliff, Haggett, and Smallman-Raynor 2004, 41).

Source: Courtesy of Cliff, Haggett, Smallman-Raynor and reproduced by permission of Hodder Education.

In this he contributed greatly to national and international understanding of the pandemic and the then current, more general debate on modes of disease diffusion and transmission. His argument for the potential of interpersonal transmission was one Snow had made decades before. It was McClellan's brilliance to make it diligently and city-by-city, at the scale of the epidemic that spread up the Mississippi, town to town. The result extended the techniques of Snow and his contemporaries, integrating local, regional, national, and international scales of address in a way that was ambitious and in its day unique. Cartographically, the maps McClellan produced for his report became a type of standard into the twentieth century. The map of an 1893 smallpox outbreak in Australia recently reproduced by Cliff and Haggett (2004) gives graphic evidence of this debt that later researchers owed to McClellan's mapping *(figure 7.8)*.

The result was a document that at once distilled the state of international knowledge about cholera and advanced that body of knowledge through a close analysis of the U.S. experience. Finally, the whole announced that the United States was a nation that could stand with others in the international community of disease investigation. McClellan's report shouted "here is the state of our knowledge about the disease that traveled from the world to the nation in 1873." The subtext of Congress's request for the report was to insist upon America's place in the community of scientific nations as a full player, up-to-date and eager to present its data. Historically, McClellan's report is thus an overture, the announcement of what, by the mid-twentieth century, would become the United States' aggressive involvement in the study of disease ecology and medical investigation.

East Africa

While McClellan's work was exceptional in its scale, as demonstrated by the extent of its bibliography and the number and type of the maps it represented, it was not unique. Indeed, it was representative of the manner in which a number of researchers were considering disease spread and diffusion. Another example is the work of Dr. James Christie, a Scottish nonconformist minister trained in Glasgow, who in 1860 abandoned his ministry for medicine and in 1865 abandoned Scotland for Zanzibar. An abolitionist, he was said to be the "last white man whom David Livingston saw as he set out on his last travels, and Livingston's body was embalmed by an assistant trained by Christie" (Davies 1957, 2).

In 1876, Christie published an exhaustive 508 page book on *Cholera Epidemics in East Africa: An Account of the Several Diffusions of the Disease in that Country from 1821 till 1872, with an Outline of the Geography, Ethnography, and Trade Connections of the Region through which the Epidemics Passed* (Christie 1876). Like McClellan's opus, Christie's combined attention to geography, ethnography, and trade in a study of the continental diffusion of cholera and its relative severity in his study area. Christie began practicing in Zanzibar in 1865 and from that post was "in the habit of meeting natives from all parts of the country between Arabia and Madagascar, and also from the interior of Africa" (Davies 1957, 3).

He was, in other words, perfectly situated to consider and study the dynamics of the diffusion and incidence of the cholera that, as a physician, he was called upon to treat.

In his early chapters he made derogatory comments on the general sanitary state of the region similar to the laments of the practitioners reporting to McClellan in the United States. Limited sanitary infrastructure and unprotected water supplies were at least as prevalent in the towns where Christie served as they were in those McClellan's informants described. Despite these deficits there was, however, no evidence of "undue prevalence of diarrhoeal disease before the outbreaks of cholera" (Davies 1957, 3) in the 1860s. The statement assured that in his work epidemic Asian cholera would be clearly distinguished from the endemic diarrhea with which it was often confused in England and the United States.[6]

Christie then noted that earlier East African outbreaks (1836–1837, 1858–1859) had occurred in Arabian and Red Sea ports to and from which pilgrims to Mecca traveled. These pilgrimages were, he believed, a principal vector by which the disease traveled to his neighborhood and country. That the routes taken by pilgrims were those used as well by other travelers brought him to a state of excited prose. "Fleeing from the pestilence but with death clinging to them like the shirt of Nessus, they journey at the utmost speed through the deserts and their track is marked by the dead bodies of men and of beasts of burden fallen from disease and from exhaustion" (Davies 1957, 3).

Over land and by sea, Christie mapped the course of the epidemic's envelopment of East Africa. It moved more slowly in the least accessible countries, faster in those with railway systems or access to the sea. Where cholera festered, its effect was uneven, attacking poor villagers more than colonial Europeans and Americans resident in separate compounds. Most affected were the slaves whose living conditions were abysmal and for whom adequate sanitary facilities were virtually nonexistent.

He argued that this was true of *every* cholera epidemic in Africa, including that of 1868–1870, the precursor of the U.S. epidemic of 1873. In short, Christie attempted to do for East Africa what McClellan did for the United States, to use the local experience as a means of advancing a general proposition of disease diffusion. Christie's attempt was the more ambitious. After all, he was a largely solitary researcher while McClellan had a federal bureaucracy and a significant infrastructure of physicians and public health officials to draw upon.

It was no accident that Christie and McClellan both mapped their studies at different scales presenting international patterns of diffusion, regional chronologies of incidence, and local conditions where outbreaks occurred. The approach was one familiar in the literature and familiar, too, to attendees of the Vienna conference. Maps were shared there between researchers from a number of countries, the state-of-the-art cholera research. Mapping was a necessary and expected tool for disease specialists, a means of distilling arguments and sharing the results of research. It would have been surprising if Christie or McClellan had not included maps and the spatial thinking they distilled in their respective reports.

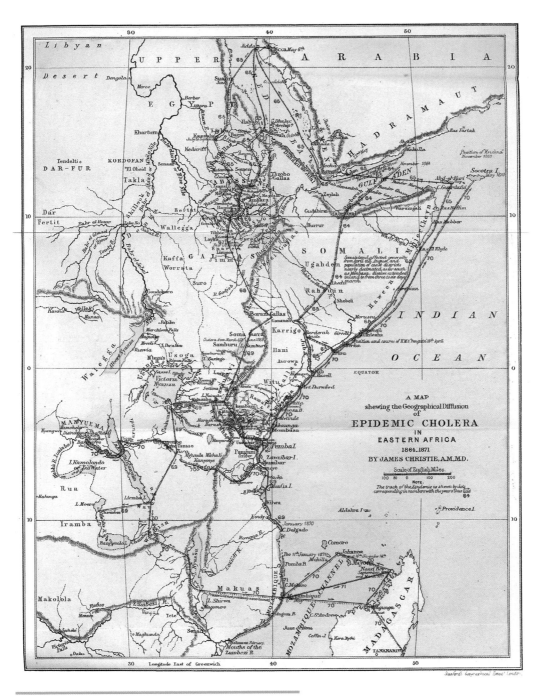

Figure 7.9 Christie's map of cholera diffusion in East Africa. Sequential numbers are used in the text to describe the diffusion of the disease by caravan, religious pilgrimage, and sea routes.

Source: Reproduced courtesy of College of Physicians of Philadelphia.

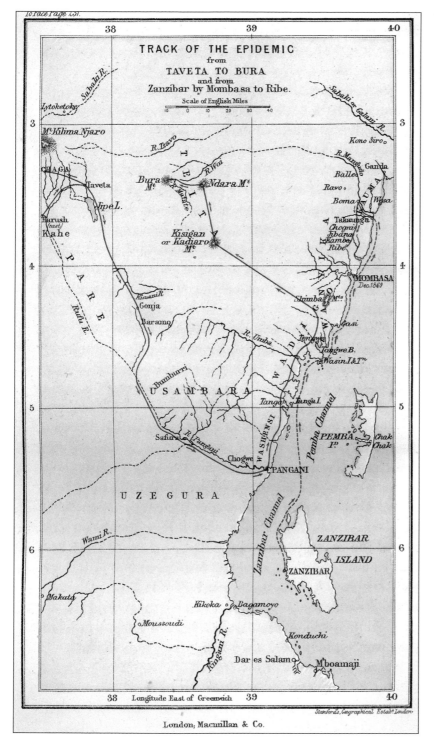

Figure 7.10 Christie's map of cholera diffusion in Zanzibar.

Source: Reproduced courtesy of College of Physicians of Philadelphia.

Unlike McClellan, Christie was not content to permit his argument to coexist with that of a miasmatic, airborne transmission. The body of his substantial work was offered in part to refute the theories of a statistical officer then attached to the government of India's Sanitary Commission, a Dr. Bryden. In his "Report on the General Aspects of Epidemic Cholera in 1869" Bryden had claimed to have proven that a "special meteorology," a bad air, was responsible for cholera's international progression. Worse, from Christie's point of view, the report, published in Calcutta by the Indian government in 1870, focused on the incidence of cholera in Christie's own territory, East Africa (Christie 1876, 457).

Bryden's argument, preserved in Christie's text, was clear: "At the beginning of the cholera season of 1869, I deduced, that from the geographical situation of cholera, a certain sequence of events would happen at certain dates; and since the sequence of events did occur as anticipated, I recognize that what was then recorded is entitled to a place, not in the province of theory, but in that of legitimate deduction" (quoted in Christie 1876). What he had deduced was an "aerial highway" carrying the miasmatic disease across Africa without any reference to local sanitary or migratory referents. Christie was furious. Anger almost drips from his pages when he first details and then methodically takes apart Bryden's theory.

In a book with more than five hundred pages of maps, charts, and text in ten-point type Christie laid out the case for a diffusion of the disease based not on atmosphere but on the travel routes of the people he served. The whole was exhaustively considered and mapped in an attempt to disprove the views of an influential and, in retrospect, wholly wrong-headed official. "Dr. Bryden's 'southern aerial epidemic highway,'" covering 'Arabia, Eastern and Northern Africa, and the shores of the Mediterranean generally,' studied in the light of the detailed history of the great diffusions from Western India in 1864–1865, here summarized, and of the secondary diffusion from Mecca, in the latter year, has no existence; for the disease moved solely along the highways of human intercourse, and in certain definite relations to that intercourse" (Christie 1876, 174).

In his text, Christie argued not only against Bryden's airborne theory in specific but, unlike McClellan, against the theory of cholera as an airborne disease generally. His pique took him to endorse a Snow-like theory of cholera that, while certainly argued at the Vienna conference, was not wholly endorsed by it. The result is, according to some researchers, a confirmation of the distinct theory of cholera as a disease resulting from ingested agents rather than those that might be inhaled. "Christie agreed with the views of the majority of the workers of the time, namely that there is a 'generative agent' in the alimentary canal of the sufferers from cholera and the spread is by faecal contamination, usually by waterborne infection" (Davies 1957, 6). That is modernity speaking, however, not Christie's contemporaries. As we have seen, not all in Vienna, or elsewhere, accepted this view, which perhaps is best thought of as contending but not yet dominating the medical theory of the time.

Medical geography: Determinism

Despite Christie's critique, the idea of an "aerial epidemic highway," and more generally of an environmental determinism represented here by Bryden's work had a number of advocates at this time. The sanitarian concern with the urban environment was more typically married to a Galenic assumption that disease incidence was at least in part a result of geographical and climatologic factors. In 1881, for example, Hirsch published the second edition of his *Handbuch der Historisch-Geographischen Pathologie*, translated into English between 1883–1886, in a much revised version, as *Handbook of Geographical and Historical Pathology* (Cliff and Haggett 2003, 11–12). A manifesto for the consideration of the relation of location and environment to disease, the text was encyclopedic. Its three volumes covered infectious diseases (like cholera), chronic diseases (tuberculosis, for example), and diseases of specific organs (cancer) (Barrett 2000a, 105–107). Also published in this period were Lombard's four-volume *Traité de Climatologie Medicale, Davidson's Geographical Pathology* (1892), and in 1903, Clemow's *The Geography of Disease.*

The importance of mapping to the medical arguments these books offered varies with the author. Clemow, for example, maps only nine of the diseases his book describes. For every disease discussed, however, he gives a brief etiology and a historical note followed by sections on (a) the geographical distribution of the disease and (b) factors governing and possibly encouraging its distribution. The latter were principally environmental: soils, winds, dampness, and so on. In all these works social contributors were sometimes mentioned, but it was the environmental, and at this time that often meant the climatological, that was important.

The general idea was as old as Hippocrates and Galen. Good airs (and good soils) promoted well-being while bad airs and bad soils encouraged this or that illness. It had been the idea behind the formidable, if inconclusive, charts compiled by Acland in an attempt to discover which physical factors (barometric pressure, wind speed and direction, rainfall) might explain Oxford's cholera epidemics. It was, too, the bedrock on which early attempts at medical geography were based. Systematized in the late 1880s, the promise was of a "historical-geographical pathology," eventually shortened to "medical geography," correlating patterns of climate, settlement, and temperature to the incidence of specific diseases. In much of this work, data on the location and incidence of disease was collected and then correlated with local physical and climatic characteristics. In some, however, researchers mapped general, environmental determinants and then considered the states of health or disease within them (Barrett 2000b, 300–301).

In some ways, the result was a last stand for the Hippocratic focus on local, physical environments as determinants of health and disease. After all, hadn't Hippocrates himself written "On Airs, Waters, and Places," a treatise on the effect of physical surroundings on health and disease?[7] In another and more favorable light, however, in play was an evolving experiential and experimental perspective that was ecologic as well as disease-agent specific. Hirsch, who insisted on the importance of studying diseases *in situ*, explained that his approach joined the social perspective of earlier decades with the climatologic and geologic knowledge then accruing. The result was a focus on "the geographically dependent factors (such as race, nationality, soil conditions, climate, social factors, etc., that have to be considered essential for the occurrence and distribution of individual diseases" (Hirsch 1883, Vol.1, 2). Lombard made a similar point in the long subtitle to his opus, describing the field as "the study of physiological, pathological, prophylactic and therapeutic influences of climate upon health."

This medical geography based on soil and climate as well as social realities demanded a mapped approach. How else could one easily distill the broad patterns of the air and the variations in soil and geology that were assumed to be determinants of health and disease? What better way to consider simultaneously social patterns of settlement and economic behavior? Nor did it hurt that the late nineteenth century saw an explosion in ever more detailed geological and climatologic mapping. Physical sciences were ascendant, and so was the evolving discipline of cartography.

Haviland and Great Britain

At the same time, better, faster presses were making less-expensive, more detailed maps ever-more available. Weather maps were being reproduced in newspapers, geological maps in textbooks. Color mapping was slowly winning acceptance, if not in the common press, then in specialty publications. Why not use maps in propositions equating local environmental conditions and the incidence of disease?

The result was a period in which illness was assumed to be largely the effect of the soils, wind, temperature, and other physical characteristics of a local environment. These factors explained both different patterns of disease incidence and, some believed, the basic nature of disease itself. "We must no longer be contented with the mere statement that certain geographical facts in the distribution of disease are coincident with certain other facts connected with the soil and atmosphere," Alfred Haviland insisted in the 1892 preface to the second edition of his *Geographical Distribution of Disease in Great Britain*. "The time has arrived when the cause of the disease itself must be thoroughly investigated, and its relation to the soil and the atmosphere ascertained" (Haviland 1892, viii). That there was a relation he and others of his day had little doubt.

Researchers like Haviland were not Luddites who rejected the evolving bacteriology that was revolutionizing clinical medicine. Instead they saw their work as complimentary to that of early bacteriologists. "The pathologists who informs us that the microbe of a given disease is shaped like a period, a dash, or a comma, without telling us what meterological donations are most favorable to its development, does only half his duty (Campbell 1885, 195–195; Mitman and Numbers 2003, 398–399). The other half of the task was to define the local conditions—geological and meterological—that would promote the pathogen's development within a specific location and encourage or inhibit the disease in the individual (Ward 1897). It was for this reason that Robert DeCourcy Ward taught climatology and the geographic distribution of disease to medical and presumably public health students

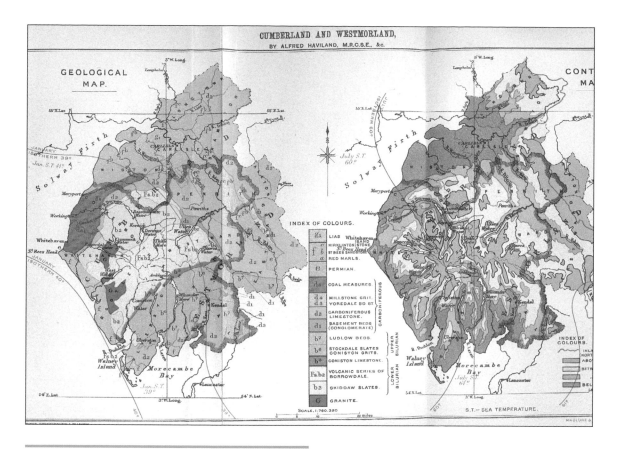

Figure 7.11 Haviland's biogeographic map of British counties. The physical characteristics of local districts in British counties were used to explain the varying rates of occurrence of specific diseases.

Source: Rare Books and Special Collections, University of British Columbia Library Haviland (1892).

at Harvard. In 1908 he would write the credo that informed his work for more than a decade: "The cause of disease is now no longer sought directly in meteorological conditions but in the effects, more or less direct, of those conditions upon the micro-organisms which are the specific cause of disease" (Ward 1908, 181).

The increasing wealth of geological and meteorological data was matched by ever-more-detailed public health records in industrialized countries like England and the United States. Together, this data permitted ever-more precise mapping of local and regional disease incidence on a national scale. The evolving physical sciences of climatology and geology offered ever-more detailed knowledge of the physical characteristics of the land itself. What could make more sense than to equate one with the other, to see in the physical environment a potential cause of specific medical conditions? In England,

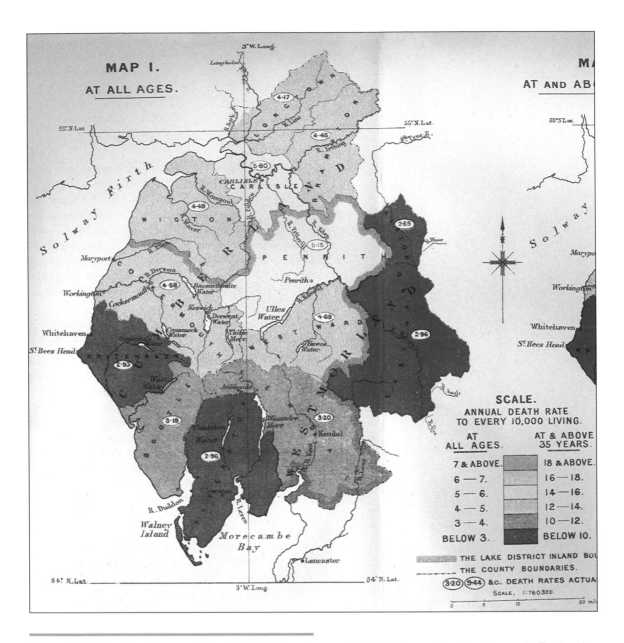

Figure 7.12 Haviland's map of the distribution of cancer in British counties for all ages in England, 1892. Differences in incidence of cancer were to be explained by geographical variants.

Source: Rare Books and Special Collections, University of British Columbia Library Haviland (1892).

Cartographies of Disease

for example, heart disease was more prevalent in the valley areas of England and Wales than coastal regions "freely exposed to the prevailing winds and sunshine." It seemed obvious that there was something in the valley's stagnant airs and nonsandy soils that somehow promoted the disease. It made intuitive sense and had the authority of the old medicine to support it, one that had yet to be fully displaced by what would become twentieth-century medical science.

This deterministic, medical geography did not typically deal carefully with social determinants of health. It was easier to point to the adverse airs in the valley than to the abysmal living conditions of the miners who inhabited it. From the perspective of officialdom, a simple correspondence of geography and disease did not require the type of social perspective earlier, one requiring expensive corrective measured, argued by Chadwick, Snow, or later, Booth. The failure was that of a science that in its enthusiasm for one type of data ignored another. It was also, however, the failure of an age whose authorities did not willingly consider socioeconomic determinants of health. The comfortable idea of a geographic determinism that could not be changed was favored over the hard idea of social factors like poverty and income inequality as criteria influencing disease in populations.[8]

It is tempting to dismiss Haviland and his contemporaries as a historical oddity, a temporary dead end quickly bypassed in the march of medical science toward its modern state of address. "Nice maps, stupid ideas," as one student sneered at the end of a lecture. While understandable, the trivializing judgment is a mistake. Yes, the climatic and geographic determinism was simplistic, an artifact of its age and the incompleteness of then-current knowledge. It did, however, identify pockets of disease and describe environments that seemed to promote this or that deleterious condition. Its understanding of the mechanisms of disease was limited, but the whole did serve to broaden what had been a fundamentally urban, social determinism (poor people are filthy and the cause of their own disease) to a more general, environmental perspective. There was merit in the physical concerns of those like Haviland who sought to consider environmental contributors in the profiling of diseases. The question would be how to enunciate that concern in a more rigorous, less-determinate fashion.

This was an age inundated with both new data accumulated at virtually every scale and of new techniques of analysis. There was, too, the increasing propogation of data in journals, newspapers, and maps that served them both. It was not simply the geology of an area, or its climatology, but the collection of those data in a way that permitted their correlation with, here, issues of disease incidence.

The result was not trivial and in time would become fundamental. The core of the argument for a "biogeographic" approach would bare real fruit in the twentieth century as researchers with better tools found new ways to consider environmental determinants of disease and health. The result would blossom in the 1950s in a more rigorous disease ecology, one in which climatic and geographic data were joined to social elements in a new approach. It would take perhaps a century for the physical as well as social constituents of health and disease to be united in a single, comprehensive theory of medical

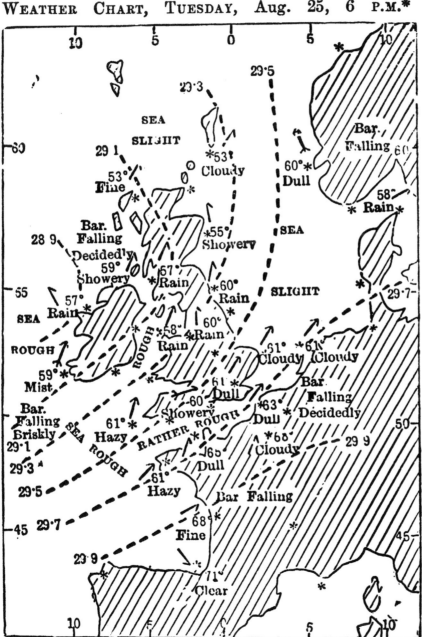

Figure 7.13 Late nineteenth century map of temperatures and barometric pressure for western Europe and England. The data collected and mapped became a component of the type of environmental analysis of disease advanced by researchers like Haviland.

Source: Reproduced courtesy of College of Physicians of Philadelphia.

ecology. But with this brief period of early medical geography, and the determinism it promoted, the pieces for that reunion would all be in place.

Endnotes:

1. Woodworth's mammoth study, *The Cholera Epidemic of 1873 in the United States,* is more widely available than most of the other nineteenth century reports discussed in this and previous chapters. A federal report ordered by the U.S. Congress, it is available through the Library of Congress, of course, and in a number of specialized collections, including that of the College of Physicians of Philadelphia and the New York Academy of Medicine. The copy from which reproductions were made for this chapter is housed at The University of British Columbia, Woodward Library.

2. The French map of "the progress of the Asiatic cholera," like the New Orleans map, is an 8.5-by-11-inch foldout inserted vertically into the book's binding. Atypically, the map has a broad border that reduces the size of the map itself to approximately 5 by 7 inches. Its reading thus requires, in the original, use of a magnifying glass if the names of individual ports are to be read.

3. The authorship of both this section of the report and of the map itself is a bit unclear. Because McClellan did not sign the map, and because it is far less detailed than those whose authorship he claimed, the assumption is that Erskin submitted it with his report. In addition, while the section of the report that describes it appears to be by Erskin, his text refers to areas not on the map. McClellan was in the habit of annotating his contributors' texts, and, of course, their maps. Finally, McClellan's concentric rings were a cartographic and an editorial device, a technique McClellan was far more likely to be familiar with than a river practitioner in the interior of the United States.

4. The Boston map is cited and briefly considered in Haglund (2002). Geographer and urban historian Arthur Krim brought it to my attention, and the Boston Public Library kindly provided a copy for use in this work.

5. It is tempting but inappropriate to think of the Boston odor map, or others of its kind, solely as amusing artifacts of an unscientific age. In August 2004, the Associated Press reported that the city council of Las Vegas, Nevada, was considering a $100,000 consulting contract aimed at finding the source of the offensive smells in its downtown. The smell along Freemont Avenue in downtown Las Vegas required the city officials to do something. "A tiny closed-circuit television system would be

used to examine the downtown storm drains, smoke would be pumped into the system to identify outlets and dye would be used to follow water flows."

Presumably the city's existing maps of its sewer systems will, eventually, be overlaid with data from their closed-circuit inspection and the smoke symbols invoked to identify specific outlets (Associated Press 2004).

6. The New York Academy of Medicine has a copy of Christie's book. It lacks Christie's maps, however, and is in fragile condition, the pages quite literally falling apart in my hands. Fortunately, a pristine copy in superb condition exists at the College of Physicians of Philadelphia. In that copy, the maps and text are well-preserved and available for close inspection.

7. While it is tempting to make fun of the determinists who believed biogeography was the modern answer to a Hippocratic medicine, it is useful to note that Howe quotes at length from "On Airs, Waters and Seas" in the 1960s in the introduction to his *Atlas of Disease Distribution in Great Britain*. The reference there, however, is nostalgic rather than clinical. Contemporary studies briefly reviewed here in chapter 11 and 12 detail new ecological studies that present a detailed and increasingly dynamic understanding of environmental determinants of disease.

8. It is tempting to draw parallels to current initiatives against HIV/AIDS, drug-resistant tuberculosis, influenza, and so on, currently epidemic diseases whose socioeconomic roots are broadly ignored by public officials and many health researchers. For discussion of this see, for example, Wallace and Wallace (1997), and for HIV/AIDS, Wallace and Wallace (1995).

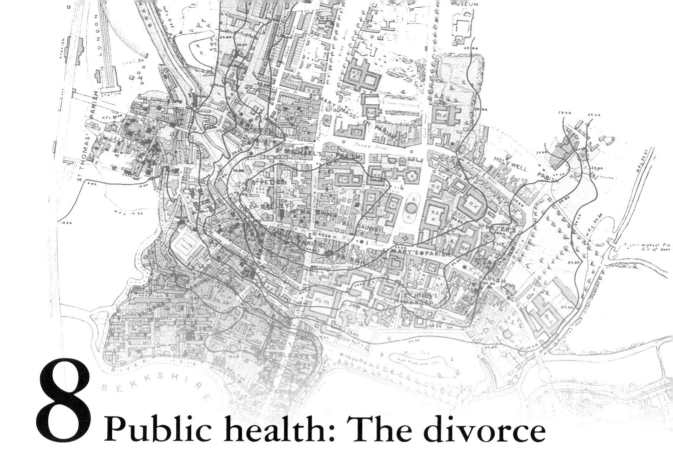

8 Public health: The divorce

In the late nineteenth century, the disciplines of public health and sanitary science were ascendant. The lessons of Snow and his colleagues, the work of McClellan and his contemporaries, had had their effect. Increasingly, developed countries accepted the idea that public health was a public interest and that medicine needed a specialty whose experts, while often not physicians, would consider issues of disease prevention and public health. Within this evolving field interest in mapping as anything but a simple, descriptive tool rapidly declined. The reasons for that are various, but the fact is indisputable: At the turn of the century medical mapping as anything but an illustrative adjunct to public health concerns was almost wholly eclipsed. The reasons say much about the discipline, and even more about issues of publication and production, than it does about the work of those, like Booth, who were mapping so effectively.

In this context, the work of W. T. Sedgwick is instructive. First introduced here for his distortions of Snow's Broad Street map, Sedgwick was the author of an influential text, published in 1901 and reprinted several times in the first two decades of the century, on the *Principles of Sanitary Science and the*

Public Health. A professor at the Massachusetts Institute of Technology, Sedgwick's goal was the education of future public health professionals schooled in sanitary science and equipped to assist in the development of healthy urban environments. His textbook was a casebook that used earlier examples, like Snow's, as instructional examples for this new class of professional. His casework explains much about the exile of mapping from the environs of public health.

"One of the most instructive epidemics in the annals of sanitary science" (Sedgwick 1911, 200), Sedgwick wrote in the book's fourth edition, was a typhoid fever epidemic in Plymouth, Pennsylvania, in the spring of 1885. Then a mining town with about eight thousand inhabitants several miles downriver from Wilkes-Barre, Plymouth fell victim to a violent outbreak of typhoid fever in early April that was to affect, before it ran its course, 1,104 people. The mortality was unusually heavy: 114 people, or slightly more than 10 percent of those affected, died.

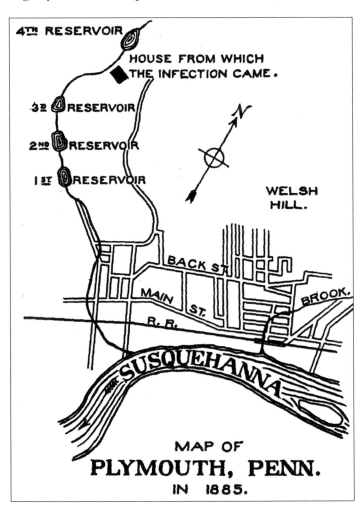

Figure 8.1 Sedgwick's simplified map of a typhoid fever outbreak in Plymouth, Pennsylvania, 1885. Compare this map with figure 8.3 on which it is based, the map by L. H. Taylor for the Pennsylvania Board of Health.

Source: Reproduced courtesy of University of Toronto Library.

Quoted verbatim in an article by reporting physician Dr. L. H. Taylor (1886), Sedgwick briefly reviewed possible sources of the outbreak, anticontagionist and contagionist. The first was "the accumulated filth of the town which, being acted upon by the warm rays of the April sun, had suddenly become noxious and the emanations, therefore, had caused the disease" (Sedgwick 1911, 201). But since Plymouth was no dirtier than other, neighboring towns, and the only one affected, a simple origin from filthy miasmatic sites was rejected.

Attention then turned to the city's two principle sources of water, the Susquehanna River, drawn to city wells by the Delaware and Hudson Coal Company, and "water of remarkable purity" from a neighborhood mountain stream on which the Plymouth Water Company had built four storage reservoirs. Since those residents whose water came from the former were unaffected by the outbreak, the assumption was that the mountain stream had become somehow contaminated. "A glance at the accompanying map will show the location of this stream and of the several reservoirs. Above the starting point of the water pipes there is but one house situated upon the banks of this stream, and one upon the banks of the fourth reservoir" (Taylor 1886).

The occupant of that house contracted typhoid fever in Philadelphia, returning to his home January 2, 1885. He recuperated in February, relapsed in March, and slowly recovered in April. The nurse who cared for him described to Taylor how she emptied the house's chamber pots on the snow and frozen ground between the house and the downhill stream that was yards from the house, and its privy that was within thirty feet of the stream. When the snows melted in the spring, they carried with them the patient's wastes from the privy in the snow outside his house into the stream. From there it flowed directly into the third reservoir.

To make matters worse, on March 26, the water company superintendent had found the first two reservoirs almost empty because the pipe joining the second to the third, upstream reservoir was frozen. The upstream reservoir, however, was filling with dangerous rapidity. To get the water flowing "he caused a fire to be built to melt the ice in this pipe and then stopped the river pumps. The honest act of an honest man, and simply in the discharge of his duty and with kindliest intent" (Taylor 1886). Unfreezing the pipes also heated weeks of snow melt, including the frozen wastes of the typhoid patient, pouring it into the city's lower reservoirs. For Sedgwick, the lesson was the sanitarian credo: "the great necessity for perfect cleanliness—a lesson which mankind at large is slow to learn" (Sedgwick 1911, 205).

Sedgwick's report includes a vastly simplified map of Plymouth based on a more detailed map referred to in Taylor's article. Sedgwick's is not a map of either the outbreak or its investigation but rather presents in a pedestrian, editorial fashion the critical geographic features of Sedgwick's tale. Its sole purpose is to orient the reader to the environment in which brilliant public health officials deduced, without use of a map, the source of the disease outbreak. The large lettering and boldly drawn river give it the appearance of an authority Sedgwick did not invest in the map. "It's the water!"

the whole suggests. But then, it's *always* the water in this period of public health, if only one can ascertain precisely which water and where. The map can be compared not only with one by Taylor but also with a map by Dr. W. S. French. He was asked by William B. Smith, then mayor of Philadelphia, to "visit the scene of the epidemic and examine into the causes of the disease, its character, condition of the sufferers, and such information as will convey the exact situation of affairs at Plymouth" (French and Shakespeare 1885). Dr. E. O. Shakespeare, a Philadelphia Hospital pathologist, joined Taylor in this study.

The first step was to determine definitively what disease was rampant in Plymouth, a question to be answered post-mortem by Shakespeare. "Our investigation began by making the first post-mortem examination that had been performed. This autopsy proved beyond dispute that the patient died of perforation of the bowels, caused by the intestinal ulcerations of typhoid fever. The results of these autopsies [two others are reported] succeeded in convincing those physicians of the town who had up to that time firmly believed that the disease was not typhoid fever" (French and Shakespeare 1885, 10).

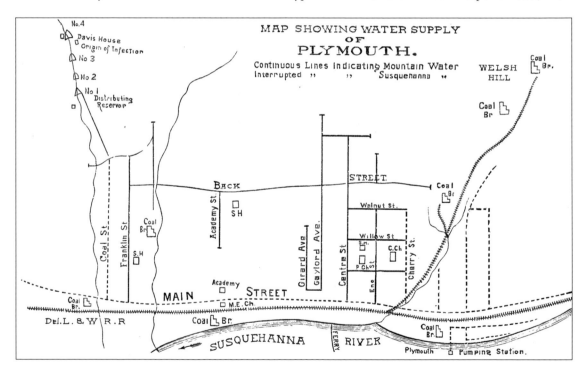

Figure 8.2 French and Shakespeare sketch map of the typhoid outbreak in Plymouth, Pennsylvania, used to show relative water sources in the typhoid-affected area. Citizens in the Welsh Hill area, whose water came from the Susquehanna, were relatively free of the disease affecting those whose water was drawn from the mountain stream reservoirs.

Source: Reproduced courtesy of College of Physicians of Philadelphia.

Having made that decision, they then considered possible disease sources ending with a conclusion similar to Taylor's. They, too, included a simple sketch map in their report to the mayor, one that was privately printed after submission. "In the subjoined map of the town the distribution of the two kinds of water is indicated. The source of mountain water is also pointed out, as well as the location of two dwellings upon the banks of the mountain stream. It will be noticed that Welsh Hill is not supplied from the pipes of the town of Plymouth" (French and Shakespeare 1885, 9).

Welsh Hill's eight hundred residents took their water from the Susquehanna at a point nearer to Wilkes-Barre than the rest of the town. Of the nine residents who became ill in the Welsh Hill area, "five of these used water, while at work or at school, from the pipes of the water company in other parts of the town. Two of the remaining cases used well water and are recent cases, in all probability infected from those first" (French and Shakespeare 1885). In other words, Welsh Hill represented an area whose water source was distinct from that of the outbreak, and whose residents, excepting those who took water from elsewhere, did not grow ill.

Here the map served both descriptive and analytic functions. The location of urban water sources and their relation to different Plymouth populations was considered graphically. Different sources were linked in the report to different wells used by residents. The outbreak was centered in the district whose water came from the mountain streams and reservoirs while a control population whose water was drawn directly from the river, the residents of Welsh Hill, were free of the disease. The French and Shakespeare map organizes two propositions, or perhaps a proposition and its null variant. If the typhoid outbreak is waterborne, then citizens whose water is drawn from the infected area should be sick while those whose water came from other sources would be free of the disease. Those in the latter group who became sick must be shown to have taken water in the infected area. Here was Snow's careful system of investigation transformed into common practice, albeit a practice not well considered by Sedgwick's overview of the case.

French and Shakespeare investigated for the mayor of Philadelphia who presumably was concerned that typhoid would somehow diffuse to his city. Their report laid that fear to rest. The most comprehensive study, however, and the most comprehensive map, was Dr. Taylor's report to the Pennsylvania Board of Health. Like French and Shakespeare, Taylor began with two questions: "What is this terrible sickness that is upon us?" and "What is the cause of so unusual an outbreak?" Typhoid fever was a frequent visitor to Pennsylvania towns, but the intensity of this outbreak, and its unusually high mortality rate of more than 10 percent, made this outbreak especially significant.

At first, local practitioners thought the disease might be malarial, or a type of meningitis, but "in a very short time its nature was made manifest and the doubt no longer existed that a true epidemic of typhoid fever was hanging over the doomed borough of Plymouth" (Turner 1991, 177). That caused some hard thinking. "Various theories were put forth, some declaring it to be due to the filth of the town;

some that it was due to drinking polluted well water; others polluted river water; others polluted mountain water; and still others that it was do to a peculiar condition of nature by no means explainable."

But as French and Shakespeare had proudly explained, post-mortem examination definitively named the disease the citizens of Plymouth were confronting. Taylor then mapped the major streets of Plymouth and distinguished them by their source of water from (a) reservoir, (b) river, (c) local brooks, or streams (d) a combination of reservoir and river water. The Plymouth Water Company typically pumped water from the Susquehanna into a 30,000–40,000 gallon reservoir near the Lance breaker (no. 11) that was full on March 26, just days before the epidemic started. Approximately thirty-five people living in town used that water and none of them became ill. Similarly, families living on Broadway, whose water also came from the Delaware and Hudson Coal Company remained healthy. So, too, did those who lived on Ridge Row, all of whose water had come from wells and springs since a Delaware and Hudson supply pipe (river water) had frozen and burst the previous January.

The principal water supply for almost all the 1,104 typhoid victims during the epidemic was the supposedly pure mountain stream and its downstream reservoir.

Before investigating the nature of the river's complicity, however, Taylor considered other theories. Might the disease have come down river from Wilkes-Barre, for example, three miles upstream of Plymouth? But not only were there just a few cases of typhoid reported in that town, and almost none in Welsh Hill, the flow of the current and the location of intake and outflow water pipes in the Susquehanna in both cities made contamination from Wilkes-Barre highly unlikely. The *only* likely source was the mountain stream, and the *only* possible source of stream contamination was the house of the unfortunate Mr. Davis who lived near the reservoir.

How much credit is to be given to French and Shakespeare and how much to Taylor is unclear at this remove. Certainly, Taylor's committee was first off the ground. He described the possibility of a contaminated reservoir in a communication to the *Wilkes-Barre Record* on April 29. The Plymouth Water Company, concerned with the suggestion, immediately struck a committee of physicians led by Taylor to investigate the outbreak. That committee's conclusions, presented to the company on May 7, were published in the following week in the *Philadelphia Medical News.* French and Shakespeare's involvement came a bit later but, at least from their report, was early involved through the first autopsies. There was, as well, an independent panel struck by the Philadelphia County Medical Society that later reviewed Taylor's conclusions. Finally, "a fourth investigation was made by a committee from the Buffalo Board of Health, Dr. A. H. Briggs being chairman" (Taylor 1886, 189), that similarly affirmed the findings of Taylor and his colleagues.

The map Taylor submitted first to the Plymouth Water Company and then with his report to the state's Board of Health distilled his argument and his careful search among possible sources of contamination. Unlike Sedgwick's, it includes the river pumping stations and the four different water sources that served the town at large. A compass rose and meridian line are added, as are, more

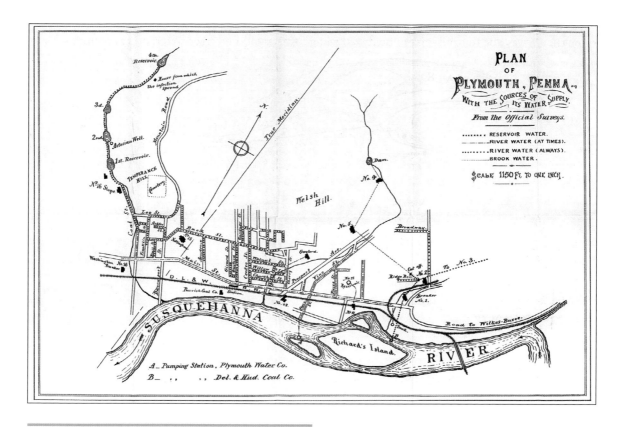

Figure 8.3 Taylor's map of a typhoid fever outbreak in Plymouth, Pennsylvania. Sedgwick later modified the map for his textbook on public health.

Source: Reproduced courtesy of College of Physicians of Philadelphia.

importantly, current lines for the Susquehanna. After all, the speed of the river current and location of sewage outflow and water intake pipes in Plymouth were potentially important data if, as some originally believed, the epidemic originated with contaminated Susquehanna River water from nearby Wilkes-Barre.

Taylor's report to the state board described the Plymouth outbreak as "one of the most remarkable epidemics in the history of typhoid fever," a phrase Sedgwick used without attribution. What was remarkable to Taylor was that "the origin of all this sorrow and desolation occurred miles away, on the mountain side, far removed from the populous town, and in a solitary house, situated upon the bank of a swift-running stream" (Taylor 1886, 104). This flew in the face of the general model inherited from those like Snow who had worked with localized water sources. For Taylor, the lesson was not Sedgwick's general sanitarian argument for cleanliness, but the manner in which diseased material may be sufficiently potent to contaminate urban cites that are geographically distant.

Taylor's map does not include the location of individual cases of typhoid. To add over one thousand by home address would have been time-consuming and difficult. The resulting map would have been unintelligible in its central section, a dark mass of dots or bars where water was received from the contaminated reservoir. It would be years before mapmaking progressed to a point where a complete dataset of disease incidence, including hundreds of cases, could be mapped.[1] Case location in this map is therefore inferred, drawn from the text into the map that worked with the text, drawing upon it.

What the map did was distill the text's general argument, its various propositions about possible sources of contamination in relation to the dense neighborhoods of epidemic outbreak. It presented a basic topology of the outbreak in a manner permitting different theories of contagion to be considered through an examination of the multiple water sources and their relation to the dense areas of disease incidence. The topology is the argument Taylor unveiled to insist upon the source whose distance Sedgwick announced as if it were obvious and clear to any sanitarian.

Sedgwick reduces both French and Shakespeare's sketch map and Taylor's careful mapping to a line art illustration, their measured investigations to a simple and perhaps simplistic sanitarian thesis. With Sedgwick's simplification the map becomes the punch line but not the story. Students reading his textbook must have shaken their heads in wonder. Remarkable? It was obvious. "Of course it was the mountain stream," they told each other. "What makes all this so special?" Nor was Sedgwick's simplification of Snow's work any less egregious. It reduced hard science to a *Classic Comic's* rendition of the Broad Street outbreak. "Snow may have been a great man," students must have told each other, "but even an idiot could have seen the complicity of the Broad Street pump, hey?" This is the limit of the simplified teaching case, in which complex reality is leavened to the cartoon-like obvious. That's what Sedgwick did with his maps and what others would do as well.

Ignored by Sedgwick was the importance of Taylor's report appearing in the first annual report of the state board constituted to consider issues of health. Here was the real sanitarian impact, one distinct from the epidemiology of the typhoid outbreak itself. The very existence of the report spoke to the growing recognition of issues of urban infrastructure and the complex of diseases that an evolving nineteenth century city might face. It thus included a dot map of the state population as a means of declaring its legitimate domain of interest and individual reports on the infrastructure of specific cities. The graded circles representing different population levels distinguished clearly between urban and rural areas of the state and the very distinct health problems that occurred in both.

Taylor's study was a scientific coup for the state board of health, a way of declaring it would investigate health problems anywhere and report without fear or favor. Other maps occurred in different chapters detailing health issues in other cities and towns, of course. The section on Harrisburg, Pennsylvania, for example, was at pains to consider issues of water contamination through a mapping of the intakes and outflows of the local sewage and water systems. The first was also a potential source of odor and disease, the later the public water supply that required protection and care. Lest any misinterpret the message,

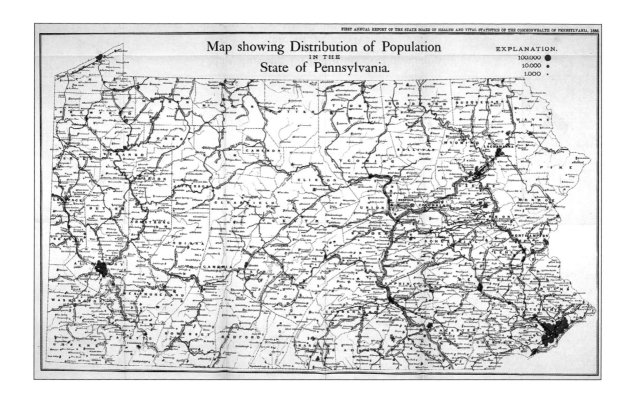

Figure 8.4   Map of the population of Pennsylvania in the first annual state report on health.

Source: Reproduced courtesy of College of Physicians of Philadelphia.

this map was juxtaposed with a map of local population. Rather, it is the same map handled differently. Here were the concerns of McClellan's correspondents transposed to the scale of statewide attention. While distrust of the federal government and its intervention in local health affairs remained, there was to be, in the future, no doubt of the necessity of state involvement in local affairs. Where there was a health problem, or a condition that threatened the health of a city, the state and its officials could be counted on to be involved.

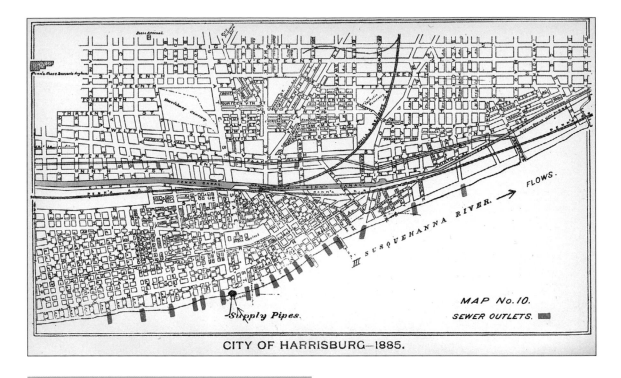

Figure 8.5 Map of sewer outlets in Harrisburg, Pennsylvania, for the first annual report of the state board of health. The map illustrates a discussion of water and sanitation in the city.

Source: Reproduced courtesy of College of Physicians of Philadelphia.

The divorce

From the 1850s into the early 1890s, ever-more ambitious maps were increasingly evident in official reports; the U.S. Congressional report on the 1873 epidemic and Taylor's report on the typhoid epidemic are examples of the greater trend. But in the evolving field of public health, their use became, by the turn of the century, more and more descriptive, less and less analytic. After the halcyon days of Snow and Whitehead, and then of researchers like Christie, McClellan, and Taylor, mapping as anything but a descriptive tool illustrating the tenets of "sanitary science" seems to have stopped. For decades, medical mapping was progressively relegated to the back burner of public health even as maps (atlases, road maps, city maps, etc.) became ever-more omnipresent artifacts of twentieth-century society.

The reasons for this are multiple and interrelated. First, after Snow and his colleagues, after the work of McClellan and Taylor, people knew where to look in their search for the locus of a disease outbreak. Water was the default culprit in an environment of "pathogenic air and corrupt earth" (Marriott 2003). In a young, if evolving, discipline whose most famous application was in the address of cholera

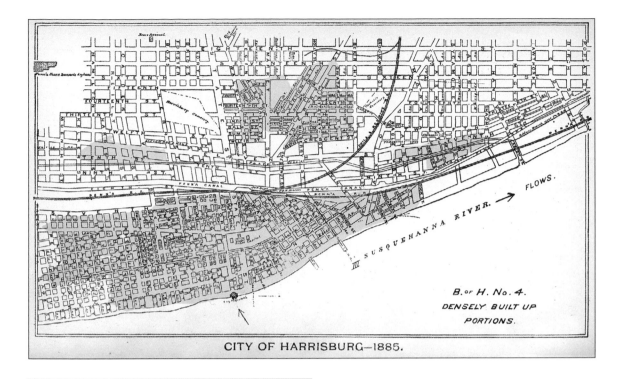

Figure 8.6 Map of Harrisburg, Pennsylvania, population from the first Pennsylvania annual report of the state board of health. This map and its predecessor of sewer outlets were used to consider sewer and water supply in relation to population.

Source: Reproduced courtesy of College of Physicians of Philadelphia.

and typhoid outbreaks, evolving bacteriology gave added weight to the assumption that contaminated water was almost always the source of epidemic disease. The sanitarian perspective, one that pointed to uncleanliness as the causative agent of most disease outbreaks, set the agenda of public health as a sanitary science. Investigators knew to look to filthy living conditions and local water supplies in the poorest areas of cities when cholera, plague, typhoid fever, tuberculosis, typhus, or any other disease occurred at epidemic levels. One did not need Taylor's or Snow's careful topography because *of course* one would find the index case occurred at or near the source of the patient's water supply.

Secondly, in the late nineteenth and early twentieth centuries, bacteriology, the ability to test water for the presence of a specific bacterium, a technique rapidly becoming standard procedure throughout the international medical community, was ascendant. "As the responsible organisms and the modes of transmission were worked out, much good and useful earlier work passed into obscurity" (Davies 1957, 1). Not only did one know more or less where to look, one also knew how to prove that the source of the outbreak was not the Susquehanna (polluted though it might be) but the area near the fourth reservoir along the stream north of town.

"It was most unfortunate that the great achievements of the germ theory carried with them an almost complete neglect of spatial and environmental analysis" (Learmonth 1988, 12). Put another way, in this period it was all germ theory that was quickly folded into the sanitarian perspective by early public health officials. The careful lessons learned earlier about the ecologies of disease seemed antiquated in the face of the knowledge that this or that bacterium was the "real" cause of a specific illness. As a consequence, Sedgwick, writing about the 1885 outbreak first in 1901 and later in the fourth edition in 1911, did not feel compelled to credit the careful steps of Taylor's investigation that considered all elements of the topology of the outbreak in attempting to identify the center of an outbreak.

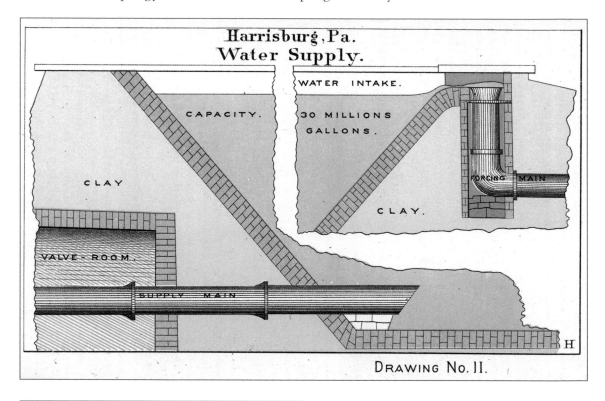

Figure 8.7 An image of the water supply for Harrisburg from the first report to the state board of health. The use of color and detail signify the pride of town officials in their water system and the importance assigned to it by the state officials who published the report.

Source: Courtesy of Cliff, Haggett, and Smallman-Raynor and reproduced with permission from Hodder Education.

A third factor was the seemingly prosaic issue of not map production but reproduction, the necessity of the clearest possible image for a mass printing whose individual illustrations would serve an instructional function. Maps loaded with names, places, arrows, and lines did not reproduce particularly well. Simple, black-and-white line drawings were easier to produce, and thus less expensive. They looked better, and they were easier to read. What to map and how to map it were issues not of scientific investigation but, for a textbook, what could be clearly and inexpensively reproduced. While public reports might squander money on multicolored images, the complexity and resulting expense of their production made them unlikely for inclusion in nongovernmental publications, especially those for teaching. The result is often startling different mapping, the difference between, for example, Taylor's map and the one Sedgwick drew based upon it.

The limits of reproduction technologies pervaded medical mapping through much of the twentieth century. Increasingly, the maps reduced arguments in a radically selective fashion that gave no hint of the thinking that lay beneath them. Compare the map of world cholera diffusion included by McClellan in his report, or those of earlier researchers, and the maps by Cliff and Haggett in their 1988 *Atlas of Disease Distribution.* The former was hard to reproduce, the quality insufficient to permit an easy understanding. Its complexity served, however, in a time when the facts about cholera's origin and diffusion remained in doubt. The names of cities and years if not days on which cholera first appeared (in Moscow and St. Petersburg, in Birmingham or London) were necessary elements of the arguments the earlier maps presented. The maps by Cliff and Haggett are clear, simple line drawings that make the progress of the disease seem obvious, a given. But by 1988, Cliff and Haggett did not *need* to map the individual cities and countries as part of an evolving argument. The facts were well known and the proposition of diffusion accepted; all they needed was the conclusion.[2]

This brings forth another distinguishing characteristic that affected medical mapping in the late nineteenth and early twentieth centuries. McClellan and his contemporaries typically drew on existing maps and did not make their own from scratch. Sedgwick's, and the maps of his successors, were typically the product of mapmakers whose principal job was to create maps for publication. Cartography as a distinct discipline was a nineteenth-century creation (Wood 2004a) whose average practitioner typically became, in the twentieth century, an illustrator of the science of others. Their medium was the textbook, the journal article, or the newspaper story (Monmonier 1989). What was lost in the process of professional, graphic presentation was the thinking of the principle investigator who was good at mapping but not necessarily mapmaking, who could use maps but not draft one that served the stringently simple requirements of textbook (or journal) publishers.[3]

Sedgwick's maps served his publications precisely because they did *not* need to serve as analytic tools. The simplified image of the town of Plymouth, Pennsylvania, is easy to read because it is illustrative of his story. His Broad Street map served because it did not consider the various elements that Snow detailed in his topology. Sedgwick's maps were tools of the authors' and publishers' trade

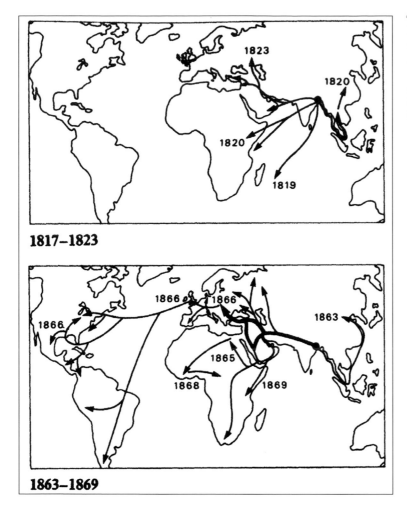

1817–1823

1863–1869

Figure 8.8 Map of historical cholera pathways in Cliff and Haggett's *Atlas of Disease Distribution.*

Source: Courtesy of Cliff, Haggett, and Smallman-Raynor and reproduced with permission from Hodder Education.

rather than those of the investigating physician or public health expert. Here one sees the process of illustrative mapmaking divorced from mapping as a way to understand the relation between a disease outbreak, its host population, and the environment that joined them both.

Of at least equal importance was that "modern statistical thinking appeared at the end of the nine-teenth century" (Gould et al. 1991, 81), supplanting the mapped approach and the resulting emphasis on spatiality that had informed the pioneers of epidemiology and public health. The advances of the "Paris School" of medical statistics began with mapping as an equal partner in the consideration of the relation of states of disease and health. In the twentieth century, a less graphic, principally numeric approach came to dominate both public health in general and the investigation of epidemic disease in particular. The assumption was that one did not need mapping if there were good statistical tools at hand, that mapping at best was a way of describing the results of a rigorous investigation whose answer was in the number, the bivariate regression, perhaps, not the interaction of complex environment factors. Mapping as a tool of medical geography, and medical geography as a subdiscipline of medical science, was yesterday's news, artifacts of a different, less rigorous age.

Nonwaterborne diseases
Plague

Sedgwick's sanitarian perspective served well enough for those relatively simple, two-step diseases (bacterium-host) whose vectors were waterborne. But at the end of the nineteenth and in the early decade of the twentieth centuries other illnesses with different etiologies appeared. In 1894, for example, a plague epidemic began in Hong Kong, entered southern China, and then progressed south through Amoy and other islands. By 1896, it reached Bombay where more than 250,000 people died from it. From there, plague traveled over land and by sea by the same routes that cholera had followed earlier, to St. Petersburg, Russia, and to Europe. In its determined course this, the plague's third international pandemic, made its way around the world, including in its travels populations in Africa, Australia, and England. Finally, in 1905, it reached the United States (Marriott 2003, 121).

At the end of the nineteenth century it was assumed that plague, like cholera, was fostered primarily by filth and unsanitary conditions, a disease "mainly conveyed from place to place by individuals in their person, clothing and personal effects" (Marriott 2003, 113). The houses and possessions of its victims were therefore cleaned and scrubbed in an attempt to stem its tide. The principal agent of the disease was assumed to be the rat whose wholesale death—they fell in the streets and in every plague house—accompanied every outbreak. The disease did strike first and hardest in areas where sanitation was minimal, living conditions overcrowded, and waste disposal minimal. Rats were a symbol of unsanitary conditions in overcrowded cities with poor sanitation and drainage. Of course they were the agent responsible. It was so obvious that in 1904, at the height of the San Francisco epidemic, a bounty was placed on rats and local residents were encouraged to kill them and bring in the corpse for a reward. This helped infect the poor who sought the bounty, permitting the true carries of the disease, rat fleas, to transfer from the rat corpse to the body of the bounty hunter.

That the rat itself was a victim of *Zenopsylla cheopis,* the flea that lived upon it and the true vector of the bacillus *Pasteurella pestits,* was a discovery that took years of study, argument, and debate. Like Seaman and Pascalis, late-nineteenth-century sanitarians and health officials missed the intervening vector. The flea-rat-human *ménage a trois* of infection and transmission was a reality too complex for a simple sanitarian argument.

Influenza

In the early decades of the twentieth century, professors of sanitary science almost reflexively blamed the victim, condemning the greater prevalence of most diseases on the squalor of the unhygienic poor, or secondarily, the failed infrastructure of the evolving city. It was far simpler than considering the complex relation between globalization, industrialization, and urbanization that were the underlying context of most epidemic and pandemic experiences. In a 1909 article on *Hygiene im Weltverkeh* (Hygiene in World Trade), for example, the Austrian, R. Pösch, "argued that it was man himself who created the most important cause for the spread of diseases throughout the world by his initiation of world trade" (Jusatz 1969, 20). Appearing in the third edition of Karl von Andree's *Geographie des Welthandels* (Geography of World Trade), an otherwise dry compendium of the general demographics, mineral deposits, and production facilities of trading countries around the world, Pösch's article did not appear in the geography's fourth edition. Even if true, trade was the lifeblood of the evolving international community, and to criticize it was to criticize modernity itself.

At the end of World War I "as the world's people were celebrating the end of war, the end of dying, and a fresh beginning, the second and most virulent of three waves of a new killer, 'Spanish influenza,' raged with a ferocity greater than all the killing power of the previous four years of war, killing tens of millions" (Duncan 2003, 7). The war was a perfect breeding ground for the new variant of the old influenza, an epidemic disease first reported in China before 1500 and well described by Hippocrates in 462 BC. The virus had mutated time and again, changing slowly as it moved through varying populations across more than two millennia. At the end of World War I it emerged in a new variant, a final murderous figment of the war.

The virus blossomed first in garrisons and barracks and then in the cities and villages affected by the war, often devastated places to which thousands of exhausted, often ill soldiers returned at the end of hostilities. Troops traveling to and returning from the Europe war provided a perfect vector for the new virus's diffusion. So, too, did the resumption of continental trade patterns at the end of the war. Railroads and ships carried goods and people across continents and around the world. With them traveled the virus that became the influenza epidemic of the century; with them traveled other bacteria and viruses, too.

Its universality can be derived from the names individual countries gave to the disease. The Royal College of Physicians in Great Britain called it the "Spanish influenza," but the British troops whose brethren died from it called it "Flanders Grippe" because it was in Flanders's Field that they (and Canadians) first encountered it. The Spanish named the disease the "Naples Soldier," an auxiliary arm of the Italian army. In Poland it was called the Bolshevik Disease, while in Ceylon it was assumed to be Indian, a "Bombay Fever" (Duncan 2003, 7). History remembers the pandemic as the Spanish flu because, as a noncombatant, Spain did not censor information on its location and spread in the manner of combatant nations.[4]

The sanitarian perspective did not serve either to describe the path of its diffusion or the ferocity of its effect. How could it? Influenza was a viral disease spread between persons, and the lessons of nineteenth century medicine had been about bacterial conditions that were largely waterborne. Plague, influenza, and a host of other diseases with different etiologies required different approaches to disease investigation, new understandings of the relation between agent, host, and the environments that promoted or inhibited their interaction. That would require a far more advanced science and an approach that returned to a dynamic but nondeterministic ecological perspective.

Sandfly fever

In the early decades of the twentieth century, a number of researchers considered a range of illnesses affecting not international but local, and typically colonial, populations. Like the work of Christie in Africa, these studies were by local researchers intimately concerned with the health of the people in their jurisdictions, populations quite distant from the evolving issues of urban centers in developing countries. This work required a type of analysis foreign to Sedgwick or the simple equivalences of the early years of infectious disease as a serious, disciplined study. Often and almost inevitably the work was mapped. The most successful examples of this period are those of relatively localized diseases whose elements could be investigated at the scale of the village or town.

Consider, for example, the work of Young and his colleagues on sandfly fever in the Peshawar district of India in the 1920s (Young, Richmond, and Brendish 1926). Understanding this condition, one that did not travel into the temperate, industrialized world, meant understanding the relation between its vector of transmission, *P. Papatassi,* and the habitat it shared with host human populations. The incidence of disease therefore was at once an entomological and an epidemiological challenge. The impetus for the work was military preparedness. British troops stationed in the district were falling ill from a fever their physicians did not understand. To control the fever—antibiotics for its treatment didn't exist, of course—required physicians first study the disease and its determinants so that its effect might be minimized, controlled.

What was known was that hospital admissions tended to peak during periods of relatively heavy spring rain, with secondary spikes in the weeks following them. Further, different populations in the Peshawar district seemed more susceptible than did others. British troops stationed in the area were at greatest risk. Gurkha soldiers were less likely to be affected, and other, local Indian troops and non-military citizenry were least likely to be affected during outbreaks of the regionally endemic disease. This data was summarized in several charts for the years of the study of which one for 1922 is a typical example.

The researchers were charged with the medical care of garrisoned British soldiers who yearly suffered from sandfly fever. Knowing when the disease peaked was useful for medical planning, but it also meant they thus knew when, and also where, to seek the fly's larva—its stage before hatching—in the weeks before outbreaks could be expected. If the fever was most prevalent in the British garrison, it made sense to search near to the barracks and common areas on the assumption that flies would hatch in the greatest number near those locations where the most people were affected.

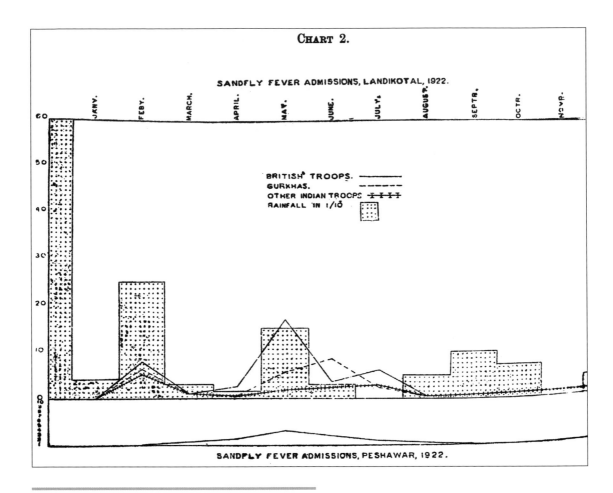

Figure 8.9 Chart of incidence of sandfly fever and rainfall in Peshawar, India, over a ten-month period. British troops were more susceptible than either Gurkha soldiers or local personnel.

Source: Rare Books and Special Collections, University of British Columbia Library.

Young and his colleagues therefore sought samples from suspected breeding grounds in Landikotal, a hutted camp grouped around the British fort. Located on an alluvial plain in the Khyber Pass at an average elevation of 3,500 feet, local temperatures ranged from around freezing in the winter months to 100 to 104 degrees Fahrenheit in the summer. This data was later also correlated with rainfall, elevation, and incidence of sandfly occurrence in a search for more specific patterns of sandfly habitat limits.

The map of local data that results carries contour lines of increasing altitude for the lands directly to the south and north of the flat plane on which the camp itself was constructed. Breeding grounds from different sites within the camp are identified in the map by their proximity to one or another military

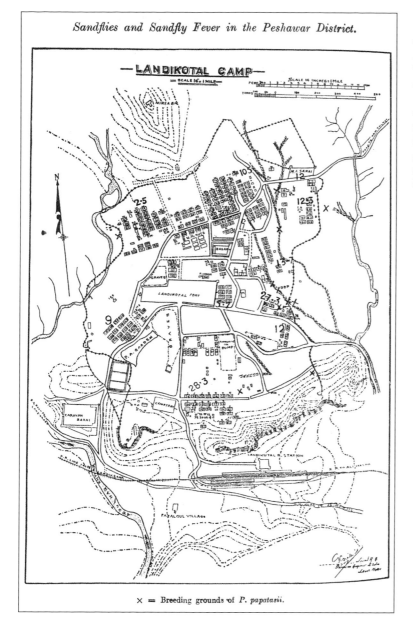

Sandflies and Sandfly Fever in the Peshawar District.

X = Breeding grounds of *P. papatasii.*

Figure 8.10 Sandfly topography in the British garrison at Peshawar, India. The "x" indicates breeding grounds of *P. Papatassi.* Numbers reflect the incidence of sandfly larvae found in the camp (Young, Richmond, and Brendish 1926).

Source: Rare Books and Special Collections, University of British Columbia Library.

group (Royal Fusiliers, Gurkha Rifles, Garrison engineers, etc.). Mapped are both the sites with the greatest prevalence of the sandfly, and simultaneously, their proximity to specific British regiments. The range of sandflies and their proximity to the general domain of camp structures and facilities is seamlessly fused to the plain of the map. The average daily catch in the area of the Gurkha Rifles was

A.	B.	C.	D.	E.	F.	G.	H.
Rajput Lines opposite Garrison Engineer's office.	Rajput Lines new Guard Room on side of main road.	Rajput Lines north of main road.	Rajput Lines alongside Fort.	Pack Battery lines.	Royal Fusiliers.	Royal Fusiliers north of road.	Gurkha Rifles Lines.
24	39	21	3	5	7	6	3
12	32	11	5	8	12	14	2
9	28	13	5	9	14	11	
9	21	8	5	12	13	9	..
14	28	10	6	8	15	12	..
9	19	10	9	10	13	11	..
15	24	11	7	11	..	..	..
TOTAL . 92	191	84	40	63	74	63	5
Average 13·1	27·3	12	5·7	9	12·3	10·5	2·5

Figure 8.11 Chart of sandfly larva counts at locations within the British garrisons at Peshawar, India. Rows describe counts on different days while columns describe the locations. Average counts summarized in the table are included in the map that accompanied the study (Young, Richmond, and Brendish 1926).

Source: Rare Books and Special Collections, University of British Columbia Library.

2.5, for example, while the catch in the area of the Royal Fusiliers was 12.3. On the road near the engineers' office the count was 27.3.

The conclusion once again seemed obvious. Since the fly habitats were found most typically in broken ground and near transport lines, "the problem of permanent material reduction of sandfly breeding in Landikotal would therefore appear to resolve itself into measures aimed at abolishing broken grounds in the sides of the nullahs [local buildings], and near the transport lines" (Young, Richmond, and Brandish 1926, 1017). They didn't think that complete eradication of the indigenous sandfly was either possible or even necessary. They did conclude, however, that a significant reduction in larvae population, and thus fever incidence, could be realized by any of several approaches their paper then considered.

What is impressive about this work is its marrying of entomology, epidemiology and "medical" or "climatic" geography in service of an attempt to understand the life cycle and habitat of the fly that carried the fever the physicians were called each year to treat. The researcher's published sketch map joined both observed fly catches and the buildings of the garrison whose individuals became ill into a composite range whose real domain was not the camp but the x-marked breeding grounds of the fly itself. All this occurred within a mapped environment that was at once physical, social, and geographic: the layout of the camp and its garrisons with the area's rivers, transport lines, and altitude contour lines. The intent of the map was to understand the incidence of sandfly fever through an understanding of the fly's occurrence within the habitat it shared with human hosts.

Compared to Sedgwick's simplistic but easily read maps, which were taken as a standard by Gilbert and his successors, Young's map was crude and difficult to interpret without the text in which it was embedded. But then its venue was an obscure academic journal, not a profitable textbook or a federally funded report like McClellan's. Nor was sandfly fever an international epidemic but a localized problem in a colonial backwater that was nonetheless an important subject to medical personnel in charge of colonial troops and local civilians. The researchers were facing a relatively unknown condition whose principal vector had uncertain habits and whose habitat had yet to be investigated. The map therefore is closer to Snow's original topography than to the maps of sanitarians in the early decades of the twentieth century.

The table whose data is distilled in the map includes basic sandfly accounts over time at specific testing locations. The average of those counts is included in the map to show relative incidence of sandflies, describing their habitat in terms of density as well as simple location. The result (mapped and in tabular form) suggests the degree to which the mapping that was prevalent in early sanitarian work became, in the early decades of the twentieth century, a tool for exploration in areas other than the established schools of public health and "sanitary science." In addition it offers evidence of the early mapping of geographic databases—incidence of rainfall and sandfly populations, for example—whose figures were then integrated into the map surface as part of an extended argument. No longer was the issue one of simple incidence, *à la* Seaman and Pascalis, but instead of density of incidence at a location and at a specific time.

What the map makes clear and what the chart does not, is the relation between the observed incidence of sandflies and of the troops most afflicted by the disease they carried. It is this general approach, albeit one with stronger mathematics and better graphics, that would come into its own after World War II as a result both of a reemergence of disease ecology and a commitment by the military of advanced nations to consider the general relation between disease and environment in the theaters of their continuing engagements.

Endnotes

1. As chapter 11 explains in a discussion of GIS mapping of the Snow data, this would eventually require, at this scale, a more three-dimensional approach with multiple deaths indicated at individual homes, towers built upon a geographical sum of incidence.

2. A more common argument would be that Cliff and Haggett's maps, and those of Sedgwick, were "better" graphics, better able to communicate. Those included by McClellan suffer because of their complexity and, perhaps at times, unfortunate symbolization. This argument (Tufte 1983, for example) perceives maps as graphic products to be judged by standards of legibility and ease of communication. It tends to ignore, however, the distinction made here between those representing the mapping of researchers, "working maps," in a disease study, and those drawn afterward solely as descriptive devices to enhance an argument made in some other, primary medium (charts, tables, text).

3. A similar phenomenon occurred again in the 1990s. At that time, however, graphic illustrators became the artisans whose function was to transform working maps of researchers into illustratively potent images for newspapers, reports, and books. In some cases these illustrators worked with digital maps themselves, with the primary software programs, and in other cases through graphics programs like Adobe PhotoShop® or the hoary Microsoft program, Paint.

4. Cliff, Haggett, and Smallman-Raynor (2004, 88–89) provide a useful and detailed review of the 1918 epidemic within a broader context of influenza generally. They note especially the effect of the military in its spread in nations like England, and internationally, Australia.

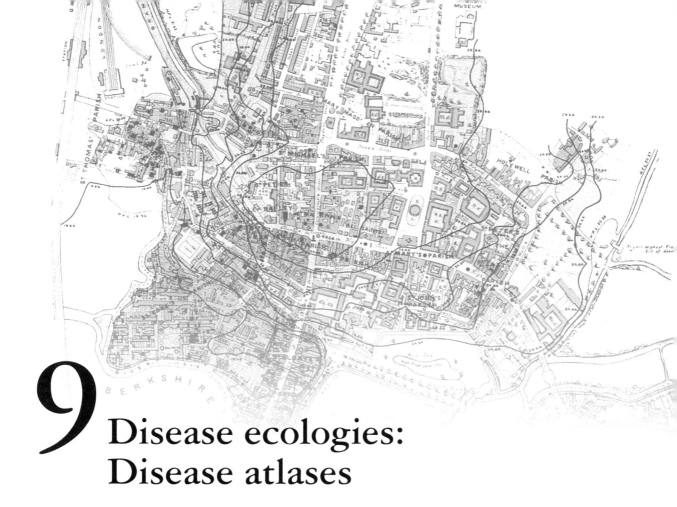

9 Disease ecologies: Disease atlases

Medicine was on the move in the years immediately following World War II. So, too, of course, were the viral and bacterial communities whose advances for a time were outpaced by those of medical science. Despite the poliomyelitis pandemic of the early 1950s (Wackers 1994, chapter 4), or the influenza pandemic that followed it in the 1950s, we do not think of this period as disease-ridden. As the world rebuilt after the war, penicillin and sulfa drugs became the base of a growing arsenal of antibiotics that promised not cures but treatments for a vast range of common, endemic diseases. A vaccine for polio was created at the cutting edge of virology, as old-style, Mendelian genetics was beginning to give way to a new, deeper understanding based upon DNA's double helix. What Lewis Thomas called *The Youngest Science* (1983) was entering adolescence. With it came new perspectives on disease and the factors that promoted or inhibited its occurrence. In the process, medical geography and medical mapping were reborn as dynamic and probabilistic rather than static and deterministic enterprises.

Jacques M. May

A former professor of surgery at the Medical College of the University of Hanoi, Jacques M. May became, in the late 1940s, the head of the Department of Medical Geography for the New York–based American Geographical Society (AGS). May was first and foremost a medical doctor, an avuncular physician-geographer who quoted this or that experience in medical school, this or that saying of a fondly remembered instructor. His focus had shifted from one typical of his medical generation—"the attention of physicians has been focused on the symptoms of disease" (May 1950)—to the broader social and physical conditions that encouraged both the generation and diffusion of endemic and epidemic diseases among human populations. Like John Snow, May's youthful medical experiences among the poor influenced his later research. And, again like Snow, those experiences made him more aware than most that "disease is a multiple phenomenon which occurs only if various factors coincide in time and space. The focus of interest widens to encompass the relationship between the various factors of this complex and their respective geographical components" (May 1950, 9).

With a substantial (for its day) $15,000 grant from the Upjohn Company, May and the AGS began the systematic formulation of a modern medical geography whose goal was to understand the interrelations between physical geography, social context, and disease pathology. "Some of these relationships are well known; many have not yet been explored in a sufficient number of cases to have statistical significance" (May 1950, 12). His goal was nothing less than to rewrite the study of endemic and epidemic disease in a manner that would expose the ecologies that fostered the relationship between agent, host, and vectors in a way that was statistically as well as experientially relevant.

To do this, May had to rewrite the definition of disease itself. "Disease is that alternation of living cells or tissues that jeopardizes survival in their environment," he wrote in the introduction to the second volume of his *Studies in Disease Ecology* (1961). The definition "is an opportune reminder that there is no function without structure," a concept that in his work encompassed the ecology promoting or inhibiting relations between a microbial agent (typically bacterial), its vector of diffusion (insect, rat, tick), and human hosts. "Disease, any disease—and let me remind you that by disease I mean maladjustment to the environment—can never occur without the combination of three orders of factors converging in time and space, that is, there must be stimuli from the environment, there must be responses from an agent, and there must be the conglomeration of thoughts and traits that we call culture" (May 1961, xvi).

By culture May meant the elements operative at a location with a specific physical profile (altitude, rainfall, soil types, temperature, etc.) as well as human settlement characteristics that encouraged or inhibited a relation between agent and host. "From the ecologist's point of view, society is an organization of living things based on a pattern of mutual tolerance that occurs for a brief period of time after the dynamism of reciprocal exclusion has been temporarily exhausted" (May 1961, xvii). A generation later, Mayer (1996, 441) would summarize May's approach: "Basic to the disease ecologic approach

[May presented] is understanding how humanity, including culture, society and behavior; the physical world, including topography, vegetation, and climate; and biology, including vector and pathogen ecology, interact together in an evolving and interactive system, to produce foci of disease."

May took the general thinking of the climatic and geographical determinists to a new, nondeterministic level. His work is most noted for its approach to a disease hazard—the propensity for a disease in a location—based on specific ecologies that sustain specific agents of individual vector-borne diseases. Thus, in considering malaria he thought of, first, the environmental conditions that were most favorable to the mosquito-carrier and, secondly, those that were most likely to assure the diffusion of the disease from areas where the mosquito was endemic. In this work he considered inorganic stimuli, microclimatic and biogeographic variables, and finally, a broad range of sociocultural behaviors by humans themselves (Pyle 1979, 81–83).

May's map of malarial vectors is a good example of his approach. On an elliptical, Euro-centric projection, the nations of the world are mapped beneath a surface of symbols describing the distribution of *anopheles* and other mosquito species known to carry the *Plasmodium* protozoa that is malaria's principal agent. It is not a map of disease incidence but of disease potential, of the sites of potential vectors of the disease. "The presence of the vector alone does not suffice to create transmission as long as only accidental introduction of the agent occurs. This is what happens in the United States, in Queensland, Australia, and in other territories where the disease has been eradicated" (May 1961, 227). In his text he considered the specific, environmental factors favorable to malaria carrying species, describing the geographical suitability of various environments for different species. The result is a careful, graphic consideration of malarial potential based on the location of disease carriers, their habitats in different geographic environments.

Those areas where the social and geographic conditions conspire to create reservoirs of endemic diseases were a special concern to May. He called these areas "foci" and was at some pains to consider in them the congregation of factors that resulted in endemic disease occurrence, for example those of plague and cholera. The mapped results of his analysis appear somewhat crude today, sketch maps of his broader argument. The "schematic map of the natural plague foci of the world," for example, attempts to distill what in his text is a detailed consideration of the complex persistence "of the causative organisms in animal hosts and the conveyance of the infection to man, as well as among the animal hosts through the ectoparasites, chiefly fleas, of the latter" (May 1961, 433).

In this map, he distinguished between areas of "natural focality" where the disease had been historically recurrent, "especially active foci" where the disease was endemic, and "little investigated foci" where the biogeographic characteristics created conditions ripe for an outbreak. The surface that resulted presented a historical summary of plague in terms of frequency of occurrence with data aggregated from regional and national health histories. The issue was not simply "plague is here," but, more importantly, "plague has been in these places more frequently than those places over time." That

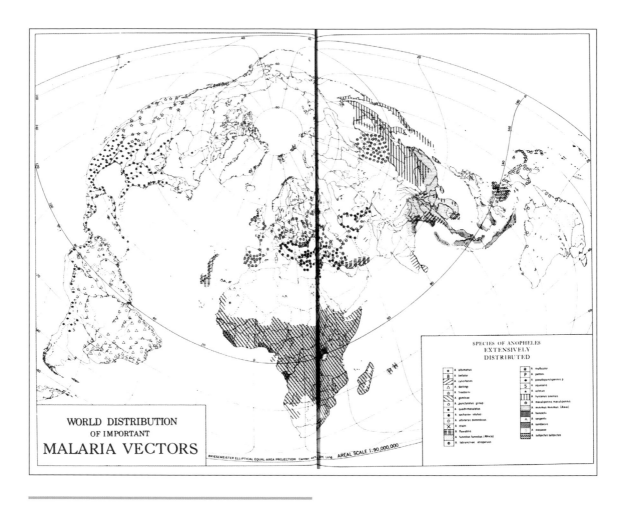

Figure 9.1 World distribution of mosquito populations carrying malaria. Note that in Africa the darkened area reflects the overlapping populations of two or more mosquito species.

Source: © American Geographical Society.

the historical correlations were crude and the mapping rudimentary does not detract from the map's importance or the importance of the data it attempted to present.

May's work reflected a self-conscious, American commitment to issues of international health that was at once altruistic and self-serving. In the immediate post-war environment "The President of the United States has declared his intention to lead the country into a new program for the advancement of backward areas of the world. When the time comes to enforce this policy, there will be a demand for facts about these backward areas. The question will be asked, what makes these people backward? What causes countries to be underdeveloped?" (May 1950, 40). For May and for others, these were questions that, in the immediate post-war years, the United States was required to ask. Its then-new position as an international superpower came with the responsibility to consider the health and economic status of less-developed, less-powerful nations. Medical geographers were among those who sought to serve the national imperative by providing answers to questions of disease causation.

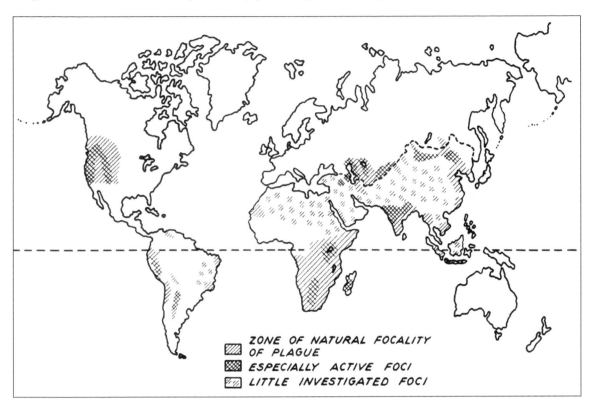

Figure 9.2 May's schematic map of plague foci, distinguishing between environments where plague was known, recurrent, and in some cases, epidemic.

Source: © American Geographical Society.

There was a measure of self-interest in this altruism. International trade was the lifeblood of the evolving post-industrial world in which the United States perceived itself a leader. This demanded, in turn, a global congregation of healthy workers employed in a manner that would permit them to harvest raw goods for American factories and to use their wages to be consumers of U.S. products. May's work was a self-conscious and very American attempt to bring "backward" people to a modern standard of living, a modern, U.S.-style socioeconomic perspective, and into a U.S.-dominated world economy. "Medical geography could become a preliminary step to the redemption of backward countries throughout the world; for, in our final definition, it is the systematic study of the correlations that exist between the diseases of the land and the diseases of the people" (May 1950, 40–41). It was the conviction of the day that health, prosperity, and a consumer-based, capitalist economy were interrelated and that the best way to advance less-developed worlds, therefore, was to urge the universal adoption of a U.S.-style socioeconomic structure. Issues of disease and health were just a piece of the greater, geopolitical puzzle.

Another way to think of May's ecology of disease is to locate it within the history that preceded it. Chadwick, Mayhew, and Booth were among the first to articulate the manner in which patterns of class, economics, habitation, and socioeconomic structure created an environment in which the spread of specific diseases was favored. Researchers like Farr and McClellan added broadly geographic attributes (altitude, the river, etc.) and human transportation systems to this social perspective. Careful local studies of disease in India and Africa added depth to the understanding of the relation of environment to disease vectors (the sandfly, for example) at a local scale. May built upon that history to craft a perspective integrating social and physical attributes into an encompassing disease ecology.

Rodenwaldt and Jusatz

May was not alone in either his ecological focus or his belief that it offered a necessary solution to the problems of international disease. Nor was he alone in his mapping of the relation between agent, vector, and host. Also in the 1950s, Ernst Rodenwaldt, E. Bader, Helmut J. Jusatz, and their colleagues at the Heidelberg Academy of Science were involved in a conceptually similar but very distinct, even more ambitious project. The principal result of their work was the monumental, multivolume *Welt Seuchen Atlas,* published with varying supplements and additions between 1952 and 1961. May's work was written, produced, and distributed by the American Society of Geographers in a format that could be easily accessed by government officials and public health officers. It was small enough to fit on a doctor's shelf and sufficiently inexpensive—its maps were in black and white—to be affordable to all. Rodenwaldt and Jusatz's large-format (75 x 50 cm) atlas was a more scholarly, less-accessible, and far more-expensive work destined for university and research libraries. Its three volumes were glorious, filled with full-page, color maps on the back of which smaller, detailed maps were included with supporting data. To this were added dense pages of text in German and English.

The coordinator for this extraordinary project, completed with the support of the U.S. military, was U.S. Navy Captain A. R. Behnke. In a real way, the *Welt Seuchen Atlas* was an offshoot of the allied victory in World War II, one building on the work of German medical experts who, after the war, were put under the general supervision of the U.S. military's medical experts. The *Welt Seuchen Atlas* of epidemic disease was begun during World War II as a contribution to the German war effort, its subject matter limited to "diseases and areas of military importance" (Cliff and Haggett 2003, 526). It was also a self-conscious attempt to advance the concepts underlying Hirsch's nineteenth-century *Handbook of Geographical and Historical Pathology.* The result was to be a modern *Atlas of Epidemic*

Diseases that would showcase the work of German epidemiologists at the Institute of Hygiene at the University of Berlin and demonstrate Germany's leadership in "geomedicine" as a principal branch of epidemiology.

In the post-war period, the *Welt Seuchen Atlas* was expanded under Behnke's supervision to include all major diseases in an encyclopedic, general ecology of endemic and epidemic diseases. In its final incarnation, the medicine it presented served the broad U.S. goals articulated by May, and not coincidentally, the need of the U.S. military for data on the medical terrain of areas around the world where U.S. forces might be sent. The result was an extraordinary primer on disease ecology at a range of scales.

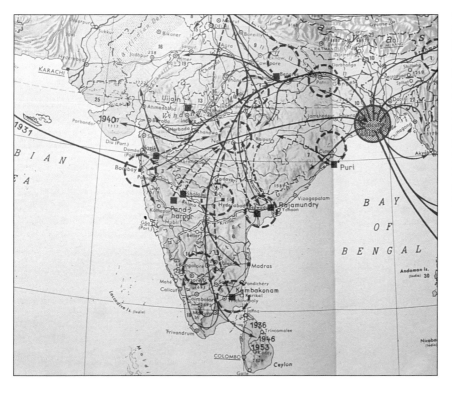

Figure 9.3 A section of Rodenwaldt and Jusatz's map of cholera in India. The map describes a "network" of disease diffusion from areas of endemic disease along commercial and religious pilgrimage routes.

Source: © Falk Verlag, Ostfildern.

Consider, for example, the *Welt Seuchen Atlas* section on cholera and its detailed color map of cholera prevalence and routes of diffusion around the world. In a portion of the map focused on India, May's general "foci" are more precisely distinguished as either areas of endemic occurrence or as secondary areas "with questionable [second-order] endemicity." The distinction reflects the relative incidence of reported cases in specific, local populations in relation to detailed vectors of cholera diffusion centered primarily on Calcutta. Through their consideration of the paths of diffusion Rodenwaldt and Jusatz create a network connecting May's foci, distilling a complex argument of not simply incidence, but of diffusion as a socially constructed outcome of trade routes and travel through specific environments.

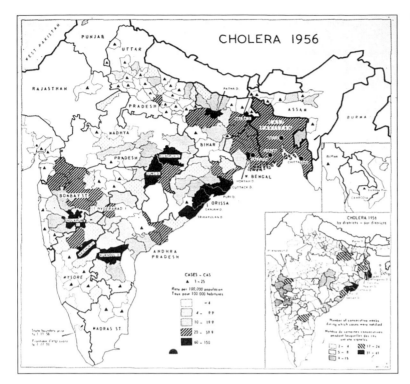

Figure 9.4 Maps of cholera incidence and distribution in India. Detail maps in Rodenwaldt and Jusatz.

Source: © Falk Verlag, Ostfildern.

In this way they advanced not only the work of Hirsch but also the nineteenth-century mapping by investigators like Brigham and McClellan. The mapped proposition fused data on trade and transportation with data on population and disease incidence within a specific environment where physical and social conditions encouraged the presence of a specific bacterium. The mapped result describes a multi-tiered network in which cholera travels between endemic (Calcutta, or Kolkata) to semi-endemic locations (Nagpur, Bombay, or Mumbai). From those locations it diffuses to other Indian cities, and internationally, by over-land and sailing routes.

The map did not spring out of thin air. It was a conclusion based on data mapped at finer scales that together gave the picture of endemic disease that in an epidemic outbreak might diffuse internationally. On the back of the color map is a black-and-white map of cholera incidence by Indian district. It was this regional data that was distilled into the disease centers in the summary map. In the world map this becomes the argument for diffusion between primary and secondary cities in the world as it is, in India at a different scale. At every level, the regional counts focused attention on the urban centers of disease. The argument begins in India, where the disease is endemic, and progresses in the map to an international scale of argument. Here was the approach that Paris school mapper-statisticians like Malgaigne earlier advanced, transposed into a more rigorous, modern study. Deaths aggregated by district became, in this work, not a final statement, but a mapped step along the road to more complete understanding.

The question rapidly became what might contribute to the variance in epidemic disease in the individual districts of India. The usual answers included population density, sanitation, and of course, water supply. But those easy answers of the early sanitarians were, in the 1950s, amenable to more careful consideration. The nineteenth-century question—how do we relate watercourse and cholera?—now could be answered with specificity.

Rodenwaldt and Jusatz considered the effect of stream flow in coastal rivers in an attempt to understand the phenomena better. Stream and river location were mapped on a black-and-white dot map of cholera cases for the Hooghly River region in southwest Bengal. The result was clear. At this scale it was evident that smaller, more turbid watercourses where flow was diminished were also areas of

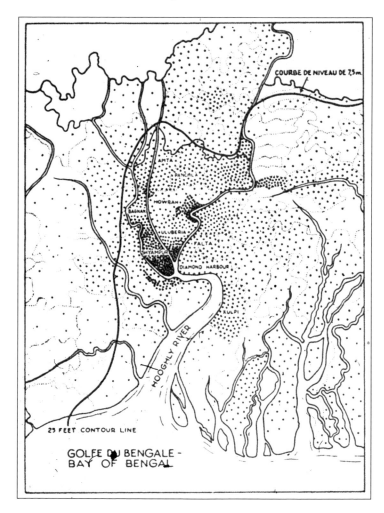

Figure 9.5 Map of cholera incidence and streamflow in the Bay of Bengal from *Welt Seuchen Atlas* page on cholera and river environments in Hooghly River delta. Dots indicate incidence of cholera, which is most dense in the more sluggish stream areas.

Source: © Falk Verlag, Ostfildern.

concentrated cholera occurrence. It was not simply the presence of the water itself, or its contamination by human effluvia, but the rate at which the river could cleanse itself that affected the incidence of the disease.

McGlashan (1972, 135) quotes Rodenwaldt's and Jusatz's conclusion in full to demonstrate how the authors associated physical characteristics with disease incidence and diffusion. "Here is a definite correlation," they state, "namely the correlation between the spread of cholera and the amount of water flow. In short, the reduction in the disease gradient of cholera stands in inverse correlation to the fall of gradient of the land and to the velocity of flow of the water." Steeper slopes means more run-off. That means faster stream velocity and less stagnant water, flushing the bacterium out of local drinking water sources. It was a solution both Farr and Snow would have accepted, a perspective missing from their work the century before. It was, too, a map they would have understood and approved.

Others attempted similar correlations between disease incidence and environmental conditions. Learmonth, for example "pioneered the use of cartographic methods to handle data of highly variable accuracy" (Cliff and Haggett 2003, 530). He not only used isolines to show contours of urban infant mortality but, in other maps, developed a simple 3 x 3 matrix to describe the variations between high and low disease incidence. This contributed, for example, to an ecology of malaria in India that attempted to understand the incidence and spread of disease in relation to specific land types (Learmonth 1957). Jungle tracks, "healthy plains" (uplands relatively disease-free), dry lands, and other environments were correlated with incidence of endemic malaria. The result was a map in which land types were correlated as favorable or unfavorable habitats for specific varieties of mosquitoes and thus as potential sites of malarial incidence. Land type 5 in the accompanying map, for example, "comprises hyperendemic hill tracts where the primary vectors are stream-breeding forest mosquitoes," while type 6 is hyperendemic lowland where the principal malarial vector is *C. phillipinensis* (Learmonth 1988, 205–207).

The result is a sophisticated surface not simply of the landforms in India, but of the interactions between the physical environment, the agents they favor, and the diseases those agents promote as they are carried to the population by specific insect vectors. In the surface is embedded the thesis that different environments promote or inhibit the incidence of the disease. More precisely, what is mapped is the range of environments that promote (or inhibit) the mosquito, now understood to be the vector for the spread of the disease agent.

Gone from the map are the urban centers, transportation pathways, and jurisdictional boundaries of other maps. It is not that these are unimportant but that this mapped proposition considers only the characteristics of the land encouraging the propagation of the disease agent and its transmission to resident populations. The result is not a complete statement but one that complements and deepens the general distillation in Rodenwaldt's network-based approach. While the *Welt Seuchen Atlas*'s map considered human vectors of disease transmission, Learmonth's map argues a relation between physical

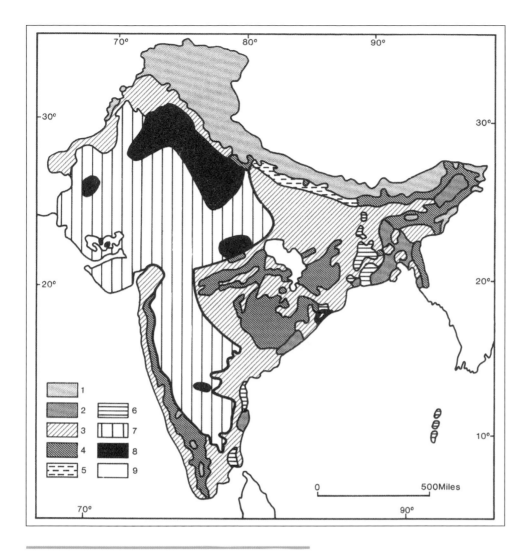

Figure 9.6 Learmonth's map of endemic land type and malaria in India. Each category distinguishes a surface type (hill, plain, jungle lowland, etc.) potentially related to malaria incidence.

Source: Learmonth (1988, 206). Courtesy of Blackwell Publishing.

environment and amenability to the disease agent. Here it was not "either/or" but "both/and" as a research methodology.

The result is not a "basemap" of environmental facilitation but of elements embedded in the greater map that serve both as a surface in its own right and as a part of the greater, mapped proposition. Thus, in a second map, Learmonth restated the urban focus of Rodenwaldt and Jusatz, adding hydrologic

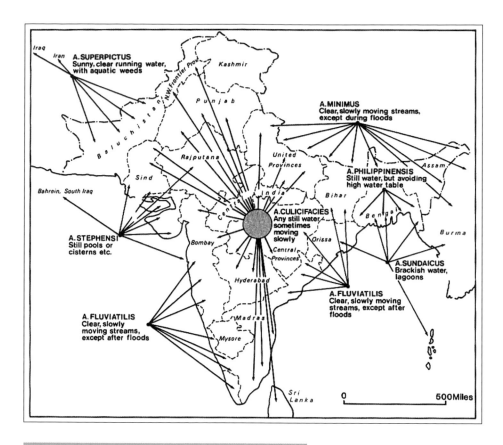

Figure 9.7 Map of malaria vectors in India based on species of mosquito and local environmental characteristics.

Source: Learmonth (1988). Courtesy of Blackwell Publishing.

data pertinent to the more general environmental analysis of the preceding map statement. The result joins Rodenwaldt's and Jusatz's mapped argument with that returned by Learmonth's more general study.

National atlas projects

In the immediate post-war period, the predilection for mapped studies of disease combining demographic, social, and geographical features led to the acceptance of the atlas as a medium for the consideration of complex health concerns. There were several reasons for this, including, in Great Britain, the movement to consider health as a governmental responsibility. A second and parallel impetus in the United States was cold-war militarism and its need for medical data on any area in the world to which troops might be sent. In both cases the result would be maps of the incidence of disease and their potential determinants.

As Mildred Blaxter,[1] the doyenne of medical sociology in the United Kingdom, put it in a letter, "the post-war plans for the 'Welfare State,' the (hopeful!) attack on the 'four evils' of poverty, homelessness, poor education, ill health, with all its rhetoric of care for the whole population 'from the cradle to the grave'—[were] hugely popular and lead to the setting up of public housing, national insurance, and universal education, as well as the health service" (Blaxter 2003). Those programs required data on the status of health in the nation, and if possible, on the determinants of health and disease.

One answer was to be Howe's well-known *Atlas of Disease Mortality in the United Kingdom,* a summary of what a national health system in Britain would have to face. Plate after plate of his atlas considered the incidence of varying cancers occurring in the country (lung, colo-rectal, stomach, etc.) as well as a broader catalog of ills (respiratory and cardiac diseases, for example) affecting many citizens at some point between cradle and grave. The result summed the incidence of disease generally, the problems a national health service would have to confront.

The need for mapping as a means of distilling data was manifest. The immense volume of data required for a portrait of national health and disease was too vast to be understood easily in its raw, statistical form. What was required was a method not simply of distillation but one that would serve to permit the analysis of the rapidly expanding database of disease incidence. "The purpose of the atlas is to show through the medium of maps the spatial patterns of variations in disease mortality in the United Kingdom. Statistical tables of the geographical distribution of disease in the United Kingdom have been available for many years but tabulated information is not directly and easily translated into a distributional pattern. The same data embodied in a map provide an instant visual impression which relates the figures immediately to their appropriate geographical position" (Howe 1963, 1).

Data mapped in the atlas was based upon standardized mortality ratios (SMRs), a statistical device that Howe lovingly, almost passionately described in his introduction. SMRs permitted accurate statements not only of the general profile of mortality (for both sexes and different age groups), but also of significant mortality resulting from a specific disease (cancer, pneumonia, etc.). Raw mortality population statistics were based upon data reported by Local Health Authorities, the descendants of the authorities created in the 1830s when cholera first rampaged, to the Registrar General in London. The result transformed the nineteenth-century idea of medicostatistical studies into a far more sophisticated and precise, twentieth-century approach.

Howe saw his atlas as the direct descendant of Heinrich Berghaus's *Physikalisch Handatlas,* and of nineteenth-century cartography generally (Howe 1963, 7). Indeed, he places his work within the Hippocratic tradition with a long quote from Hippocrates's argument for attention to environmental determinants (especially airborne) of disease. The new atlas was thus a self-conscious addition to the long tradition of environmental concern bolstered by the rigor of modern statistics and epidemiological

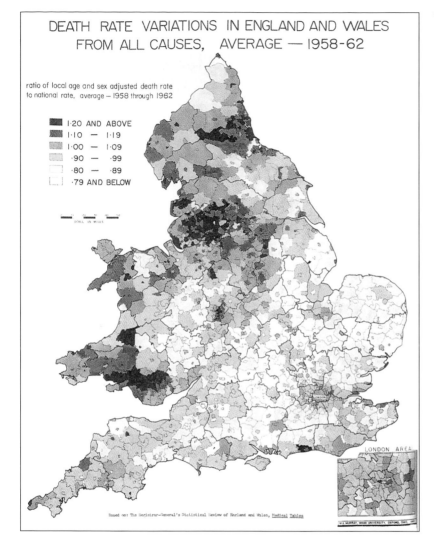

DEATH RATE VARIATIONS IN ENGLAND AND WALES
FROM ALL CAUSES, AVERAGE — 1958-62

ratio of local age and sex adjusted death rate
to national rate, average — 1958 through 1962

■ 1·20 AND ABOVE
▨ 1·10 — 1·19
▨ 1·00 — 1·09
▨ ·90 — ·99
□ ·80 — ·89
□ ·79 AND BELOW

SCALE IN MILES

LONDON AREA

Based on: The Registrar-General's Statistical Review of England and Wales, Medical Tables

Figure 9.8 Death rate variations from all causes for males, 1958–1962. A choropleth map showing relative variations in death rate based on standardized mortality ratios.

Source: Reprinted with permission of Special Libraries Association (www.sla.org) and G. Melvyn Howe, PhD.

science. In his introduction, Howe drew strong parallels between his work and the mapping of cholera in the nineteenth century, singling out both Shaptner's map of the cholera epidemic in 1832 and the work of Snow as inspirations and antecedents. There was no doubt of his intent: Howe's atlas was to be the inheritor of the tradition of medical mapping and of the more general tradition of a disease ecology that stretched, for him, from Hippocrates to Snow to May to Rodenwaldt and Jusatz.

In its first edition there was, however, a problem that limited the effectiveness of the maps that resulted. Mapping SMRs in a choropleth map whose geography was that of the individual political district lost a lot in the translation. "Such a [geographical] base gives prominence to the standardized mortality ratios of the extensive, sparsely, and unevenly populated areas but provides insufficient weighting for the limited and localized areas of dense population associated with metropolitan and county boroughs. An incorrect visual impression of regional intensities of mortality incidence is therefore created" (Howe 1969, 16).

Minor geographical areas with small populations might show a high incidence (one case in a district of two people is 50 percent) that did not reflect accurately the relevance of the data at a national scale. The SMR did not reflect local characteristics of population density, and the SMR thus became homogenized in the resulting map, hiding much that it was supposed to reveal. It was the problem of scale. At what scale can one best perceive differential incidences of a specific disease: town, parish, county, region, or the nation? The problem was (and remains) at once statistical and graphic.

Early computer mapping

One answer presented itself in the then-evolving conjunction of mainframe computers attached to plotters or printers capable of generating graduated symbols of various sizes, shapes, and patterns. The old dream of computing machines had come to pass, an unexpected dividend of World War II and the need of war department scientists to perform large calculations accurately and rapidly. ENIAC was completed in 1946, and in 1952 UNIVAC became available (Sui and Morrill 2004). In the 1950s and early 1960s, mainframe computers were large and complex "computing machines" whose service was largely mathematical and statistical. Even in this early period, however, their potential for mapping did not go unnoticed. Not only might they calculate SMRs, but with some tweaking they could also, perhaps, map the results returned by those calculations.

Engineers experimented in the 1940s with plotters and other printing devices that, joined to diagnostic tools like oscilloscopes, might provide a physical record of transitory electronic images (Longley and Batty 2003, 2–3). In the early 1960s, computers and plotter-printers had evolved to a point where outputs might be graphic as well as numerical. Here was the answer to Howe's problem. Computers could generate a map that would marry the rigor of national statistical calculations with a mapped surface that reflected not simply a geographical area but area defined by population and incidence.

The result liberated his cartographers from a reflexive reliance on geographically accurate "base-maps" of political districts, permitting instead a computerized demographic comprised of "a number of 'squares' (representing metropolitan boroughs, county boroughs, and the aggregates of municipal boroughs and urban districts of the administrative counties), the areas of which were proportional to the population 'at risk'" (Howe 1969, 18). The greater the population of an SMSA, the larger the graded symbol mapped. Different categories of population center (industrial, rural, urban, etc.) were distinguished by different sets of graded symbols (square, diamond, circle).

The landscape was transformed in the process. The result provided a way to consider in a national event the local incidence of disease without losing reference to the incidence of disease by population. The second edition of Howe's *National Atlas Disease Mortality in the United Kingdom*, (1969) included

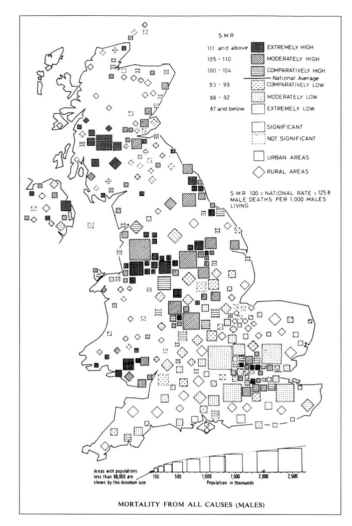

Figure 9.9 Computer-generated map of arteriosclerotic heart disease, including coronary disease in British males, 1959–1963. The map for the second edition of Howe's atlas was described in a 1969 *SLA Special Bulletin: Geography and Map Division.*

Source: Reprinted with permission of Special Libraries Association (www.sla.org) and G. Melvyn Howe, PhD.

both these new, computer-generated maps and those produced in a more traditional manner. While Howe was especially proud of those generated by computer, they are, from our contemporary perspective, hopelessly crude and needlessly confusing. A map of arteriosclerotic heart disease, including coronary disease, in British males (1959–1963) gives a sense of the mapping that resulted.

Freed of recognizable political jurisdictions, the result was difficult to interpret by any but a demographer or epidemiologist familiar with the data the map distilled and the geopolitical environment the data represented. In retrospect, the map reveals the indivisible relation between disease-related data and the context in which that data is collected and to be considered. Without the jurisdictional political boundaries all one has for context is the frame of the broad national coastline, and that is insufficient for the average reader. Lost, too, is data on the jurisdiction in which the data is collected, the context that anchors it in the map's space and in the reader's vision.[2]

However, this approach had a signal, undeniable advantage beyond its novelty, one that justified the attempt and Howe's justifiable pride in it. It presented a technology permitting the mapped conclusion of numerous calculations at various scales in a comprehensive fashion. Large databases of distinct data could be manipulated and the results plotted or mapped in a manner whose result retained existing spatial relations between different places (London, Birmingham, Nottingham, etc.) while distinguishing qualities (altitude, income, disease intensity, rainfall, or occupation) potentially relevant to disease incidence. The scale of the map could be quickly changed in a new map of a specific section of the greater database, generating a new perspective on localized incidence. Those results could be presented either in an old style map or on this new, computer-generated surface in which statistical data was fused to spatial information in a way that created or argued something about disease incidence.

The promise of this approach also attracted the attention of Dr. H. C. Hopps, chief of the Geography Pathology Division in the Armed Forces Institute of Pathology in Washington, D.C., where similar experiments in computerized mapping were underway at the same time. The goal of his department was "to develop methods by which a very wide variety of data pertaining to infectious disease may be effectively stored, collected, and computer-manipulated to yield direct print-out in the form of distribution maps" (Hopps 1969, 24). The Army's "Mapping of Disease Project" (MOD) was begun in the early 1950s, the same time as May's initiatives "to provide the means whereby the disease panorama can be quickly and effectively presented in its map form in a time context that may be either current or historic" (Hopps 1969, 25).

A complex database, including data on all locations where a disease occurred, was distilled in the resulting map. Included were details of disease occurrence, local agricultural activity, climatology, geography, soil, and population characteristics. Out of this would come "meaningful maps (and other graphic displays) that show the distribution of a disease(s) in terms of prevalence, incidence, severity, etc., along with distributions of (and interrelationships among) selected casually-related factors" (Hopps 1969, 26).

The MOD team sought to present nothing less than a "disease panorama," its renaming of May's "disease ecology," including everything and anything that would contribute to the understanding of a specific medical condition *in situ.* "We mean disease panorama to include location of the disease at a particular time in terms of prevalence, incidence, mortality, and morbidity—within the population *in toto,* also its various segments. But more than this: we mean it to include also information as to the quality, quantity, and location of those numerous environmental factors which influence rate of occurrence as well as character of disease" (Hopps 1969, 25).

Maps were to be a principal medium for the output of data accumulated by the MOD because they provided a relatively intuitive medium whereby the essential relations defining the disease panorama could be assembled, compared, and contrasted. Here mapping and geography are joined, the first a method of argument and investigation, the latter a discipline of spatial relationships. "Geographical pathology is, in a sense, a kind of comparative pathology—one in which place (rather than species) is the primary variable. Geographic pathology attempts to answer the questions: "What (disease); Where (is it)—and When; and Why (is it there)" (Hopps 1969 1:7).

The result would lay bare patterns of incidence and diffusion for those diseases "strongly influenced by a wide variety of ecologic factors, e.g., temperature, rainfall, humidity . . ." and so on (Hopps 1969, 26). The goal was the mapping of "epidemiologic relations," those in which specific environments contributed to the spread of disease. The mapping program was dedicated to a single goal: "to utilize to the fullest extent the data that are available, recognizing the many limitations of these data, and present the best information possible, concentrating upon the distribution of disease/environmental factors within a precise time/location framework" (Hopps 1969, 26). As research statements go, this one is remarkable for its modesty and completeness. It recognizes the limits of the data, asserting only the best results possible within the context of current methods. And it limits its investigation to a type of relation that is both temporal and locational in its environmental address.

That the push for disease mapping in the United States was military rather than civil is not surprising. In the nineteenth century, Congress turned to the military for answers to the cholera epidemic of the 1870s. The nation was under attack . . . who better to coordinate its defense than the military? May's work was part of a U.S. initiative to advance and remake the world, economically and socially, in its own image. Rodenwaldt's and Jusatz's post-war work was supported from the start by a United States military that had learned in World War II the necessity of understanding the medical conditions in areas in which its troops were stationed. With Korea in the 1950s, and in the cold war generally, the United States embarked on a period of international military activity that would see its troops dispatched more than seventy times to nations around the world by the millennium.

In the 1950s, military medical experts knew that to fulfill their role they would need to be versed in the health risks to troops in Asia (especially China, Korea, and Taiwan), Southeast Asia (Vietnam, Cambodia, Laos, etc.), the South Pacific (Philippines, and Guam, as well as Central America (Guatemala, Honduras, San Salvador) and South America (Colombia, Chile, etc.). Hopps insisted from the start that, to be useful, the military needed not simply an international database of disease incidence but one that considered environmental contributors to disease. This meant the data his department collected had to include demographic and geographic data pertinent to all the diseases occurring in all the areas where U.S. military personnel might someday serve. The medium of the map was "ideally suited to a consideration of multiple factors simultaneously" (Hopps 1969, 27), if only the computer technology of production could be adapted.

To explain how he would carry out the enormous challenge of mapping a database of both the incidence of disease and the factors that contributed to it, Hopps used Burkitt's analysis of an African

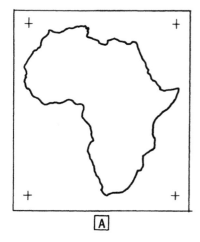

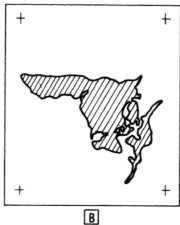

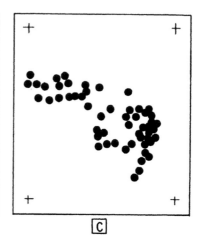

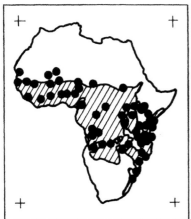

Figure 9.10 Maps showing the ideal of computerized mapping by Hopps (1969). Map A is the geographic domain, map B the regional domain. Map C is a dot map of incidence on which map B is dependant. The final map combines these three layers into an integrated statement.

Source: Reprinted with permission of Special Libraries Association (www.sla.org).

lymphoma as an example. On (A) the outline of Africa, the territory under consideration, (B) areas that met specific physical criteria for disease potential were mapped. In this case, they were those areas with an altitude under five thousand feet, a seasonal mean temperature exceeding 60° Fahrenheit, and an annual rainfall greater than twenty inches. A third map (C) of observed disease incidence was added to the mix. The result was (D) a map in which the incidence of Burkitt's lymphoma is shown to occur within a specific environment defined by altitude, temperature, and rainfall.

Hopps's use of Burkitt's map was more for show than for practice, an illustration of what could be done and not an example of what he and his colleagues in fact were doing. Hopps and his colleagues experimented in the 1960s with early mapping programs like SYMAP (SYnagraphic MAPping) run on large mainframe computer systems with clumsy, plotted graphic capabilities.

Early results of the MOD project were little more successful than Howe's. The thinking was there, but the technology had yet to catch up. In an attempt to map the incidence of schistosomiasis[3] in

South America, for example, they used an IBM® 7090 to plot variations in incidence on a hand-drawn outline of the continent. In one version, disease incidence was mapped using contour lines. The results were crude at best, at least at the continental scale. In another map of the same data, areas of greatest intensity were distinguished by progressively darker hatching roughly drawn by a plotter. While it served to show large areas of variation, the approach was too crude—and the printing too primitive—to permit even relatively fine distinctions between areal incidences. The promise was there, but the images returned were too coarse to be of real service.

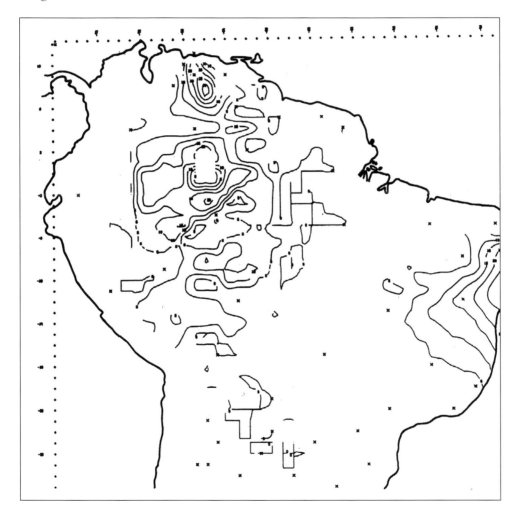

Figure 9.11 Maps of computer-generated contour lines for infection rate of schistosomiasis *(s. mansoni)* reported plus estimated points.

Source: Reprinted with permission of Special Libraries Association (www.sla.org).

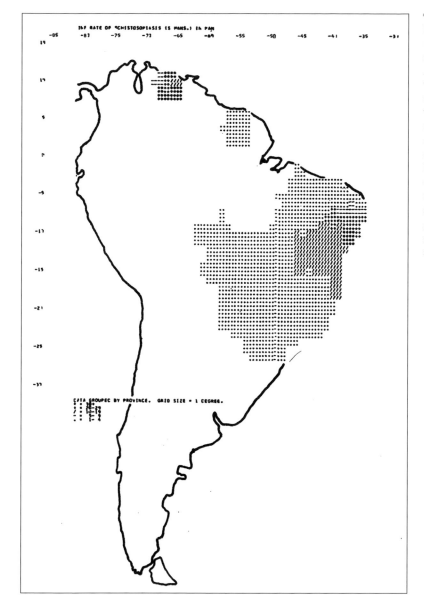

Figure 9.12 Computerized map of density gradient schistosomiasis in South America. The map on the left is a contour map using a 1-degree grid, the map on the right is a density gradient map using overprinted characters for shading. Both were built in an IBM 7090 mainframe computer environment using two different plotter systems for output.

Source: Reprinted with permission of Special Libraries Association (www.sla.org).

More interesting, perhaps, and certainly more successful was an attempt to map the incidence of schistosomiasis as a surface in which variations would be seen as altitude on the hand-drawn outline of South America. The algorithm that generated the map was relatively complex and the computing time costly, but the results, in its day, were spectacular. Here was the visualization of data, the transformation of the geographic surface into one representing synthetic data that the other maps hinted at but did not really provide

The ability to generate a surface map whose peaks and values reflected the relative presence or absence of an attribute in space had myriad potential uses. It would simply take time, better computer languages, faster machines, more sensitive computers, and of course, better printers to realize the potential of the technology. And as both Hopps and Howe insisted in their respective works, that potential was important. There was simply too much data available, too many potential variables and too large and populated a world to attempt an understanding of the location and diffusion of disease without the assistance of computing machines and a mapped representation of their analyses. This early work by the British atlas project and the U.S. MOD program signaled a general confidence that computing machines with their voracious memories would permit a more detailed and statistically rigorous ecology of disease, one whose natural output medium was mapping.

The roughness of the maps that resulted from the MOD masks their historical importance. The system of map generation was inferior and the computer programs both cumbersome and difficult to manipulate. In time, however, the simple SYMAP-powered plotter would be replaced by dot matrix, ink jet, and finally, laser printers. Mainframe computers would evolve into desk and then laptop computers of extraordinary power. Early computer programs would evolve into sophisticated systems capable of precise analysis and detailed presentation. These were early days for the technology, a first

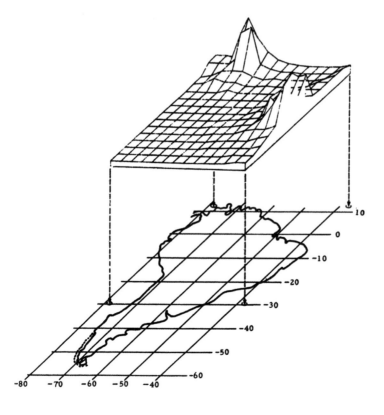

Figure 9.13 Early three-dimensional computerized map of schistosomiasis data in South America using altitude to indicate intensity of occurrence.

Source: Reprinted with permission of Special Libraries Association (www.sla.org).

attempt at a new application of the mainframe computing machine not simply to store but also to manipulate vast arrays of data that could be distilled graphically and then easily printed.

Burkitt's tumor

The atlases were largely about diseases whose etiology was understood. Where it was not—cancer, for example—it was less investigatory than descriptive. Here we see this type of cancer in the nation; there others can be found. At the same time, a parallel stream of work on diseases of unknown etiology, including specific cancers, was being carried out with a similarly ecological approach. An example is Burkitt's studies (1962a; 1962b) of a primarily African lymphoma named after him, the example Hopps used in describing how computerized medical mapping might best serve medical science and the military.

Langlands (1969, 9–15) argued that Burkitt's work exemplified the map-rich work of the period's African health administrators and investigators whose district health officers, like Young and his colleagues in India in the 1920s, were faced with understanding diseases not well known in the developed world.[4] Certainly, Burkitt's studies serve today not only as an example of the ecological approach developing during this period but also of the way in which relatively simple mapping was used to good effect. That the work was done without the benefit of computers and yet was held up as an example of what computerized mapping would eventually be able to do is one of the minor ironies of this history.

Burkitt's attention was drawn to a childhood lymphoma resulting in a disfiguring tumor that occurred in the jaw of children in Uganda, where he practiced, and was also broadly reported in eastern and central Africa. The tumor gives the type of geometrically asymmetrical facial appearance

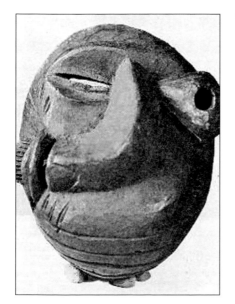

Fig. 9.14 An African mask of person with Burkitt's lymphoma.

Source: Courtesy of Dr. Maurice Reeder, USUHS.

that many associate with African sculpture. In the early 1960s there was no clear clinical understanding of the tumor, no bacterial, parasitic, or viral rationale for its appearance in some areas and not in others. Unlike Snow, whose research was a part of an international effort to understand a pandemic disease, Burkitt was relatively alone in his study of this ill-understood, localized lymphoma occurring only in parts of Africa. Determined to understand "the strikingly distinctive jaw tumors that cannot readily be mistaken for any other lesion" (Burkitt 1962a, 379), Burkitt first sent an illustrated leaflet "depicting the characteristic features of these jaw lesions, and containing a brief description of the other presenting features" to medical units across Africa. Data returned indicated a generalized pattern of occurrence from the coast of Kenya and Tanganyika to the coast of Senegal. Tantalizingly, however, it was almost unknown in South Africa and north of the Sahara.

The result was a map of general occurrence with dense clusters occurring in West Africa. Burkitt then mapped, on the basis of data returned in his questionnaire, a research trip that would take him from areas of minimal incidence through areas of dense occurrence in an attempt to "define as accurately as possible some portion of the apparent boundary of the tumour belt" in hopes that the result "might provide valuable clues as to the etiology of this condition" (Burkitt 1962a, 380). The goal was to visit "as many [responding] hospitals as possible along the 'negative' side of the assumed 'edge' and then along the 'positive' side." Hospitals he hoped to visit were notified a year in advance "so staff might look out for these lesions and refer to their hospital records." In effect, the map answered the practical question how best to investigate known locations of lymphoma incidence by mapping the relation between incidence (by reporting hospital) and roads amenable to automobile travel.

Burkitt's hospital questionnaire returned a general description of the extent of the lymphoma whose secret, he suspected, lay in the environments of the villages in which those with this condition lived. "At every hospital visited, we endeavored to portray, with the aid of an album of illustrations, the various features of this tumour syndrome affecting children. Our purpose was to discover the localities from which these patients came, rather than to determine in which hospitals the condition had been recognized." Thus, while the first maps of incidence reflected the location of reporting hospitals, the fieldwork was self-consciously aimed at finding common characteristics in the villages in which the hospital patients lived. Given the huge service range of African hospitals, the difference between home location and hospital address could be significant.

In his field research, Burkitt discovered there was a clear, geographical profile to the tumor's incidence. "In four areas fairly sharply defined 'edges' to the tumour-bearing area were detected" (Burkitt 1962a, 384). These edges were defined by altitude and by temperature, although the range of altitude and temperature in which the tumor occurred shifted as one moved from equatorial to subequatorial regions.

Along the coast the villages from which tumor patients came were all in lowland areas (white areas) with an altitude less than three thousand feet while communities existing at higher altitudes (shaded

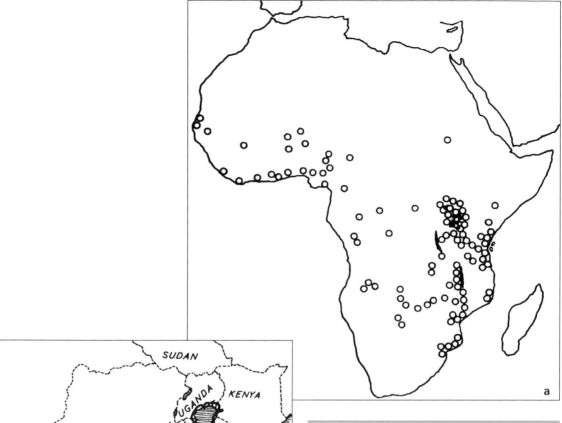

Figure 9.15a and b Map (a) of lymphoma incidence reported by medical professionals. Map (b) of disease route based on reported incidence.

Source: © Nature Publishing Group. Burkitt, D.N., *British Journal of Cancer* (1962), 16.

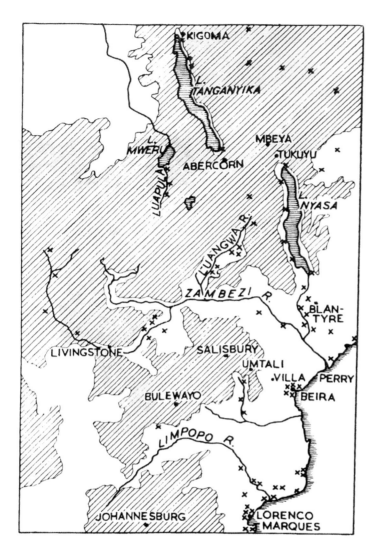

Figure 9.16 Burkitt's map of incidence of lymphoma in lowland as opposed to highland areas. Shaded areas indicate altitude relative to river course in lowland areas.

Source: © Nature Publishing Group. Burkitt, D.N., *British Journal of Cancer* (1962), 16.

areas) were typically tumor-free. Where cases were reported in highland areas, interviews revealed the families of affected children had moved from lowland villages. Similarly, mapped occurrence of the tumor based on temperature showed a clear edge at a temperature gradient of approximately 64° Fahrenheit. In Burkitt's map the shaded areas are those in which temperatures may fall below that level while the white areas, occurring along lowland riverbanks, were areas of higher temperature.

Finally, Burkitt noted, when comparing data from locations visited on his research safari, as one moved away from the equator the altitude range in which tumors were found diminished. Where three thousand feet of altitude was an upper limit of the tumor belt near the equator, in subtropical South Africa that altitude dropped to one thousand feet. It was not that tumor occurrence was dependent on

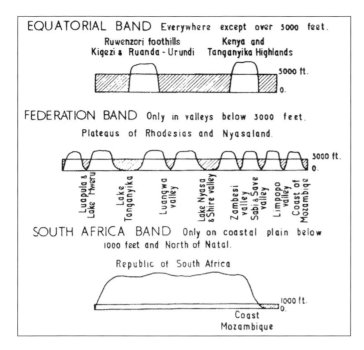

Figure 9.17 Burkitt's diagram of the relation between altitude, temperature, and incidence of Burkitt's lymphoma near the equator, in subequatorial zones, and farther south, in South Africa. Distance from the equator corresponds with differences in temperature and rainfall.

Source: © Nature Publishing Group. Burkitt, D.N., *British Journal of Cancer* (1962), 16.

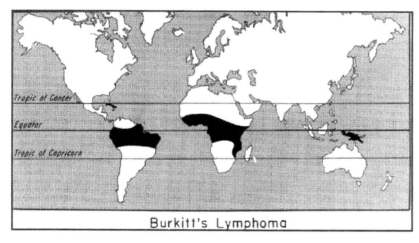

Figure 9.18 Burkitt's lymphoma (all types): 2003 distribution.

Source: © Nature Publishing Group. Burkitt, D.N., *British Journal of Cancer* (1962), 16.

altitude (*á la* Farr) but that altitude was perhaps a surrogate for other related attributes, for example, rainfall and temperature, defining the boundaries of the habitation of a parasite or other vector. "The actual limiting factor appears to be a minimum temperature of about 60° Fahrenheit," Burkitt concluded. The relationship between altitude and tumor incidence as one moved away from the equator also reflected consistent differences in temperature and rainfall as one moved away from the equator.

While suggestive, Burkitt's work was not conclusive. The lymphoma named after him was and remains something of a mystery. What he demonstrated was that the occurrence of this "unusual tumor" was ecologically dependent, reflecting temperature and perhaps rainfall patterns at specific altitudes that were favorable to an agent he could not identify and more modern researchers have been unable to name. The whole "implies that some vector be involved in its transmission. This in turn suggests the possibility that a vector is implicated." Almost in passing Burkitt noted that the range of the tumor was roughly the same as that of malaria that "in recent years swept through Uganda, Southern Tanganyika, and Northern Nyasaland . . . .. This may point to comparable vectors transmitting the causative agent" (Burkitt 1962a, 385).

Others considering Burkitt's work in recent years have confirmed a relation not simply between incidence and altitude (and thus temperature) but also with rainfall. There is, in addition, a general correspondence between Burkitt's lymphoma and the conditions in which malaria is endemic. Precisely why this is remains unclear, as does a positive correlation between incidence of the lymphoma and the Epstein-Barr virus.[5] Not the least fascinating element of the problem is the now recognized, relative universality of the lymphoma once thought to be specific to Africa. An international "lymphoma belt" appears to exist within a specific temperature range. Wherever it appears, the lymphoma also tends to be more common among poor than well-to-do children, suggesting a socioeconomic weighting of contributing factors, whatever they may eventually be discovered to be.

It is important to consider the manner in which the mapping was an indivisible characteristic of Burkitt's research. First, he mapped the incidence of the disease, using questionnaires to hospital officials, to determine the incidence of the lymphoma. This data was loaded onto a general map of Africa to plan his "research safari." On that safari he collected data on a range of potential contributors to disease incidence in the villages of patients with the disease. In the end, his travels suggested a relation between altitude and associated temperatures as defining. He mapped the correspondence of disease incidence and occurrence. Others later noted a correspondence between the zones of occurrence of the lymphoma and those of malaria—endemic among the affected population—and later yet, Epstein-Barr virus. At every stage of the research, from data sampling to hypothesis generation and conclusion, mapping played a part, as did statistical analysis and old-fashioned, shoe-leather research. Local data returned by the questionnaires was aggregated to a national map at the first stage of work. Local attributes were then investigated in the fieldwork that returned a general environmental frame within which the lymphoma seemed to occur.

Cancer in West Devon

In the 1960s, the focus of medical research in the developed world was shifting to viral disease from those that are parasitic or bacterial. The latter had been well studied, at least in the developed world, and the former were only beginning to be understood. The interest reflected the fact that, in the developed world, cancer had become the number one cause of death among citizens who no longer died frequently of the old killers: cholera, malaria, polio, pneumonia, tuberculosis, typhus and typhoid, yellow fever, and other once-common diseases. While informed by national perspectives like those in Howe's atlas, these new studies tended to the localized scale of John Snow's analysis and its focus on local topologies in areas of high incidence. They return as well to the work of people like Haviland who sought physical as well as social constituents of disease. In this new iteration, however, the statistics and science were far more rigorous, the mapping more detailed.

One of those most frequently cited studies at this scale[6] has been Allen-Price's consideration of the uneven distribution of cancer in West Devon, England. He began with an apparent anomaly: while cancer was responsible for an average 16.5 percent of all deaths in West Devon, a rate roughly equal to the nation's (16.8 percent), "local 'folklore' has it that certain parts of West Devon are rife with cancer (Allen-Price 1960, 1235). Was this the case, he asked, and if so, what might explain it?

To consider the problem he first compared the incidence of cancer by West Devon parishes, using death rates per one thousand people living for the years 1939–1958. He then analyzed the percentage

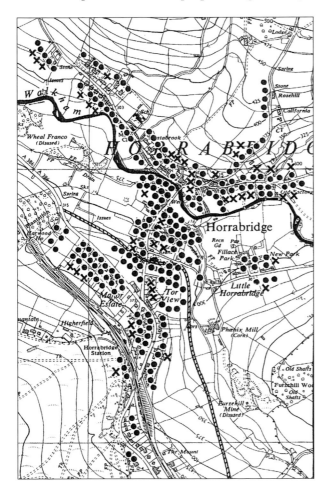

Figure 9.19 Map of cancer incidence in the Horrabridge area where rates reached 46 percent of all deaths. The x's describe deaths from cancer while circular symbols indicate locations of noncancer, "normal" deaths.

Source: Reprinted with permission from Elsevier, *Lancet*, 4 June 1960, 1235–1238.

of all deaths attributed to cancer in the area's parishes by population and found an enormous variation with the lowest level of parish mortality at 4.5 percent and the highest in Bere-Ferrers parish at
22 percent. The adjoining parish, Buckland Monachorum, had a mortality rate for cancer of only 14
percent with a comparable population. Clearly, something was going on. There were areas of unusually
high incidence masked at more general scales of analysis that were evident at the local parish scale

"Having investigated the cancer incidence in a general statistical way, which did not yield any really
positive result, except those set out in the above tables, the situation was plotted on a map. The 5,547
deaths were depicted on a six-inch-to-the-mile Ordinance Survey map. A cross on the map marked
deaths from cancer, those from other diseases by a circle. The extraordinary unequal distribution of the
disease at once became apparent. For example, in one hamlet the ratio of crosses to circles is 1 in 12,
while in an adjoining hamlet of comparable community [population] the ratio is 1 in 3" (Allen-Price
1960, 1235).

The "cluster," as it would now be called, thus revealed is certainly startling, especially at the village scale of Horrabridge, "a compact village of about 1,200 people," where cancer rates reached the
exceptional level of 46 percent of all deaths. The section of the Ordinance Survey map reproduced in
black and white in his article provides contour details, springs, well sites, and the River Walkham
along whose northern branch a marked number of cancer deaths (x's) can be seen beside noncancer

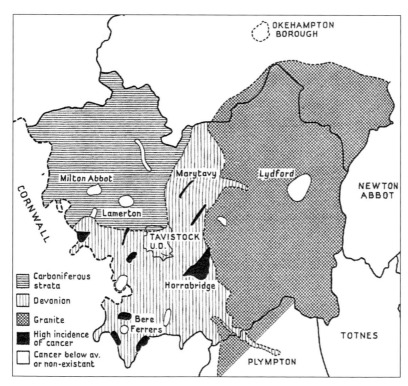

Figure 9.20 Map of
West Devon geology
used by Allen-Price in
his consideration of the
unusually high incidence
of all cancers in the area.

Source: Reprinted with permission
from Elsevier, *Lancet*, 4 June 1960,
1235–1238.

deaths. These classes of deaths, cancer- and noncancer-related, are integrated within a domain of urban settlement and gross physical features (altitude rivers, springs, etc.) that together defined the parish's physical environment.

After considering the relation between circles and crosses, between deaths from cancer and deaths from all other conditions, the question became: what generally distinguished domains of greatest cancer deaths from those where deaths from cancer were far less frequent? To answer that question Allen-Price mapped incidence of deaths by cancer per population on a rough geological map of the region. On this more general map the blackened areas of high cancer mortality (including Horrabridge) and light areas on the map—holes, really—in the surface of cancer incidence distill relations between incidence and the geology of the study region. Areas of higher than normal incidence occurred in regions of Devonian strata (shale, grits, and limestone) "which has, during the course of time, become highly mineralized" (Allen-Price 1960, 1236). Communities in which cancer was below average or nonexistent were built upon granite layers of igneous matter that was less mineralized or carboniferous systems whose composition was also less mineralized.

This was certainly suggestive. Where for Haviland and other nineteenth-century researchers it would have been decisive, however, for Allen-Price it was only one step on the analytic road. "A series of two-fold correlations were then undertaken" to quantify the results. At this stage Allen-Price compared incidence of specific cancers in relation to local geology. The result was a statistically significant correlation in which cancer in towns located in the Devonian strata was found to be positive ($r = 0.4972$ with S. D. ± 0.153) while, for those in the carboniferous strata, the results were less significant ($r = 0.0843$ with S. D. ± 0.193). "The inference is that some cancer-provoking agent is more active in one area than in the other. It is suggested that this agent is a trace element occurring in sufficient concentration on the Devonian stratum to be capable of detection" (Allen-Price 1960, 1236).

Allen-Price then went back to the Ordinance Survey maps to see if he could discover in the clusters of cancer deaths occurring in specific locations a grouping that would explain how, in highly mineralized areas, a cancer-causing agent might *move* from the soil to the population. The answer was (of course!) the water supply. In most areas water came from two sources, either underground through the aquifer or from surface waters collected in reservoirs. With some more research, and more statistical analysis, Allen-Price was able to argue that "the parishes with the highest incidence of cancer, and the highest death-rate, derive their water-supplies from wells and springs, which with two exceptions, are all in a highly mineralized strata, Devonian or granite."

Unfortunately, while his mapping gave weight to the theory, the inability to publish the map in color limited his ability to describe adequately the relation of geography, water source, and cancer incidence. "It is not possible to convert this color presentation [of the physically larger, Ordinance Survey map] to black-and-white symbols and still maintain complete accuracy" (Allen-Price 1960, 1238). Lost were lines of demarcation distinguishing water sources (including wells), for example. The problem was neither in the mapping nor the mapmaking generally—color mapping had been around for more than a century—but in the prohibitive cost of color reproduction for journals like *Lancet*. Black and white remained the default for illustrations reduced and simplified to fit the journal's page size and production limits. It would be a generation and more before techniques of electronic production and reproduction would easily permit coloration of maps like Allen-Price's.

Still, the mapping was a critical step, and the mapmaking his technology permitted innovative, even brilliant in its simplicity. As interesting, perhaps, is the use Allen-Price made of mapping and statistics as allied tools of exploration. Here we see the nineteenth-century marriage of statistics and mapping reborn. At first, a purely statistical review of cancer incidence did not yield "any really positive result." Mapping of statistically rigorous data at a local scale did, however. That led to more analysis and different maps, and they in turn lead to more focused statistical consideration. At every turn mapping informed statistics that informed more mapping in a project whose result was an ecological exploration of local variants in cancer incidence. At this point in the post-war period medical mapping and statistics again were growing together to provide a more comprehensive, multimedia approach to disease as it was to be considered at different scales of incidence.

Conceptually, the whole built upon Snow's early idea of a topography of disease and the work of those, like Haviland, who had sought to consider environmental determinants in the generation of disease. But by the 1960s these themes were transformed in a complex ecological consideration of the constituents of disease that were more rigorously considered and more carefully defined. Gone was the optimistic nineteenth-century assumption that one can simply take a single variable (the air, the water, the soil) and explain disease behavior based upon it. Gone, too, was the simplistic sanitarian perspective. In its place was an increasingly rigorous, mapped approach involving both graphical and statistical analytics whose goal was the consideration of disease incidence as a complex outcome of geographic and social variables. In this period mapping and statistics were advancing together—in health studies and elsewhere—thanks to the increasing computerization of data and the evolving flexibility of computerized systems of data storage, analysis, and presentation.

Endnotes

1. Mildred Blaxter has not only served as a preeminent medical sociologist seeking an understanding of social determinants of health, she has also lived through these years and speaks eloquently about them. The passage quoted is from an e-mail she kindly sent in answer to a query about the impetus to national health plans in the last century.

2. In the 1980s, Openshaw considered the problematic nature of such jurisdictions, and their relation to data, in his articulation of the "moveable area unit problem," or MAUP. The essence of the problem is the manner in which aggregation of data to a specific (and often arbitrary) areal unit in the end effects consideration of the data itself.

3. Schistosomiasis is a tropical, parasitic disease caused by the pathogen *Schistosoma* living in one of five species of worms that invade the bladder or intestines of humans who encounter the worms while wading, bathing, or working in polluted water. Snails serve as intermediate hosts for the worms as may certain waterfowl. Interest in the disease stems in part from its global prevalence: Africa, Asia, China, India, the Middle East, and South East Asia. Learmonth (1988) devotes a full chapter to studies in which the incidence, distribution of hosts, and national diffusion of the disease were mapped by various researchers. Indeed, it may be among the most frequently mapped conditions of the 1960s. For a contemporary review see Cliff, Haggett, and Smallman-Raynor (2004, 120–122).

4. Langlands (1969) gives a representative bibliography of Burkitt's writings in a range of journals, including the *East African Medical Journal*. He also is at pains to put Burkitt's work within the more general context of African medical geography and medical writing. I am obliged to Harry Steward, Clark University Department of Geography, for a copy of Langland's essay in the *SLA Geography and Map Division Bulletin,* courtesy of Special Libraries Association.

5. What is now becoming understood is that the Epstein-Barr virus (EBV) is responsible for a range of conditions, including Burkitt lymphoma (the possessive has been dropped). Current thinking suggests microRNA mediated gene suppression in EBV contributes by complex pathways to tumor formation and a bypassing of immune system protection. See Pray (2004).

6. For two decades authors like McGlashan (1972) and Learmonth (1988) were fond of citing—and praising—Allen-Price's work in textbooks reviewing ecologic, medical geographic studies. Surprisingly, perhaps, more contemporary textbooks on medical geography do not include a review of his work even though its mapping of disease clusters and analysis of them on the basis of environmental factors remains important.

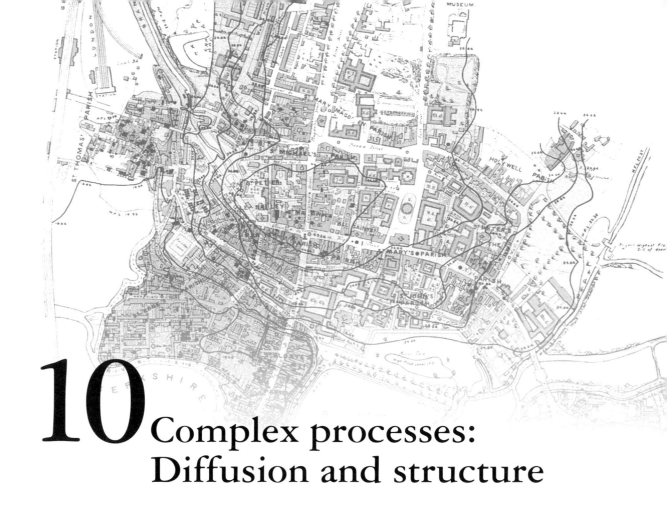

10 Complex processes: Diffusion and structure

The mainframe computer's potential to manipulate vast amounts of digitally stored data transformed almost every branch of science and social administration. Economists could run ever-more complex models based on ever-greater accumulations of digitally stored data. Epidemiologists could create beautiful algorithms calculating likely trajectories of this or that disease over time if not necessarily in space. However, those calculations typically lose the thick reality of place, abstracting without attention to the topographic variations that were Snow's greatest contribution to an understanding of epidemic disease and community health. Urban theorists could manipulate data on rank and relationship in a way that previously would have been prohibitively time consuming. Matrix analysis, factor analysis, and a range of other tools entered social science and the health professions, and calculations that would have taken months or years by hand now could be performed in days or hours. It was this evolution of computers that also enabled individual credit cards and computerized school records, and which would, experts promised, lead to a digital and paperless world. The full transformation of science and society to a computerized base took at least two generations. In the 1970s, that transformation was under way.

In the health sciences two streams of work advanced as a result. The first was that of the public health expert, trained in epidemiology, whose modeling was typically aspatial. "Professional epidemiologists appear oblivious to where the epidemic is," geographer Peter Gould et al. would complain (1991, 82), "asking only when numbers will appear along the time horizon" of an epidemic outbreak. This lack of spatial thinking in their otherwise sophisticated computations seriously limited the effectiveness of the models. Opposed to this were the mapping tradition and that of a medical geography that in this period came into its own. "During the 1970s, 'computer cartography' in health studies became quite popular . . .. Extensive collections of computer maps [were] produced by public agencies, often with little or no interpretation or pattern" (McGlashen and Blunden 1983, 85). It fell to medical geographers rather than epidemiologists or public health experts to use increasingly sophisticated, mainframe-computer-based mapping programs to interpret the spatial patterns of disease occurrence and diffusion as another step in understanding their occurrence in human populations. The result married increasingly sophisticated statistical analytics with ever-more readable and legible mapping.

Influenza 1970

In 1971, Hunter and Young published a major paper on the diffusion of influenza in England and Wales, one that took as its subject the incidence of a new and virulent strain of the disease appearing first in the 1957 flu pandemic. Influenza had been a recurrent concern of international health officials, especially since the 1918 pandemic, which is remembered as "the greatest single demographic shock that the human species has so far received" (Cliff, Haggett, and Smallman-Raynor 2004, 88).[1] The virulence of the 1918–1919 pandemic was followed by a series of less deadly but still serious epidemics and pandemics into the 1950s when another serious pandemic, an H2N1 "Asian Flu" killed millions internationally. Influenza thus presented a constant and recurring challenge to public health officials with the 1957 dataset representing, in 1970, the best and most complete record of epidemic (and pandemic) influenza then available to researchers.

There was no question about the nature of the disease. It was viral. Nor were its ecological determinants at issue. The disease spread from person-to-person without the necessity of an intervening vector (rat, flea, mosquito, or tick). The ecology of the disease in a single location was therefore less important than understanding influenza's dynamic progression in space over time. The antecedents to this stream of work are the nineteenth-century maps of cholera's national and international progress in the second and third pandemics. The work done in the 1970s on disease diffusion was far more complex, however, and far more rigorous. It was as if Victorian portrait artists had been given moving picture cameras and told to do a life documentary.

In Britain, the 1957 epidemic began with the docking of infected seamen, Pakistani naval personnel whose vessel was berthed at London's Tilbury Docks on June 13. Almost simultaneously, physicians treating air travelers reported flu cases among travelers returning to England from areas like Pakistan where influenza had been reported. Over the next three weeks a series of boats with crewmen infected abroad docked at a series of British ports: Bristol, Jarrow, Liverpool, London, and Sunderland, where the cholera epidemic of 1831–1833 began. "A total of thirty-five infected vessels arrived in port[s] between August 19 and the end of October" (Hunter and Young 1971, 638).

Week by week the epidemic grew until it peaked in the sixth week, its numbers diminishing slowly over the next six weeks in the familiar, bell-shaped pattern of epidemic occurrence described by cholera researchers in the 1850s. Within England, the disease spread across the nation's sixty-two individual counties, affecting different counties at different times across three months of epidemic occurrence. The question Hunter and Young considered was how to map this progression, how to understand the dynamics of the disease over space and time.

The problem was not calculating incidence by population but, as Howe and Hopps had discovered, how the resulting calculations might be appropriately mapped and then understood. In 1971, Hunter and Young used computer-constructed cartograms to solve the problem in a manner both more elegant and more legible than any previously attempted. The "simple accretion technique" Hunter and Young employed resized county polygons to reflect not area but population size. The result retained the spatial relationship between counties but varied their size to reflect population. On this surface, called a "cartogram," disease incidence was then mapped using a choropleth technique to describe relative disease incidence by county population at a specific time. Multiple maps of disease incidence, each representing another week of the epidemic, resulted in a type of stop-frame mapped sequence of the disease's progression over time in British counties.

Seeing the sequencing is easier than describing it. In the accompanying map, consider area 11, London. It is geographically small, an almost invisible polygon in the map's southeast corner, almost insignificant in relation to Greater England's total landmass. But London's population assures it will dominate a map in which population and not area defines district size. If one includes the well-populated neighboring counties of Essex, Middlesex, and Surrey, Greater London looms even larger on the cartogram. The result is an interpretative and synthetic distillation, a reconstructed population space that permits the incidence of disease to be presented within each reporting jurisdiction. Into this surface, Hunter and Young mapped the progress of the disease week by week. The resulting pattern leaps out to the researcher. "The heavily populated industrial counties . . . explode in size and reveal the true weight of the epidemic in the north, and elsewhere. The worst hit county was the East Riding of Yorkshire [numbers 55–56], where influenza incidence reached a level of 31 percent [of the population] for the twelve-week period" (Hunter and Young 1971, 644).

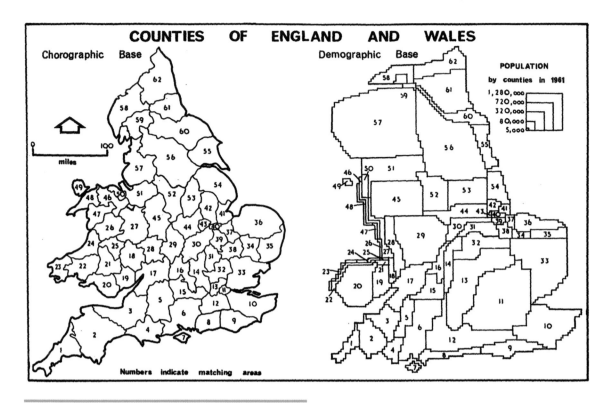

Figure 10.1 Cartogram of British population by district. On the left is a hand-drawn image of the districts by geographical attribute. On the right each district is redrawn to reflect population. Hunter and Young, 1971.

Source: Courtesy of Blackwell Publishing.

For perhaps the first time one could see the *progress* of a disease over time and in population space, profiling its diffusion week by week across the population-adjusted districts of the map. Before this, one could use arrows and lines, with dates of occurrence written over them, to suggest when and where an epidemic began and subsequently spread. Or one could write tables coordinating time and occurrence and population. However, those are difficult to read and the results, at best, are nonintuitive. Hunter and Young achieved a more detailed understanding of the epidemic's progress than had been possible in May's work, or in that of Rosenwaldt and Jusatz. Analyzing the data for the hard-hit counties of Lancaster and Leeds, Hunter and Young were able to identify primary foci, predictably the port of Liverpool and the large town of Hull, and secondary foci as the epidemic wave expanded inland (Leeds, Sheffield, Blackburn, and Manchester). As importantly, Hunter and Young were able to assess the effect of one particular attribute, "population potential" on the epidemic's progress. Based upon county data in the then-current 1961 census, population size was used to uncover the pathways of the

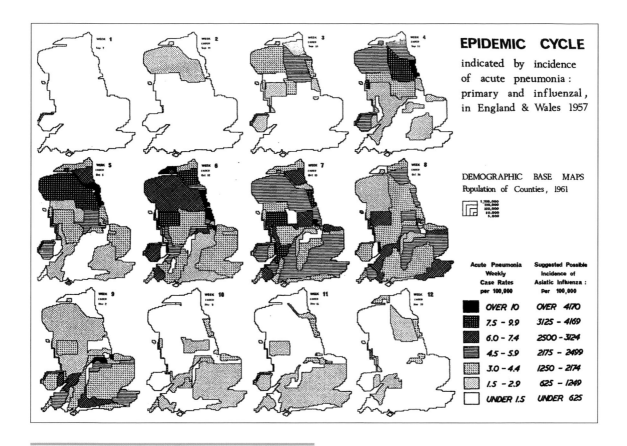

Figure 10.2 Serial maps of influenza in England using the cartogram approach by county over time. Cartograms are used to regularize incidence data by population.

Source: Courtesy of Blackwell Publishing.

epidemic, and perhaps, of future epidemic outbreaks, too. "A broad ridge of high potential extends from Lancashire and West Yorkshire southeastwards toward London. The advancing epidemic wave of influenza . . . followed the ridge way of high potential" (Hunter and Young 1971, 651).

Once it had taken hold in Britain's industrial north, the disease's center of gravity shifted toward the populated counties of the southeast, along the seven hundred case-incidence isoline. This idea of epidemic gravity, of a moving center of highest incidence progressing across a hierarchy of populated areas was the result. Down the center of the map are points on a track like those that show where a storm center has been. They end in the contours congregated in the London area, the endpoint of the epidemic's passage from north to south. The point is no longer simply the incidence of influenza by population but the dynamics of an epidemic's viral progression over time through the populated space of England itself.

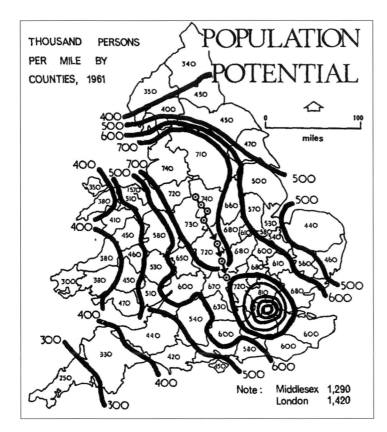

Figure 10.3 Progression of influenza over time in England as the center of the epidemic shifted from the northern to the southern counties. Contour lines reflect incidence by county population.

Source: Courtesy of Blackwell Publishing.

Diffusion

The idea of gravity, of a hierarchy of population centers affected by the epidemic whose progress it influenced, of a "moving front" of disease diffusion, were importations to the study of disease from geography, a field then in a period of rapid development. A "quantitative revolution" was underway as geographers empowered by the computer's computational abilities mapped a range of dynamic processes, especially that of diffusion. In 1969, Alan Pred translated from the Swedish Torsten Hägerstrand's landmark text, *Innovation Diffusion as a Spatial Process.* First published in 1952, Hägerstrand's work made its way into English first through the work of those like Everett Rogers (1962) who saw the potential of rigorous, computer-enabled diffusion studies that modeled the way everything and anything moved in time and space from a point of introduction through a community or the world.

Hägerstrand began with a simple model to describe the decision of an adopter, or potential adopter, to an innovation. A grid, a "mean information field (MIF)," was floated over the mapped population surface. In each pass of the grid, a person who had adopted an innovation became the central cell in the MIF. Surrounding cells would either adopt or reject the innovation depending on the rules of the program. A Monte Carlo process[2] was used to determine the probability that any contact with the

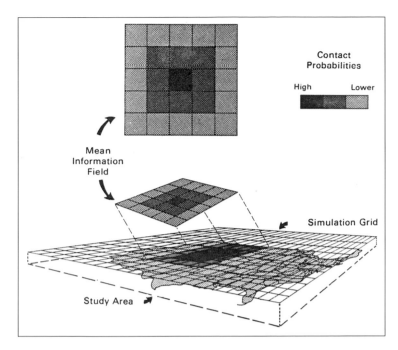

Figure 10.4 Mean information field as a means of spatial analysis in which the mean information field floats over the simulation grid surface in a manner that considers probability of disease or innovation adoption by those nearer or further from an agent.

Source: Courtesy of Rowman and Littlefield Publishing, Inc.

innovation agent by a potential adopter would result in acceptance by the second person. The simple rules of the program (there were in the original model, all told, only four) included one that said increasing distance from an adopter (being at the edge of the MIF grid) diminished the likelihood of acceptance.

Hägerstrand's genius lay in his perception of diffusion as a multidimensional, dynamic process. Trend lines could be extended statistically and spatial patterns predicted. While Hägerstrand's own interests were economic, the idea was generally applicable. The same rules applied, the same process was in force whether what was being transmitted between persons was an idea, a new widget, a bacteria, or virus.

For those interested in health and disease, Hägerstrand's work presented an opportunity to self-consciously advance May's 1950s-style medical geography, one that was environmental but static, to one in which "an increased amount of attention some geographers were lending to the concept of disease causation through cartographic knowledge" (Pyle 1976, 98). That knowledge was at once statistical and graphic, an attempt to map the etiology of disease through an understanding of the relations between incidence and environmental factors on the one hand and processes of diffusion and adoption in those environments on the other. To understand this synergy, it is necessary to pause for a moment and review briefly the simultaneous expansion of studies of urban structure as a part of the broadly environmental focus earlier advocated by May at a very different scale of analysis.

Bronchitis

In the 1960s, the study of urban structure and the networks that joined cities of varying sizes was in a period of tremendous ferment. In the 1930s, the Chicago School came to perceive urban structure as zonal, with the city built out from a central core surrounded by a ghetto to different and increasingly affluent communities. These insights were then tested in the analysis of a range of data, including, for example Federal Housing Administration mortgage insurance records. That application resulted in an observed pattern of residential urban growth that was, in fact, more axial than concentric (Badcock 2002, 184). This work on urban structure was complemented by that of central place theorists who advanced an understanding of urban structure in a general, quantitative approach to the spatiality of the urban world (Haggett 1966).

Not surprisingly, given the increasing urbanization of economically developed nations like the United States and England, urban studies were quickly adopted by medical geographers seeking to understand issues of urban illness. Consideration of the hoary conception of the "unhealthy city" took on a new and more complex cast as illness gain was considered as an outcome of urban demographic structure.

An example of this work from an urban perspective was Girtz's "urban ecology" of chronic bronchitis. His goal was "to estimate the basic spatial structure of simple chronic bronchitis . . . and to attempt to derive a complex of factors which might be responsible for the generation of this pattern" (Girtz 1972, 212). At that time, two theories of chronic bronchitis were being considered. The first assumed that air pollution was the principal cause of bronchitis irrespective of social or political factors. The second "indicted city conditions" (Girtz 1972, 212) for the high incidence in some rather than other areas. Girtz's argument certainly echoes Snow's from the cholera debates: "If air pollution does cause bronchitis the disease should show a similar spatial pattern. On the other hand, if bronchitis is more a result of socio-economic factors than the contemporary physical environment of the city one should expect a sectoral tendency in the distribution of morbidity" (Girtz 1972, 218).

He tested the theory in the British industrial city of Leeds. First, Girtz divided the city into thirty distinct quadrats, square or cubic spaces, to assure a range of physical and socioeconomic environments. Between seven hundred and eight hundred female residents living in each were randomly selected for interview. Women were chosen "because it was thought their occupational histories would be simpler and shorter than males" (Girtz 1972, 216). The statistical evaluation of bronchitis based on this analysis suggested a strong and obvious spatial element in the incidence of bronchitis among women in Leeds.

A simple probability analysis of occurrence of bronchitis gave a "less than 0.05 probability of the extreme prevalence in the quadrats occurring through a Poisson process and, hence, it was concluded, that the significant spatial variation in bronchitis prevalence did exist between the places included in the sample" (Girtz 1972, 218). That difference clearly suggested any explanation based on airborne

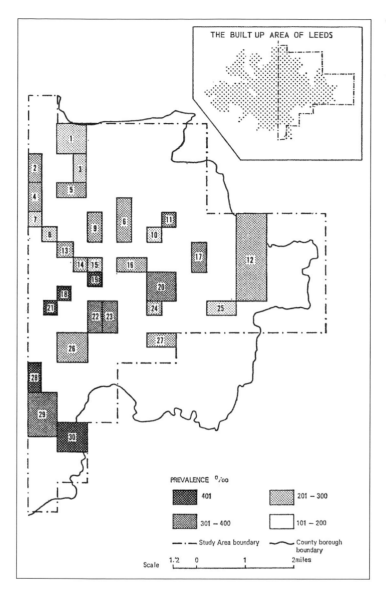

Figure 10.5 Map of bronchitis among women in Leeds using sample quadrats for population testing. The result shows areas of greater intensity not randomly distributed. After Girtz (1972, 216).

Source: *Medical geography: Techniques and field studies.* N. D. McGlashan, 1972, Routledge.

vectors alone would be incomplete. The question then became how to involve other factors in a more complete description of bronchitis.

In the next stage of his study, Girtz used then-current urban theory to consider his results based on the assumption that (a) a city expands and (b) is organized around both concentric and sectoral zones (Learmonth 1988, 93–94). "Inhabitants of a city tend to be distributed into sectors according to socioeconomic status around the center, each sector growing concentrically outwards as the city grows"

(Girtz 1972, 218). Assuming that to be true, Girtz reasoned that variations in bronchitis among women in his study might reflect differences in socioeconomic conditions in different urban sectors.

The result suggested a socioeconomic rather than a simple atmospheric profile of bronchitis. It was more frequent in sectors where income and living standards were lower when compared with those in which income and socioeconomic factors were higher. The correspondence was not a simple, one-to-one correlation. Environmental factors, including air pollution and housing density, clearly contributed to bronchitis incidence. So, too, however, did socioeconomic factors that in turn were determinants of the housing environment in which people resided. There was no single, simple explanation, only an ecology whose social and physical elements interacted, together contributing to the likelihood of bronchitis in the population. Those living in sectors of the city that were poorer—where density was greatest—were more likely, irrespective of other factors, to suffer from the condition.

In this and other studies of the period statistics and medical mapping were conjoined. Mapping was not ephemeral to this and other contemporary studies but central to an evolving understanding of the relation between disease incidence and the environments that promote it. Pyle (1976, 98) argued that this ecological focus, understood through mapping, had its origins in the 1960s when the "cartographic point of view" departed from May's "more conceptually oriented works" to those which self-consciously sought to present "the interrelationship of human disease and natural environment." Girtz exemplified this new focus, mapping a statistically appropriate sample of neighborhoods, his quadrats, and then extrapolated from that to a citywide profile of bronchitis. Using a simulation program, he then filled in the urban map with numbers of presumed incidence, of the likely occurrence in areas for which data was not known based on what was known. To this he joined a schematic map of urban structure, one whose general theoretical basis was well considered,[3] in an attempt to fuse urban theory to the mapped differences his study had uncovered. The mapped results were tested for their significance using modern statistics. Mapping and statistics were entwined from the start of the project as they had not been since the early experiments of the Paris School in the 1830s.

Cholera redux

Not surprisingly, perhaps, others used the new interest in urban studies, and what might be called a revitalized or perhaps reborn procedure for statistical mapping to revisit issues raised by the historical incidence of disease. Pyle, for example, used evolving theories about the historical relation between cities to reconsider nineteenth-century cholera epidemics in the United States. In this work, he compared the pattern of the 1832 epidemic with the one occurring in the 1860s. In the first, cholera typically entered the country through northeastern seaports and from Montreal, Canada. From these concentrated points of introduction the disease traveled down the maritime eastern coast and west along the Erie Canal to the Great Lakes, and from there down the Mississippi to New Orleans in mid-November.

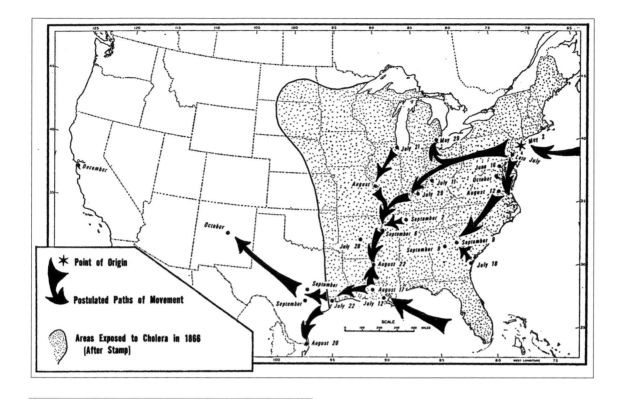

Figure 10.6 Map of the diffusion of cholera in the United States in 1866 showing the growing effect of the maturing transport system (river, rail, and sail) on the diffusion of this disease compared to the 1832 epidemic.

Source: Reprinted from "The Diffusion of Cholera in the United States in the Nineteenth Century" by Pyle. *Geographical Analysis* 1(1):59–75. © 1969 by the Ohio State University Press. All rights reserved. Reprinted with permission.

By 1866, however, there were two very distinct points of disease introduction: northeastern industrial cities, especially New York, and New Orleans. This time the disease traveled by both rail and river systems from these distinct entry points, diffusing in a very different pattern across the developing nation. In 1866, a maturing transportation system linked cities that were hierarchically related. The disease tended to flow from both port cities by rail, river, and sea route to smaller cities in a manner detailed by McClellan in his cholera report of the 1870s. Unlike McClellan, however, Pyle was able to order the progression generally following a rank-order formula of urban size.

The rank-order law, articulated by Zipf in 1949, formalizes an observed and general regularity: while there are typically a small number of large events, there are as typically a large number of small events of the same class (Longley and Batty 2003, 329–332). The relationship between ranks is ordered with each being one-half size of the next. Pyle reported a general coincidence between city size and the path of cholera occurrence in the 1866 epidemic that flowed from the largest U.S. city

(New York) across the country. This underlies Pyle's map of the general paths of cholera's U.S. diffusion from New Orleans and New York between July and September in 1866.[4] For an understanding of the relation of rank order to cholera diffusion, Pyle used a graph that abstracted the cities from his general map and showed the relation between size and diffusion of cholera over time.

By 1977, cholera had become both a metaphor for the determinants of infectious disease and the index case of modern pandemic disease. In a review of the lessons learned from more than almost 150 years of study of successive pandemics, Jusatz (1977) was able to tie it together into an ecological perspective that included climate, commerce (trade routes), hydrology (of individual streams), geography (altitude), sociology (of populations), and population migration. The study was a historical review whose topical application was the then-current pandemic of cholera's most recent evolution, the *El Tor* variant. In 1961, this new serotype began its migration around the world that would last to the end of the century. In this incarnation it was not the fearsome, unknown killer but known, a familiar whose origins and pattern of spread from city to city and nation to nation had become almost comforting in its constancy.

Hepatitis

Neil McGlashan's 1977 study of an outbreak of viral hepatitis in Tasmania presents another, more graphic, example of the analysis of disease diffusion in terms of urban infrastructure. Like others, including most notably Peter Haggett, McGlashan recognized the value of studying disease diffusion on an island. "By choosing islands for study, leakage will be reduced to a minimum and, importantly, these tend to occur at well-defined times when ships and/or aircraft bond the islands to continental [disease] reservoir areas" (Haggett 2000, 32). McGlashan studied the spread of hepatitis in the municipal network of Tasmania in an attempt to test the idea that hepatitis diffused from larger to smaller cities, as Pyle's work suggested it must. "While not returning completely unequivocal results," he reported "a simple analogue model is here illustrated" (McGlashan 1977).

The island's forty-seven municipalities were mapped and weighted by size of population. Here, however, the result was not a cartogram but a series of larger or smaller circles representing population centers of different sizes *á la* Rosenwaldt and Jusatz. To this were added transportation links between the cities, the network that permitted people and goods to travel throughout Tasmania. Using simple network theory, McGlashan calculated the circuitry between different municipalities to give an idea of the network's robustness. He then mapped the occurrence of viral hepatitis, week by week, for a period of 163 weeks as it worked its way through the system. In this, he paid careful attention to the effect the disease's incubation periods might have on the result. What resulted was a map of the effect on disease diffusion of population size and urban transportation networks linking cities of different sizes at national, regional, and local scales. The map of these relations described the pathways of infectious diffusion. In the map, cities of different sizes are joined through a network whose connectivity is

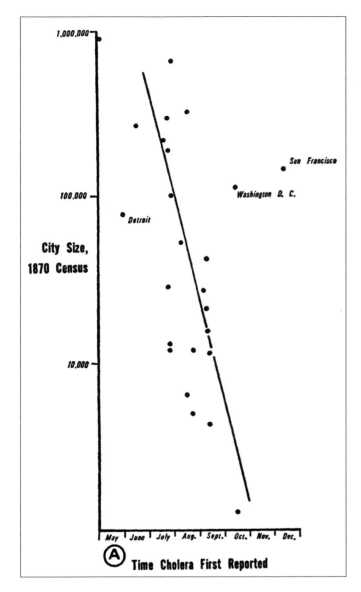

Figure 10.7 The relation of city population size to the diffusion of cholera in the United States in 1866. Larger cities with maturing transportation links tended to earlier introduction of an epidemic. In later models, distance from the epicenter of an outbreak was added to population density in modeling of diffusion.

Source: Reprinted from "The Diffusion of Cholera in the United States in the Nineteenth Century" by Pyle. *Geographical Analysis* 1(1):59–75. © 1969 by the Ohio State University Press. All rights reserved. Reprinted with permission.

clearly related to the diffusion of the disease and its dynamic. In this way, population, transportation theory, urban rank order, and diffusion theory were united in a single study of the spread of a disease over time and in space.

Embedded in the maps are several distinct themes. First is the incidence of hepatitis over time and in space, its progress through the hierarchy of towns and cities of Tasmania. The outbreak traveled from larger to smaller towns just as cholera had moved from ports to smaller service centers, New Orleans to Memphis, and human immunodeficiency virus (HIV) would, in the 1980s, move from Boston and New York and Washington, D.C., to smaller towns like Johnson City, Tennessee. Second, these two elements, the scales of diffusion over time and in the urban hierarchy, are linked by the transportation and interpersonal links that carried the human vectors of the disease from one place to another within a process of general urban exchange and interchange. The results are strong linkages at some times and between some nodes, the transmission clear, while at other times the linkages between cities is weaker, reflecting a different stage of disease spread. The subsystems of regional and local diffusion are most clearly seen here, at this level. In this work, the outcome is based on urban hierarchy, network links, and human interaction together. All work as elements in the ecology of a disease that finds purchase in urban reservoirs from which it spreads along transportation systems that serve as vectors for contamination by urban carriers who travel between cities.

The model for this work was Peter Haggett's now classic study of the spread of measles in Cornwall, England (Haggett 1966). Data on the time and incidence of measles in the study area (identified in

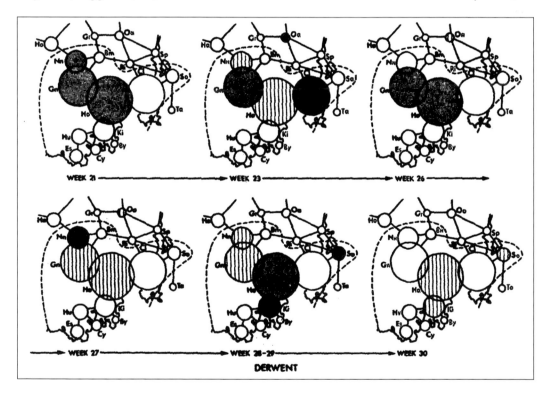

Figure 10.8 McGlashan's map of the outbreak of hepatitis over time. White circles are urban centers free of the disease, striped circles are those where the infection is waning, and black circles are new sites of epidemic outbreak.

Source: *Medical Geography: Techniques and field studies.* N.D. McGlashan, 1972, Routledge.

map "A") for the period October 1966 to December 1970 was abstracted into a cell coding (infected or not infected) for twenty-seven towns based on data in the *Registrar General's Weekly* return, Farr's reportorial legacy of disease occurrence. The towns were themselves abstracted into a "planar graph," a network of the towns in the area with size reflected in larger or smaller circles. The result permitted the spread of diffusion to be mapped and analyzed week-by-week and town-by-town within the network of urban relations in the district.

Statistics: "The poverty syndrome"

In these years increasingly sophisticated mathematics were used to consider a range of phenomena as computers enabled new statistical approaches. Sometimes, the mapping of problems considered statistically distilled the results of complex computations, commenting on them and orienting their results spatially. Other times, statistics served to critique an incidence map and advance the argument it presented or proposed. Either way, mapping and statistics were reunited in a fundamental fashion in this computerized approach to medical geography.

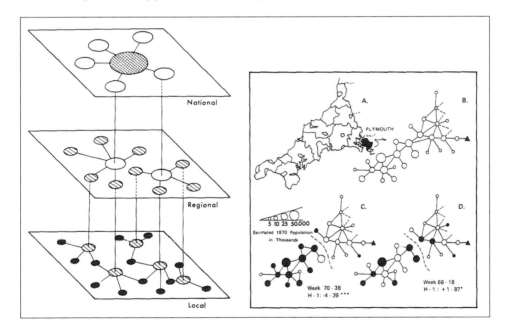

Figure 10.9 Examples of weak (C) and strong (D) relationships in a network map (B) of urban centers in a section of England during a measles epidemic. The result is a graph analysis of disease diffusion through a twenty-seven-node urban structure located in map (A).

Source: Permission to reprint courtesy of *Economic Geography*.

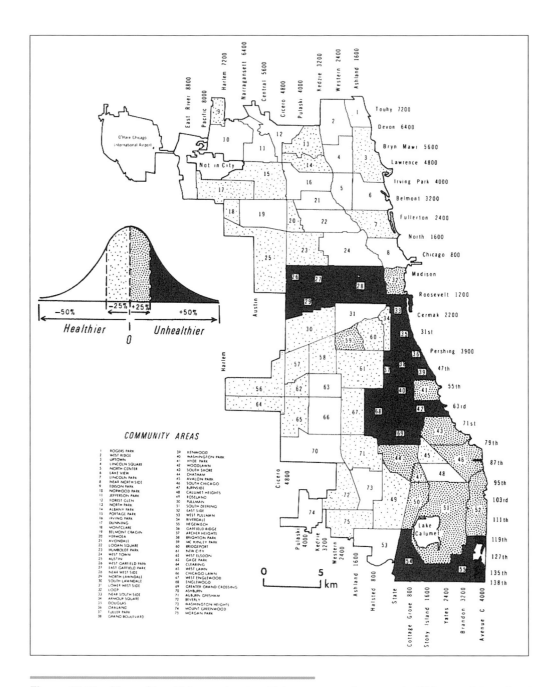

Figure 10.10 Map of healthier and unhealthier community areas in Chicago determined by factor analysis. Maps based on specific factors and a nineteen-variable disease index yield different, specifically detailed maps.

Source: Pyle and Rees, 1971. Courtesy of Economic Geography

Too often, perhaps, mapping hid the analytics that powered the conclusions that a map sought to reach. This was especially true with spatial analyses that were being developed during this period. In a map of "the poverty syndrome," for example, Pyle mapped the Greater Chicago area, labeling different electoral districts as healthier or unhealthier. Here was a map of disease and health, one that showed an extraordinary spatial variation in the incidence of disease or its absence within adjoining jurisdictions within a single urban environment. It was also a statistical surface of spatial data manipulated "behind the scenes" to create a powerful result: large but explicable variations in the incidence of healthy and unhealthy persons *á la* Chadwick within a single urban metropolis.

The assignment of relative health or disease in individual Chicago districts was determined using a multivariate analytic factor analysis. In Pyle's map eighteen disease variables, including population density, were analyzed in this fashion. Those that are typically associated with poverty (employment, income, etc.) showed up as the most important factors, accounting for more than 40 percent of the variance between healthier and unhealthier Chicago districts. Other critical indicators included population density within a district and the combined incidence of three childhood diseases (mumps, whooping cough, and chickenpox).

Mapping each of the principal factors individually makes for a series of maps, each with a distinct profile. Pyle's work relates population to disease incidence and then joins them both (through the database) to the map of Chicago's districts. The map included here is that of the principal factor of socioeconomic determinants (poverty, density, etc.) of disease incidence. There are echoes of Chadwick's maps of Bethnal Green and of Leeds, of Booth's famous complex set of variables whose many constituents (income, schooling, health insurance, etc.) create a social and statistical space that informs an urban map of health and disease.

Geographical analysis engine

In this period, the "justification for spatial analysis," the reason for building one or another disease-related topography, was "the more traditional objective analysis of map patterns itself" (Openshaw et al. 1987, 335). That is, the mapping of data using computerized approaches generated maps whose distillation and organization were themselves revealing. Simply, the work was in the map which was neither illustrative nor representative but instead the very medium of analysis and exploration. Nowhere is this clearer, or the effect of the mainframe computer more evident, than in Openshaw's Geographical Analysis Engine, or GAM.

The goal was to "generalize the locational aspects [of a problem] by examining circles of all sensible radii for all possible point locations in a given study region" (Openshaw et al. 1987, 338). If the question was the incidence of a disease within an environment and the theory was one of contagion from a specific source (the Broad Street Pump, for example), then a mainframe computer could test that theory using a series of circles to reveal the probable source of a disease cluster, a concentration of cases. Because the computer is powerful, dumbly iterative, every point on the map, all potential points across its surface could be tested. To keep from having a map whose test circles overwhelmed the page, a test statistic was needed to weed out clearly irrelevant data circles, those that were just noise in the signal. Openshaw choose the Monte Carlo simulation procedure for this because it "shifts the decisions back in the direction of the specification of a particular null hypothesis regarding an underlying generating process" (Openshaw et al. 1987, 240).

To demonstrate the approach, Openshaw and his coworkers tested for clusters of cancer incidence in Northern England using case data for the years 1968–1985 from the Newcastle and Manchester cancer registries. The assumption was that cancers would cluster, be more evident in areas near radiation-releasing centers. At the time, the effect of radiation was a very contested subject. On a total of 853 cases of leukemia and 163 cases of a specific tumor, Wilms's, Openshaw's program ran its simulation to test 1,625,986 possible correlations. The whole process took just under eight hours of computation time.

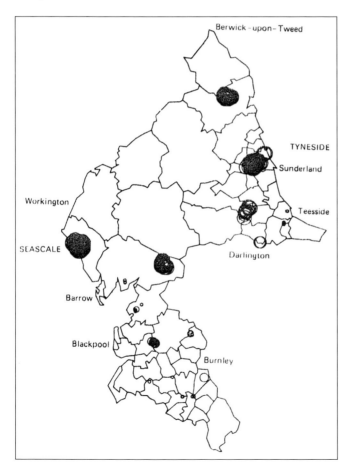

Figure 10.11 Openshaw's map of leukemia clusters in England using the Geographic Analysis Machine (GAM).

Source: Courtesy of Regional Science Association.

The resulting plot of circles of significant relation at the p=0.002 level showed several significant clusters of lymphoblastic leukemia. "The results are surprising, not because they confirm the existence of the cluster at Seascale [where a reactor was located], but because of the much larger cluster that seems to exist in Tyneside focused on Gateshead" (Openshaw et al. 1987, 348). The absence of any radiation site in the Gateshead area where another cluster occurred suggested, "a common non-radiation link might be responsible for both Seascale and Gateshead."

The advantage of the result was that "the combination of Monte Carlo testing and geographic interpretation of the map pattern . . . offers some hope of being able to identify all the major clusters which are sufficiently robust and persistent to stand out from a background of random noise" (Openshaw et al. 1988, 100). The combination of computerized statistics and mapping generated a surface in which the circles would show clusters of disease related to specific locations embedded in political jurisdiction in a way that had been unavailable before. Simulation testing identified statistically significant, "sensible radii" that were mapped. Each circle was mapped graphically and tested statistically, graphics and statistics joined in a single testing procedure.

There were limits to this approach, however. First, the results were dependent on the length of the radii of the circles that needed to be set manually by the operator. Second, the computing time—eight hours to run this study—was expensive and limiting. Finally, the resulting plots created a crude surface that while suggestive were imprecise and difficult to read. The significance of the results, and their comparison with other nongraphic, statistical forms of cluster analysis, were hotly debated for years (Fotheringham and Zhan 1996). But the basic problems of computing time and clarity were soon solved as computer programs became more sophisticated, and with increased power, more able. The limits of the map itself were to be resolved with modern laser printers, online graphics, and the newer programs whose graphical solutions would be more precise.

Surface analysis

Measles, an illness used by many epidemiologists and medical geographers in studies of disease diffusion, is the simplest disease to model (Haggett 2000, 16).[5] But influenza, a virus as persistent but more adaptable than humankind itself, is the real challenge. Unlike measles, influenza is a rapidly mutating virus that year-by-year changes its configuration to accommodate to the human environment. To begin to understand the pattern of its diffusion, we again have the work of Pyle to consider, albeit work from the 1980s, not the 1970s. Gained across that decade was an increased sophistication in statistical and graphical thinking. This would not have happened, however, were it not for the simultaneous advance in the 1980s in computerized printing and the computers whose software directed the output. Finally, one began to see maps capable of relatively subtle black-and-white gradations, maps whose lines were sharper and whose curves were smooth and consistent. The result was not

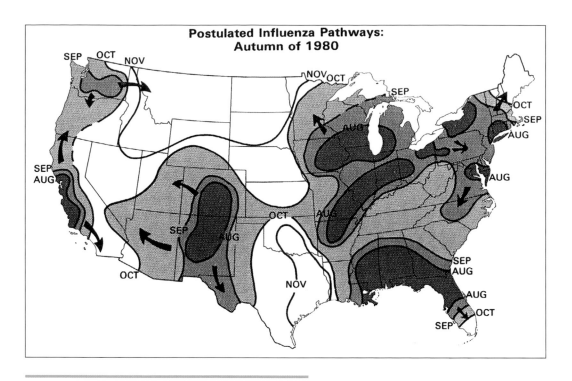

Figure 10.12   Map of pathways of the 1980 U.S. influenza epidemic. This epidemic had multiple centers of diffusion suggesting an epidemic of an endemic disease rather than the single center model of diffusion more typically representative of an epidemic of a new strain.

Source: Courtesy of Rowman and Littlefield Publishing, Inc.

simply the ability to complete more complex calculations but to map data as a dynamic surface and to do so with increasing clarity and sophistication.

Pyle (1986, 172–174) used harmonics to distinguish between different waves of influenza, an approach requiring computer power and computation expertise unavailable even a generation earlier.[6] In this manner he transformed mapped data of disease incidence (by month and by year and by city) into a generalized map of influenza over time. Using deaths per one hundred thousand people per month for the 1977–1978 and 1980–1981 seasons, he calculated "postulated influenza pathways" of the disease's spread over time from various centers. In any month (the time frame of the map), influenza is developing (numbers low but climbing), peaking (its numbers high), or waning (its numbers dropping) somewhere in the United States.

The resulting surface distills a lot of data marked, point-by-point, on lower-order maps. With this approach researchers were able to look at the diffusion of influenza in a number of ways, comparing the patterns of new strains with single index cities of introduction with those of older strains whose spread appeared to begin at several points simultaneously. The approach also served for retrospective analyses in which data from epidemics (1917–1919, 1947, etc.) could be expanded, mapped, and compared as medical geographers struggled to understand this most recurrent and persistent of epidemic diseases

This type of surface analysis, and the calculations it depends on, also opened the door to more powerful predictive analytics. Demographers knew with some precision not only the number of deaths per epidemic, but also the relative mortality of different age groups within those coarser number sets. Since seniors are the most likely age group for whom a severe respiratory infection will be fatal, by considering the distribution of seniors a map of probable mortality in future epidemics could be created. Relying on census data, Pyle calculated population over 65 years of age for a city, divided the distance between one city and another (the distance a disease would have to spread), and multiplied by a factor describing the potential for infection of the urban location. What resulted was a map of future, probable mortality based on the location of not just general populations but more specifically populations at risk in cities mapped within the general, observed pattern of disease diffusion.

HIV-AIDS: Peter Gould

"Epidemiologists searching for definitive explanations to spatial-diffusion procedures should initially consult the long-standing expositions of Gould," Pyle wrote in 1986 (195). Peter J. Gould was a geographer who, with Cliff, Haggett, and earlier, Hägerstrand, focused his attention on the process of how things spread across space and over time. In the mid-1980s he became passionately concerned about the problem of HIV in the United States. The Pennsylvania State University professor focused his attention on the potential for HIV infection among the student populations he encountered. The best estimates of infection rates in the mid-1980s meant, Gould et al (1991, 81) pointed out a likelihood of 111 cases at Pennsylvania State (student population 37,000) and nineteen at Carnegie-Mellon University (student population 6,500). With a then largely uninformed student population that was presumed to routinely engage in unprotected sex—a 1980s population unaware of the risks—Gould perceived a potential epidemic of HIV within the student populations he taught.

Gould was angry at the failure of medical and public health officials to educate sexually active people—homosexual and heterosexual—about the disease's potential. "Education is all we have to fight further transmission of the virus. Education, particularly anything touching upon sexual education, is notoriously difficult in this country" (Gould et al. 1991, 81). They were not doing enough, he argued, to educate people in a way that was comprehensive and convincing. He set out to address the problem using his skills as a geographer expert in diffusion studies. The result was not simply educational, however, but fundamental.

Gould believed his background made him a natural researcher in this area. "For a geographer, a fascination for things spreading over space through time, no matter what they are—viruses, innovations, fashions, fads, etc.—seems not only natural but inevitable, almost what it means to be called to the geographic way of seeing the world" (Gould 1993, 61). Shocked to discover that epidemiologists

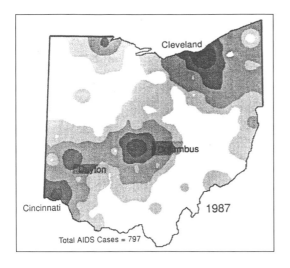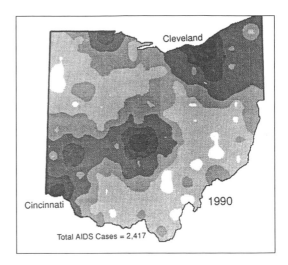

Figure 10.13 Maps of the active AIDS cases in Ohio, 1987 and 1990. Gould mapped the progression of the disease from its inception into the 1990s, developing a predictive model of its future advance. These were two of a series of maps of AIDS history and its future.

Source: Gould (1993). Courtesy of Blackwell Publishing.

typically modeled temporality at the expense of spatiality, Gould and several colleagues set out to map not simply the diffusion of HIV but also its probable rate and direction of spread. Gould wanted the results to be understood not only by epidemiologists and public health officials but by the students he taught and thought of as his critical audience. They might elect to participate in risky sexual behavior but should not, he believed, do so out of ignorance. For this reason, he was adamant that the results be mapped in a way that would be generally comprehensible.

The task was formidable. The spread of AIDS is at once "spatially contagious," moving out in a predictable pattern from an initial source of infection, and hierarchical, appearing "to jump from place to place, usually city to city and town to town, without necessarily touching down at places in between" (Gould 1993, 63). Worse, it had not a single point of diffusion but appeared to spread from many points simultaneously. Every person infected with the disease was a carrier. The North America index case was eventually traced to an Air Canada airline steward, Gaetan Dugas, "patient zero" (Verghese 1995, 287) who infected men with whom he had relations in every city he visited, introducing the virus to North America as those he infected unknowingly infected others.

Gould was interested less in that level of epidemiology, studying the initial introductory phase of the disease, than in the resulting pattern of disease spread. That was what he sought to understand and then map. First, he mapped the diffusion of HIV, year by year, using data from the U.S. Centers for Disease Control. The data for incidence in individual cities was generalized on a raster surface whose

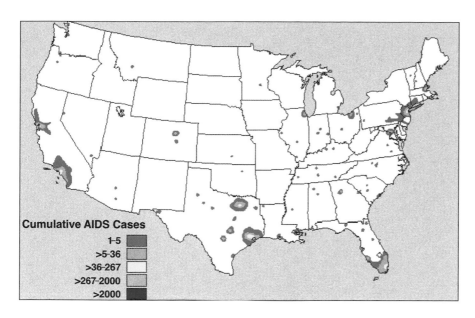

Cumulative AIDS Cases

1–5	
>5–36	
>36–267	
>267–2000	
>2000	

1982

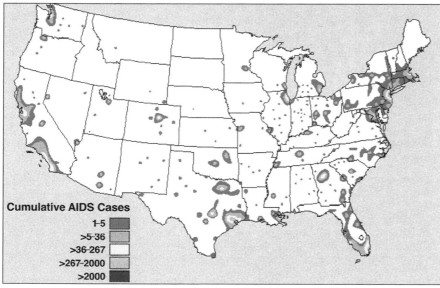

Cumulative AIDS Cases

1–5	
>5–36	
>36–267	
>267–2000	
>2000	

1984

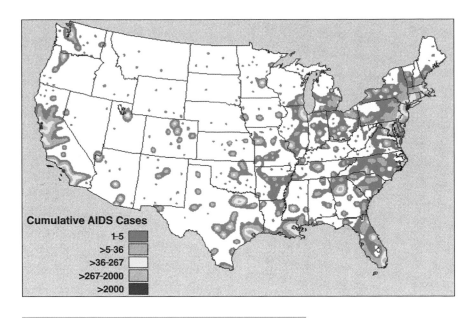

Cumulative AIDS Cases

1-5	
>5-36	
>36-267	
>267-2000	
>2000	

1986

Figure 10.14 Gould's maps of AIDS in 1982, 1984, and 1986. The diffusion of the disease is gravity dependent, moving between larger cities and from there to smaller.

Source: Gould (1999). Courtesy of Blackwell Publishing.

space was divided into discrete cells, each of which has an attribute value depending on the number of cases reported in it. In this way Gould was able to show the spread of HIV over time in a way that was graphically explicit and comprehensible to any student who might think HIV would not come to his or her city or town.

This in itself was an important corrective. "Despite millions of dollars spent on the AIDS epidemic," he told *Science Magazine* in 1991, "we have virtually no picture . . .[of] the geographic dimensions of this deadly virus" (Walden 1991). Gould gave the world a picture of HIV as it spread across states and across the nation. To drive home the point, he then decided to map the probable spread of HIV, its likely future diffusion across the hierarchy of cities and towns. The resulting maps exposed a "very good general and overall relationship between AIDS and population" (Gould 1993, 184). One could see its growth, plot one's own home on the greater map of Ohio, or the nation. Here again was the rank size that Pyle had used in his retrospective study of cholera, an ordering of potential nodes by urban population size. In this transformation, however, it is part of the equation, a factor in the complex of relations distilled in the resulting maps.

Gould next developed a "geographic bloodhound" as a predictive tool, a spatial adaptive filter something like Hägerstrand's MIF but more sophisticated. Think of it as a modern computer 'bot designed to search the map surface in an attempt to gather sufficient data to predict where AIDS

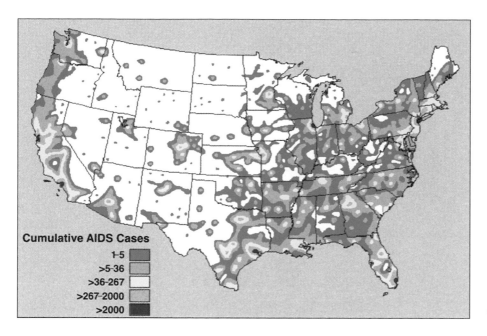

1988

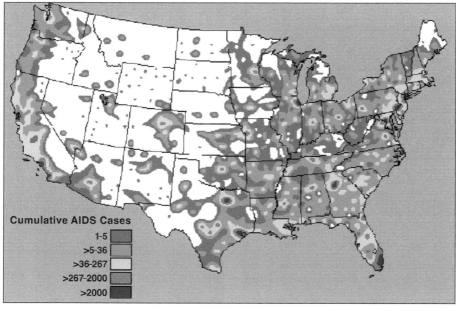

1990

Figure 10.15 Gould's maps of AIDS diffusion, 1988 and 1990.

Source: Gould (1999). Courtesy of Balckwell Publishing.

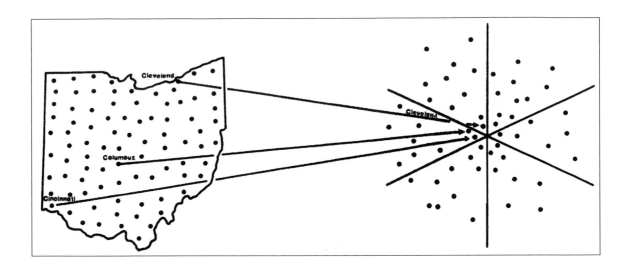

Figure 10.16 Map of the attraction between cities based on population and distance brings them closer in mapped space than they are in a traditional map-basing relations on Euclidian distance.

Source: Gould (1993). Courtesy of Blackwell Publishing.

would next appear. The filter took the coefficient of AIDS historical incidence in individual cities to build a pattern of coefficients whose principal components were latitude, longitude, and time. When mapped, the result could "track very smoothly over time, changing in highly regular and predictable ways" (Gould 1993, 185). That predictability permitted prediction, the next step in the x, y, t coordinates of Gould's map of the future.

The predictive algorithms by which the x, y, t of future location in cities of different size was to be built were based on "gravity model thinking," on the observed relationship between population, distance, and the diffusion of disease. Gravity is a core concept in locational geography that argues movement between two centers is "proportional to the product of their populations and inversely proportional to the square of the distant separating them" (Haggett 1966,35). The result is a tendency to go to larger cities for specialized services and goods; the larger the city, the greater its stock of those things one cannot find in one's own hometown, including HIV. For his predictive modeling Gould used gravity to reorder the relations between places relatively distant in space that, because of gravity attraction based on size, might effectively be closer in "AIDS space."

The idea permitted Gould to transform the geographical map of HIV-affected areas into a place map of cities and towns based on their gravity. In Ohio, for example, the nearness in "HIV-space" between Ohio's largest towns—Cincinnati, Cleveland, and Columbus—was very different from nearness in Euclidian space. Based on their gravity—their size and attractiveness to at-risk persons—Gould's study showed how each would become reservoirs from which the infection would spread back to the smaller towns from which their visitors were drawn. Here McGlashan's Tanzania network (and Haggett's seminal measles network) is refocused and recalculated, the simple links between places redefined in the modeling of population and distance as related factors in a single equation. Gould did not need to show the network, the roads, and highways. They were there, however, assumed in the work. What he really needed was to map the result of the analysis in which this map served as a waypoint in his thinking.

The precise execution of the computational model Gould and his colleagues developed required a relatively complex algorithm run on a mainframe computer to apply Gould's "geographic bloodhound." That was the type of calculation that required large blocks of computer time for numerous iterations as the basic algorithm was fitted to the data. The maps had 96 percent accuracy, Gould said

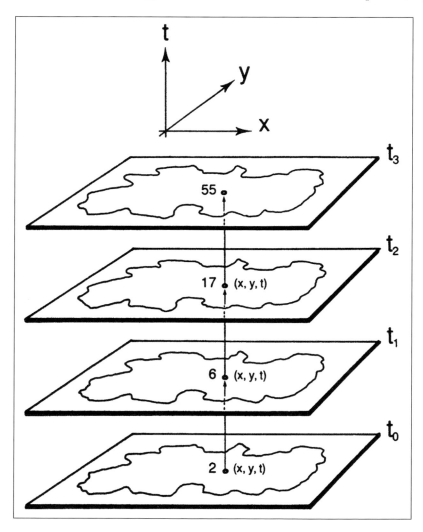

Figure 10.17 Gould's map of locational data aggregated over time helped create a predictive map of disease diffusion in the future. Historical data showed regularities that permitted a future prediction of the diffusion of AIDS cases

Source: Gould (1993). Courtesy of Blackwell Publishing.

with satisfaction in 1999 (Gould 1999, 227). That is, his approach accurately predicted the disease's diffusion in ninety-six out of every one hundred cases. The result was not only a boon to epidemiology, the best predictive map of AIDS that had been done, but its mapping was clear enough for a layperson to understand. When the map sequence was shown at an international conference of AIDS researchers, which had never seen the like, "one epidemiologist in the audience got up and said, 'I believe we have a new paradigm here!'" (Gould 1999, 187). Nothing new, Gould said, at least not to geographers for whom modeling in space and time was second nature.

The progression of the disease Gould mapped was animated and shown to students more likely to watch a video or a film clip on the evening news than to read a technical paper on HIV diffusion. "Upon reviewing the AIDS explosion in the carto-geographic domain, many people are persuaded for the first time that AIDS is not something 'out there,' remote and far removed from them, but may well be all around them" (Gould 1999, 188). Under Gould's joining of epidemiology and geography, the moving presence of AIDS, the sum of its victims over space and time across the United States could be shown, movie-style through the animation of his maps.

As important clinically, the map showed the probable future of contagion, the disease's likely progression across the map, over time. Not only was this interesting to epidemiologists but its message to his intended audience, his students, was clear. Embedded in the maps was the message that the disease's predicted spread would happen if people do not protect themselves against the disease by using protection during sex and not sharing needles. The map empowered the viewers, Gould's students and strangers alike, challenging them to change the map, to modify the probable future it presented by changes their own behaviors.

A clinician's perspective: Verghese

It is easy to assume that by this point mapping was all about computers, computer printing, and the power they brought to geomedical research. Obviously the work of Gould, Haggett, Hägerstrand, McGlashan, Pyle, and others would have been almost impossible without the computer. To do the computations and then map the result would have taken not days or weeks but months, maybe years, had modern computing machines and their printers been unavailable. As important, computers permitted a kind of thinking, graphic and statistical, that invited the address of complex problems in a way that demanded complex algorithms and advanced analysis.

But while the computer facilitates the computations, and more efficient printers improve the map-making, and computing machines and well-designed software assist map thinking, they are not the thinking itself. The work of Abraham Verghese makes this point in a powerful fashion. A young specialist in infectious diseases who moved to Johnson City, Tennessee, in the early 1980s, Verghese had seen the occasional AIDS patient during his residency in Boston. It never occurred to him when he took up a post in eastern Tennessee that the disease would dominate his professional career in the coming years. In the first years of his relatively insulated, semi-rural practice, he saw an increasing number of patients who were HIV positive. Many were gay men who had moved away in young adulthood and come home when the disease was well progressed. Others were local men who had contracted the disease in anonymous encounters at truck stops or elsewhere. Some of them passed the disease on to their wives. In addition, there were hemophiliacs whose disease resulted from contaminated blood transfusions in the days before HIV testing was developed. The medicine Verghese practiced with his patients was one that Snow would have understood, a frustrating battle to treat the symptoms of a disease whose etiology was unclear and whose result was inevitably mortal.

Verghese had access to modern medical journals, but those were the days in which knowledge of the virus was as limited as was its treatment. How could he understand the disease, the persons it affected and the pattern of its spread? Like others who had attempted to solve medical puzzles, Verghese

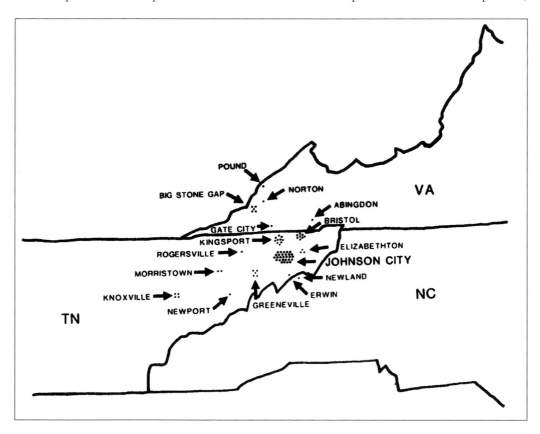

Figure 10.18 Verghese's tracing of the HIV patients he treated in the Johnson City hospital catchment area.

Source: Courtesy of *Journal of Infectious Disease*; Verghese, Berk, and Sarubbi (1989); and the University of Chicago Press.

looked for patterns in the records of the patients he treated, the knowledge he had of their lives. "I compiled a list of every person with HIV that we had seen in the office, the VA [Veteran's Administration Hospital], the Miracle Center [hospital] or the hospitals in our neighboring communities. I made a line-listing with three columns: patient name, address, and a blank column in which I penciled in what I knew about each patient's story, how and where he or she had acquired the disease" (Verghese 1995, 392).

In search of a pattern, Verghese took a U.S. wall map from his son's bedroom and in pencil traced the four-state area (Tennessee, Virginia, North Carolina, and Kentucky) that defined his practice. On it he marked in red the residences of the patients he had treated. "The dots clustered around Johnson City and included Bristol and Kingsport—the Tri-Cities. But the dots also spilled over the ledge of upper east Tennessee into southwest Virginia and Kentucky and across to North Carolina, Big Stone Gap, Blackwood, Wise, Pennington Gap, Pikesville, Whitesburg, Norton, Pound—our HIV-infected patients were tracking down from the small mining towns of southwest Virginia and Kentucky; they

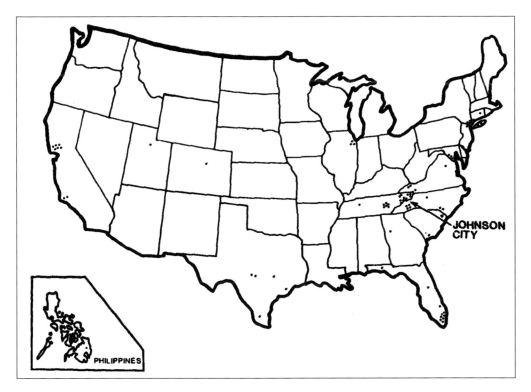

Figure 10.19a Verghese's map of where his Johnson City patients were infected with HIV before returning to their family homes in his region.

Source: Courtesy of Verghese, Berk, and Sarubbi (1989); and the University of Chicago Press.

were coming from the farming towns of east Tennessee like Greenville, Morristown, and Tazewell. They were even coming across the mountains from North Carolina" (Verghese 1995, 393–44). This map he labeled "Domicile."

Verghese next traced the outline of the continental United States and on it located the places where each patient had lived between 1979 and 1985, the period during which they had likely contracted the disease. Johnson City's sentinel patient had come back to Johnston City from New York City. Another returned after a prolonged period in Jacksonville, Florida. Yet another had lived in San Francisco. What resulted were clusters of former residences, many in areas where AIDS had been most active. The maps told more than the tale of "here" and "there," of his practice and the locations where his patients had contracted the disease. The tale they told him was more detailed, and more poignant.

"The dots on the larger map, the 'acquisition' map, were no longer confined to the rectangle of Tennessee and its neighboring states as they had been on the 'domicile' map. Instead they seemed to circle the periphery of the United States, they seemed to wink at me like lights winking a roadside sign. Here was a tight cluster around New York City. Below that, a few dots around Washington, D.C., and then scattered dots on the eastern seaboard down to Florida, where a clump of dots outlined Miami, and single dots pointed to Fort Pierce, Orlando, Jacksonville, and Tallahassee" (Verghese 1995, 394). Other dots cropped up in more distant cities as well: Chicago, Denver, Houston, San Antonio, and San Francisco, for example.

What Verghese perceived was that the disease was largely imported into his area by "native sons who had left long ago and were now returning because of HIV infection" (Verghese 1995, 395). But if that was true, how could he explain the infection of the patients who had never left? The answer was on the map and in the patient list he had constructed. "Here in our little corner of rural America, my patients, trickling in over the past several years in ones and twos, had revealed a pattern to me. Their collective story spoke of an elaborate migration" (Verghese 1995, 394–396).

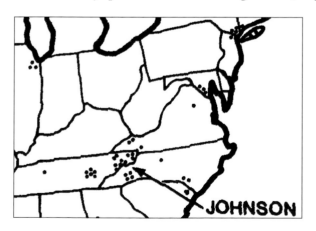

Figure 10.19b Detail of the eastern United States in map of the infection sites of HIV patients treated in Johnson City. Clusters occur near Miami, Florida, Chicago, New York, and Washington, D.C.

Source: Courtesy of Verghese, Berk, and Sarubbi (1989); and the University of Chicago Press.

The migration was of men driven from their homes by prejudice based on sexual preference and then driven back home by the effect of the disease and the need for family care. Implicit in the map was the result of that prejudice and its effect on both the young gay men who left and the families who cared for them in their last months or years. Here, too, however, was the history of the diffusion of the disease, of its travel among host populations—gay and hemophiliac—through the homosexual and heterosexual populations affected by it.

The result of Verghese's thinking was two crude maps eventually published in the *Journal of Infectious Diseases* that distilled the argument traced on the map from his son's bedroom. The maps themselves were rough, more like the early computer maps of Howe and Hoppe than those of Gould. But in the end they provided a similar portrait to Gould's, a complementary perspective from the clinical perspective, an almost equally detailed understanding of the diffusion of AIDS from the viewpoint of a doctor in Small Town, USA. They did this not from the point of view of the analytical geographer but from the narrower focus of the practicing physician whose concern is the patients he or she sees, the illnesses they bring to his or her attention.

It was with the epiphany of the mapping, and the lesson of the rough sketch maps that resulted, that Verghese began to write about the disease, to tell the story of his practice, "the story of how a generation of young men, raised to self-hatred, had risen above the definitions that their society and upbringings had used to define them. It was the story of the hard and sometimes lonely journeys they took far from home into a world more complicated than they imagined and far more dangerous than anyone could have known" (Verghese 402–403). It was that voyage he mapped, the migration away from home to find an identity and then the return of the prodigal son.

Endnotes

1. Both the bubonic plague and the world wars that plagued the last century killed higher percentages of specific populations, but the 1918–1919 influenza pandemic was both truly global, killing people everywhere, and so concentrated in its timing (a six-month period) that Cliff, Haggett, and Smallman-Raynor (2004, 88) give it prominence as a historical killer.

2. The Monte Carlo simulation was a creation of 1940s computing. It was first developed at the Los Alamos project to cut down on the mathematics required to assure that a nuclear explosion, if detonated, would not cascade into the end of the world, but would stop and not continue to involve the whole of the atmosphere, ending life as we know it. While its calculations were challenging in the

1940s computing environment, by the 1970s the simulation could be easily run on a university's mainframe computers.

3. In fact, the sectoral and concentric city organization, based on work by the Chicago School, did not easily translate to many European cities whose long history had resulted in different structures and patterns. Those advancing this approach therefore had to pay careful attention to a range of distinct urban models that together were part of a more general urban taxonomy based on varying geographic and historical patterns.

4. Pyle did not extend his study to the 1873 epidemic that spread up the Mississippi from New Orleans. Perhaps he did not know of McClellan's work or, because the disease's path was not centered on the eastern seaboard, seemed to him too different an epidemic to include in his study.

5. Haggett makes clear there are a number of reasons for measles to have been a marker disease for diffusion studies. These include the fact that its diffusion is always by direct transmission, not through an intermediate agent, its clear wave-pattern behavior, structural stability, and clinically, its distinct rash which makes diagnosis relatively easy. For ease of study, Haggett's studies of its diffusion tended in the 1970s to island populations where the disease's introduction could be easily noted and its diffusion more conveniently studied (Haggett 2000, 16–21).

6. Gerald F. Pyle was that rarest of birds, a first-rate geographer who understood the epidemiology and etiology of the diseases he studied. While Pyle's work today is less well remembered, perhaps, than that of Peter Haggett and Peter Gould, it is still worth reading and studying, especially Pyle's 1979 text on applied medical geography.

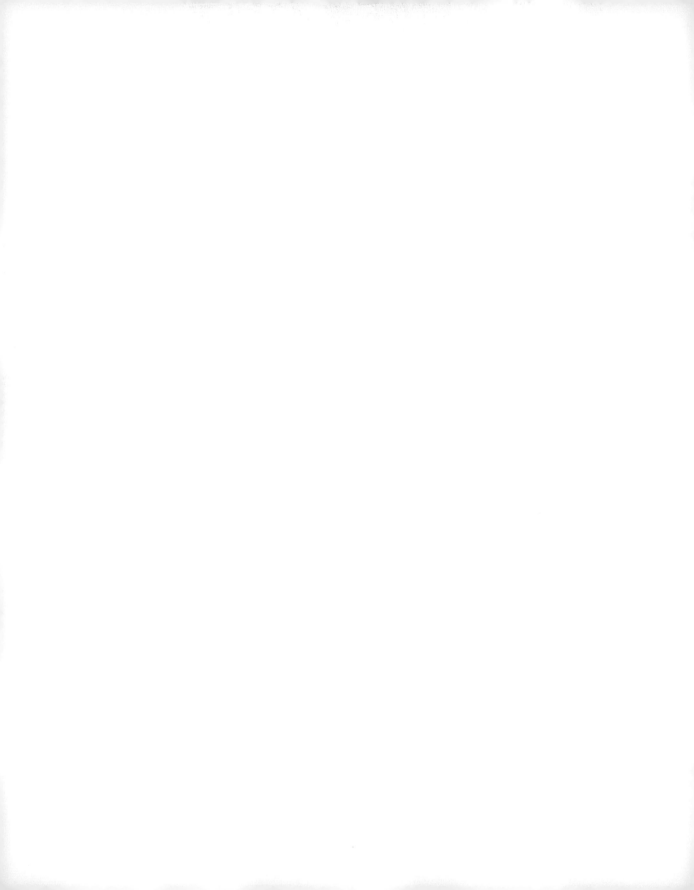

11 GIS and medical mapping

In 1970, I struggled through George McCleary's undergraduate course, *Introduction to Cartography*, at Clark University, earning an undistinguished C+. Among the laboratory exercises was one in which we were instructed to make a map of a U.S. state by creating computer punch cards for each point defining the state's boundaries. These were the days in which Hägerstrand's work was generating enormous excitement and central place theory was contributing to cutting-edge urban studies. The mainframe computer was becoming the tool of choice for geographers engaged in the discipline's "quantitative revolution." In fact, geographers had been quantifying for years but only with the mainframe could nonmathematicians complete advanced and complex calculations in a timely fashion.

Because of my general incompetence as a cartographer and as a quantitative geography student—my interest was in third-world development and especially healthcare—I was assigned to map North Dakota, a state with almost perfectly regular borders. The exercise required, as I remember it, that I prepare six punch cards. Each card carried data on the latitude and longitude of the points that when joined could be plotted to map the outline of the state. Displacing a card in the stack and incorrectly entering data on another, the result was that my North Dakota looked more like Rhode Island. Traumatized, I swore off formal mapmaking forever.

In 1988–1989, I spent the academic year at Ohio State University where I had the inestimable good fortune of working under transportation geographer Howard Gauthier, Jr. He required everyone in his undergraduate course to perform a regression analysis on the Euclidian distances between urban service centers. For the exercise we all were given a page and a half of computer instruction and told to go to the university's computer center and enter the program with our data. I asked if I might do it not on the mainframe but on my Apple® computer and the new laser printer, one of the first generally available, that I had purchased that fall. "You can't do this on a personal computer," Howard said. "You need the mainframe for this work." When I insisted my Macintosh® computer was up to the task, he laughed and invited me to try. "This I have to see," he said. The spreadsheet called *Multiplan* had regression as a basic function and Howard was startled when, the next day, I showed him the results. "I never would have believed it," he said. Personal computing had arrived.

In 1998, I began an analysis of the U.S. graft organ transplant organ distribution system. On my desktop computer I tried linear programming, then used for certain types of locational problems, but the results returned were unsatisfactory. I knew I needed computerized mapping if I were to consider issues of justice and efficiency in an organ transplant system which included 164 heart transplant-performing hospitals serving the population of more than 4,500 cities and towns in the United States. With the assistance of University of Hawaii geographer Matthew McGranaghan, I learned the basics of ArcView® 3.1 and began to map the U.S. system of graft organ distribution. Where the required calculations exceeded its capabilities, I used the Microsoft Excel spreadsheet program. Within three months the first maps were accepted by a professional journal (Koch 1999a), and over the next several years the mapped analysis of systemic inequalities grew into a book (Koch 2002).

This was not the mapping George McCleary tried to teach me. Or maybe it was, albeit with methods accessible even to those like me who had struggled with the older punch-card-based, computer-assisted cartography. In the 1990s, a series of off-the-shelf mapping programs designed to run on personal computers became available for a price roughly equal to that of the Microsoft Office software suite. Despite differences in design and execution, all shared several critical characteristics. ArcInfo®, ArcView, EDRISI, Manifold®, and Maptitude®: all presented geographical data in a standardized format that could be manipulated graphically as well as statistically; all relied on spatial databases (of cities, provinces or states, roads, and so on) to which attribute tables could be joined. The mapped and charted results of these conjunctions could be easily printed using any of the then available desktop printers: laser, inkjet, or even dot matrix.

The move from mainframe to desktop gave to many the potential to undertake research programs like those pioneered by Cliff and Haggett, Gould, Hägerstrand, and Pyle. Embedded in the evolving software—analytic or mapping—were algorithms for a range of sophisticated statistical tests, including

Monte Carlo simulations. Buffering, contouring, and surface analytics quickly became standard tools. The popularity of these programs lay in their ability to generate inexpensive and readily comprehensible maps, charts, and tables based on the manipulation of spatially related data. However, the real power of evolving GIS systems resided in their database structure. An amateur could develop a table of disease incidence by location, analyze it in terms of census demographics, aggregate that data to the level of county, province, or nation, and then present the result in a map, chart, or graph. Indeed, one could use all three to explain the conclusions at various scales, and the way those conclusions were reached.

GIS models[1]

GIS mapping software served not simply to move mapping programs from mainframes to personal computers, but also to introduce a new stage in the history of mapping itself. In the 1960s, the first computerized mapping systems typically drew either crude vector maps or raster maps using overprinted characters like those generated for the U.S. Army's MOD program. The computer-aided design model then employed stored geographical data in binary file formats that became points, lines, and areas. Very little detail other than locational coordinates was stored in the database about the attributes themselves. It was for this reason that early, mainframe computer mapping required programs like SYMAP to prepare maps of basic geographical data.

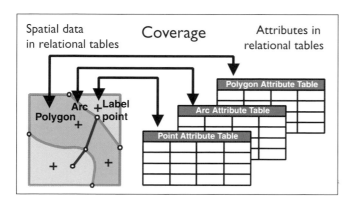

Figure 11.1 Elements of the coverage data model for GIS introduced by ESRI in 1981.

Source: Zeiler (1999). *Modeling Our World*, Courtesy of ESRI Press, ESRI.

In 1981, ESRI introduced its first commercial GIS software, ArcInfo, which implemented a second-generation geographic data model, the coverage data model (Zeiler 1999, 4). In this approach, spatial data stored in indexed, binary files was combined with attribute data optimized for display and ease of access. The attribute data was stored in databases whose rows equal the number of features in the binary tables and are linked by a common identifier (Zeiler 1999). All features were aggregated into homogeneous collections of points, lines, and polygons. In this format, topological relationships could be stored so that, for example, the locational record for a single point or district could be stored with data on the deaths that occurred at that location; a parish or enumeration district polygon could be stored with demographic and health-related data pertinent to the jurisdiction. The coverage material, correctly located, could be manipulated numerically and then projected, its data defined within one or another symbol system.

The generic behavior supported by the coverage model (a line is a line is a line, irrespective of the type of network in which it is embedded) enforced a topological integrity that lent and lends itself to certain types of medical mapping. It permitted, for example, a rigorous topology of disease incidence (points) and suspected sources (points) within an urban network traversed by citizens (lines) that was Snow's subject in his attempt to understand cholera on Broad Street, and later, McClellan's focus in his study of interurban diffusion of cholera in the United States. The mapping of data in the coverage data model facilitated consideration of specific phenomenon (cholera, influenza, yellow fever, etc.) at a range of scales and from a variety of perspectives. The buffers, contour lines, and surface analytics that had required sophisticated, mainframe computer generation progressively became basic, desktop functions suitable for disease analysis.

The evolving desktop computer provided extraordinary opportunities for what earlier had been complex analytics largely reserved for those with access to mainframe computers and the ability to use them. In the coverage data model spatial attributes (latitude and longitude) were stored with secondary attributes (address, time, number of persons, demographic characteristics) in a manner available to a range of computational approaches using algorithms built into the software or in complimentary programs like Microsoft Excel, SPSS®, SASS, and so on. GIS had develop into a medium for both graphic and statistical consideration of spatial problems whose resolution could be reported at once in charts, graphs, maps, and tables.

Finally, the evolution of GIS coincided with the broader shift, still under way, from print to digital storage of demographic and spatial data. The evolution of the World Wide Web in the mid-1990s provided a medium by which studies pertinent to disease might be retrieved from afar and then joined with files of locational attributes.

The result has been an unprecedented availability of social and health-related data that can be downloaded to the desktop and independently manipulated in GIS systems whose analytic and graphic capabilities are far beyond those that were available a generation ago to researchers like Gould and Openshaw. For example, by the late 1990s a decade of data on graft organ retrieval and use was available online (*www.unos.org*) for all transplant-performing hospitals in the United States. Where important, details of the relative status of the populations of cities and states in which those transplant-performing hospitals were embedded could be analyzed and related using official socioeconomic census data (*www. census.gov*).

In a somewhat different venue, the aggregation of data pertinent to West Nile virus (WNV) provides a similarly instructive example. For a recent study of the virus's ecological determinants, in 2004 I located on the Web site of the U.S. Centers for Disease Control data on WNV incidence by U.S.

county for all five major species effected (birds, humans, mosquitoes, large-scale mammals like horses, and sentinel flock chickens) for the years 1999 through 2003. Population data for United States cities with a population above five thousand people, and socioeconomic data for the counties themselves, was bundled with each of my desktop mapping software programs (including ArcGIS® 9.1, ArcView 3.2, Maptitude 3.5, Manifold 4.5). Also available electronically were data on a range of potentially important environmental attributes like rainfall and temperature averaged on a monthly and yearly basis. The result was unprecedented access to a wealth of data potentially critical to the understanding the spread of this viral disease.

Medical atlases

Advances in GIS mapping and map production have resulted in a spate of new health-related atlases whose maps have become the increasingly popular subject of academic and popular writing. These atlases, and these stories, take not the mapped but the geographic perspective as their *raison d'être*: "In healthcare, geography is destiny," promises the *Dartmouth Atlas of Health Care in the United States*, a "mapped compendium describing healthcare utilization based on geographic patterns" (Gundersen 2000, 161). As a class, the medical and health-related atlases created within the computerized transformations of the 1990s seek, as did their predecessors, to identify clusters of disease and where possible to correlate their incidence with potentially generative social, economic, or geographic determinants.

The pages of these atlases distill thousands of pages of data in a manner that at the least has been suggestive, generating hypotheses to explain apparent variations in incidence. GIS enthusiasts have made much of the result. Speaking of this work, for example, the lead author of the *Atlas of United States Mortality*, Linda W. Pickles, insists the result has been a quantum leap forward in the identification of disease clusters. "No one saw patterns [before] because each state had its counties alphabetized and you couldn't see what was next to what." But "once the data were mapped, people saw clusters and said, 'Aha! I know what's there.' It's really amazing" (Gundersen 2000, 164).

Perhaps. But first one has to know what one is looking for and what to map. And once those decisions are made the trick is to interpret the results of the search. Consider a map of cumulative AIDS across the ninety-three largest Standard Metropolitan Statistical Areas (SMSA's) of the United States through October 1989. First published in black and white in 1992 (Smallman-Raynor, Cliff, and Haggett et al. 1992) for the *London International Atlas of AIDS*, it was recently redrawn in color for the *World Atlas of Epidemic Diseases* (Cliff, Haggett, and Smallman-Raynor 2004). In the original, black and white shading was used to describe degree of probability of AIDS in the metropolitan centers based on SMSA population size and reported disease incidence. In the more recent map, color gradients replaced earlier black-and-white variants to articulate differences in probability of occurrence in metropolitan areas.

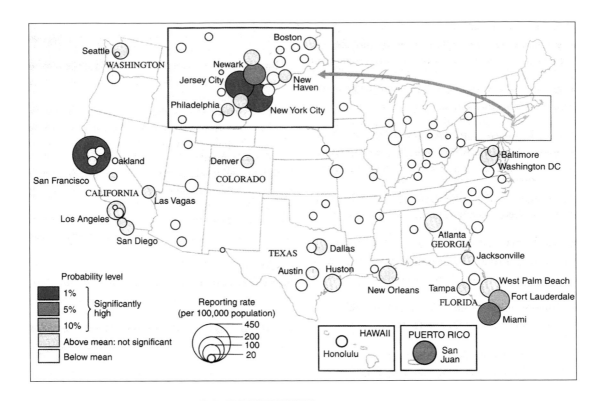

Figure 11.2 Map of cumulative AIDS in ninety-three Standard Metropolitan Statistical Areas (SMSAs) in the United States by October, 1989. Probability is measured against a poisson distribution, reflecting unusual probability, not just intensity.

Source: Courtesy of Cliff, Haggett, and Smallman-Raynor, 2004 and reproduced by permission of Hodder Education.

At one level we have, here, the urban population symbolized in a way that Hoppe and Howe had hoped for in their early computer maps. Population size is given geometric shape in a way that permits comparisons to be made and conclusions drawn. Unlike those early, in retrospect clumsy efforts, in this map the graduated circles are legible and comprehensible in a way differences in those earlier maps were not. The coloration clearly shows four centers to be hugely abnormal with reported AIDS cases (as of 1989) four times that of other SMSAs: New York, Florida, San Francisco and Puerto Rico. Is this "amazing," an "Aha!" map? What exactly are we seeing?

In both the original black-and-white version and in this updated, multicolored rendition the atlases serve not as primary tools of discovery but instead like *Cliff's Notes*® of a complex book or crib notes for a science course, as distillations of the detailed work done by people like Gould and Verghese (and of course by Cliff, Haggett, Smallman-Raynor, and so on). In the cumulative map of AIDS occurring at the end of 1989 in major USA populations we see the centers of gravity from which AIDS diffused hierarchically, year by year, in Gould's map sequence. We have, too, the population centers to which Verghese's patients had traveled and from which they returned to Johnson City. Indeed, one could to best effect overlay the Smallman-Raynor map on Gould's maps of AIDS diffusion to see the hierarchy of centers along which AIDS diffused in his map. Similarly, laying Verghese's patient map of AIDS origins onto the Smallman-Raynor map makes the general case of the specific of experiences of his client population.

This is not to disparage the Smallman-Raynor map that distilled a wealth of data and a lot of computational thinking in its presentation. Certainly Gould and Verghese both would have appreciated the result. The analytic geographer would have understood the population centers and their effect on diffusion, the physician the locus of his patients' conditions. For both, however, the atlas would have been less a tool of discovery than of summary, the "Aha!" quotient theirs and not the map's.

Contemporary atlases

Online atlases available in early 2004 include the following:

- Women and Heart Disease: An Atlas of Racial and Ethnic Disparities in Mortality
  www.cdc.gov/nccdphp/cvd/womensatlas/atlas.htm
- Health Map—Interactive maps on the net
  globalatlas.who.int;www.who.int/csr/en
- Atlas of Cancer Mortality in the United States, 1950–1994
  www.nci.nih.gov/atlas
- Atlas of United States Mortality
  www.cdc.gov/nchs/products/pubs/pubd/other/atlas/atlas.htm
- The Dartmouth Atlas of Health Care in the United States
  www.dartmouthatlas.org

By 2004, the most advanced atlas projects were providing online, interactive statistical analysis and mapping based on huge databases of local, regional, and national data. The interactive *Dartmouth Atlas* Web page (*geiger.dartmouth.edu*), for example, offered the opportunity to plot specific measures of health care resource and utilization across the United States on a graph whose vertical axis was a specific, health-related variable and whose horizontal axis included up to twenty-five specific locations for which data had been collected. It offered the opportunity to "benchmark" specific health-related variables, comparing the locations of an individual place to the national average for that attribute. In addition, a "community profile" for any local health service area could be generated.

Even more impressive, perhaps, is the USGS National Atlas of the United States whose interactive GIS Web mapping environment contains several public health data layers, including: United States mortality with data on eleven leading causes of death, eight subset causes, and all mortality causes combined for reporting Health Service Areas. Other sites—interactive and static—were available from other state and federal agencies, including the Environmental Protection Agency. In a comprehensive review of the movement of spatially grounded, health-related data from "stovepipes," largely inaccessible silos, to the World Wide Web and its mapping environment, Croner argues a fundamental change is underway. "Increasing Web resources from distributed spatial data portals and global geospatial libraries, and a growing suite of Web integration tools, will provide new opportunities to advance disease surveillance, control and prevention, and insure public access and community empowerment in public health decision making" (Croner 2004, 105–106).

None of this necessarily results in Pickles's, "Aha! I know what's there," however. Indeed, most often it does not. As Seaman and Pascalis learned, and Snow later discovered, "seeing" the incidence of disease and understanding apparent correspondences are very different. The aggregation of data in a map or atlas's map series, while typically suggestive, is rarely inconclusive. Too often, however, contemporary fascination with maps and data, out of context and without careful consideration, gives the appearance of knowing but not the reality. On September 19, 2000, for example, *USA Today* published a front-page story on variations in surgical procedures performed in the United States. "The geography of surgery," promoted the release of the *Dartmouth Atlas of Musculoskeletal Health Care*, "the latest in the eight-year [Dartmouth] series devoted to all areas of health care" (Vergano 2000, A1). The atlas mapped what had been long known: "four times more people in one region get a surgery" than do those with identical diagnoses in different parts of the country.

The map that accompanied the article—and bar charts that gave the story the appearance of authenticity—reviewed the regional disparities between surgical rates for lumpectomies, radical prostatectomies, carotid endartectomies, hip replacement, coronary angiography, and leg amputations. Its data was derived from a 1996 analysis of national Medicare data involving 38 million citizens receiving approximately 40 percent of all medical care nationwide.

The map was data-rich rather than informative. Data are the facts on which information is built; information the conclusions based on the aggregation of facts into an argument whose conclusion they support. The map said only that incidence of surgeries varies across U.S. jurisdictions, not the rationale. It said nothing about the reasons—some legitimate, some not, perhaps—for this variation. Differentiating between data and information is critical. The variations might be wholly benign, and easily explicable, suggestive of problems in the general health service or a dire warning about problems in medical diagnosis and treatment.

Did the number of operations performed represent variations in population and demographics (areas with higher incidence of surgeries being those with specific, at-risk populations), patterns of different treatment modalities, or something more ominous? Might the distinction between radical prostatectomies in Baton Rouge, Louisiana (153 percent above the national average) and Binghamton, New York (73 percent below the national average) represent the use of nonsurgical, radiation therapies in the latter not available in the former? Did the average of hip replacement surgeries in Honolulu

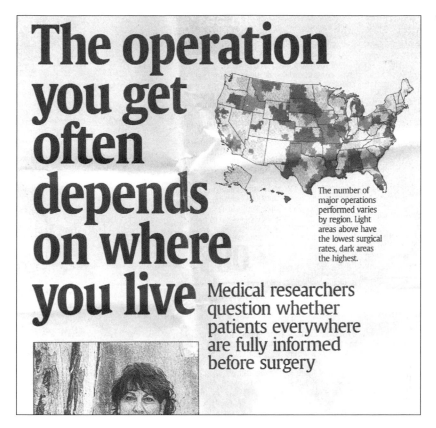

The operation you get often depends on where you live

The number of major operations performed varies by region. Light areas above have the lowest surgical rates, dark areas the highest.

Medical researchers question whether patients everywhere are fully informed before surgery

Figure 11.3a *USA Today* front-page story for September 19, 2000, based on mapping of surgeries.

Source: From *USA Today*, a division of Gannett Co., Inc. Reprinted with permission.

Hawaii, 64 percent below the national average, represent the benefit of a healthier lifestyle than the one lived by the citizens of Sioux City, Iowa, whose number of hip replacements was 63 percent above the national mean? Or, perhaps, did it reflect Hawaii's unique standing as the only state with a population base that is more than 50 percent non-Caucasian, one with comparatively large Polynesian and secondarily Asian (Japanese and Chinese) components?

The newspaper reporter asked none of these questions in his story, assuming its data was wholly informative, taking the map not as a complex statement whose meaning was unclear but as a "snapshot," a picture that might speak for itself.[2] Nor, to be fair, were these questions of sustained inquiry in the *atlas* itself. The only thing the map and the atlas that contained it say is "this" is here, that fewer or more of "x" procedure is performed in one or another part of the country. Indeed, because the data is distilled by county but without geographical references on the map, we cannot judge ourselves the rate of incidence by population, as was possible in the Smallman-Raynor AIDS map. Nor does this map offer a theory or idea or analysis of the facts. We have instead a distillation of factoids that promise a pattern whose meaning is hard to understand, a map that asks for thinking to be done rather than the announcement of thinking, hard work completed.

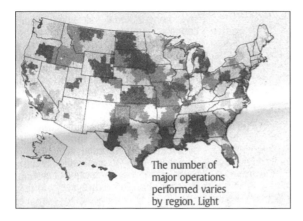

Figure 11.3b Detail of *USA Today* page including map of regional variation in surgeries. The map was based on an atlas description of regional variations in specific surgeries.

Source: From *USA Today*, a division of Gannett Co., Inc. Reprinted with permission.

The number of major operations performed varies by region. Light

To ask about what these variations mean is to ask what else might be correlated with this data, what other factors can be mapped to make sense of the variations this map presents. Do locations of higher incidence of a particular surgery or medical condition reflect variations in the rate of health insurance, of personal income, or of race? Does the map reflect the concentration of hospitals in some areas and their paucity in others? All are potentially contributing factors to be considered, elements of critical thinking that atlases (and newspapers) rarely provide. At best, the atlas is suggestive or summative, rarely conclusive or revelatory. It is more typically a collection of data rather than a wealth of information. That must come from the hard work of thinking about what the data itself, what else must be mapped—statistically or graphically—to understand the problem at hand.

GIS has made mapping easier and more accessible. The digital storage of data has made it increasingly available through a range of online sources. What neither GIS nor the online storage of potentially pertinent data do is guarantee that thinking about illness or disease will be more innovative, more penetrating. The connection between higher incidences of lung cancer in certain east coast cities to the history of asbestos exposure in World War II shipyards, for example (Gundersen 2000, 164), was not an answer that leapt from the map. That required a detailed exploration of the local environment and the individual histories of those whose lives were symbolized as a data in a disease cluster on a cancer map. Mapping may have shown where to look, where the disease incidence was heaviest. It did not show what to look for.

GIS and its critics

For this reason, and perhaps because of unreasonable claims made about GIS by its adherents, some in epidemiology and public health argue mapping is at best a minor, inconsequential tool in the struggle to understand states of disease and health. Proponents of the use of GIS in health studies are assumed to be popularizers, or worse, dilettantes. "GIS aficionados . . . see themselves as standing for the public health in the face of the jeering throng and as rushing out into the real world to save real lives while the stodgy, plodding scientists fussily demand more evidence" (Vinten-Johansen et al. 2003, 397).

The ease with which GIS programs produce their arguments inevitably leads, according to some critics, to thoughtlessness, and shallow work. One sees this, they argue, not only in vacuous maps of disease incidence generally but specifically in treatments of John Snow's iconic work, still the most popular first lesson for students in epidemiology, medical geography, and public health. As Brody put it in a study of Snow's mapping and the GIS perspective, "One sees an echo of Snow the mapmaker without the corresponding appreciation of Snow the thinker in today's 'desktop mapping revolution'" (Brody et al. 2000, 48).

The egregious errors of the map generated by the CDC in its map (see chapter 6) certainly appear to give substance to the criticism. But most of the appropriations of Snow's mapped work detailed in chapter 6 were done before the advent of modern GIS programs. And irrespective of the mapping medium, the most flagrant were by epidemiologists like those contributing to the CDC version, and public health officials like Sedgwick.

GIS and John Snow[3]

It is dangerous to blame a medium for the failings of those who seek to manipulate it. One may agree with Brody, Vinten-Johansen, and their colleagues that some who have used GIS to map issues of health and disease have done inferior work. But whether the problem is inherent in the medium or simply presents research that does not meet a standard irrespective of the medium needs to be considered. One way is to follow the critics and return once more to Snow's work, the locus of their argument, and ask two questions: "Can GIS do what he did more easily?" and "Can GIS advance the thinking beyond the point of Snow's work?"

What Snow did was create a topography of cholera that included the homes of those affected with the location of the water sources he suspected as points of contagion. These were embedded in a network of streets on which local people traveled to and from their homes and workplaces (schools, businesses, etc.). In considering the resulting map he argued (a) an unusual, nonrandom cluster of occurrence existed (b) defining a "cholera area" of unusual incidence that (c) was centered upon the Broad Street pump. If the disease was waterborne, it was the overwhelmingly likely locus of contagion. Furthermore, he argued, "off the map" no other environmental or locational attribute of the area served to explain the disease cluster (a) in the area of epidemic occurrence (b).

His argument was graphic and visual rather than statistical, a problem for modern researchers. In contemporary medical science it is not enough to say "it appears that" or "I see this" without quantifying those observations. To do what Snow did more easily it is necessary only to show, as he did, the apparent clustering of cases in the Broad Street area. To do it better requires an at least modest statistical rigor his work did not possess. Consider again the electronic map based on the Cliff-and-Haggett-

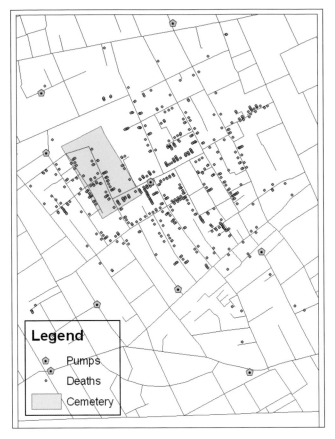

Figure 11.4 A GIS version of John Snow's 1854 map drawn in ArcGIS 8.3 based on data digitized from the Cliff and Haggett, 1988, by the author.

Source: Courtesy of Cliff, Haggett, Smallman-Raynor and reproduced by permission by Hodder Education.

derived database of cholera deaths occurring in St. James, Soho. Its stacking of the cholera-related deaths is similar to Snow's and the intent, here, is to see how careful thinking with GIS may further Snow's thinking using his basic approach. Consider the resulting map that includes the deaths, pumps, and streets Snow described but without the added locational data (schools, workplaces, etc.) he mostly alluded to but did not himself map.

Snow's essential observation in the Broad Street maps was that deaths appeared to be both centered on the Broad Street pump and densest in the area of the pump. Using a GIS program, the relation between the Broad Street pump and the set of deaths from cholera can be easily demonstrated in several ways. By creating a set of interlocked, dissolving buffers around the 578 deaths from cholera Snow recorded, a map results whose center is clearly the Broad Street pump (number 7 in figure 11.5). The "cholera area" is the lightest area centered on that pump and radiating from it in a contiguous fashion. Excluding the few deaths buffered below pumps 9–11, and those three near pump 13, the result is roughly the same as the rectangular area Whitehead suggested in his report.

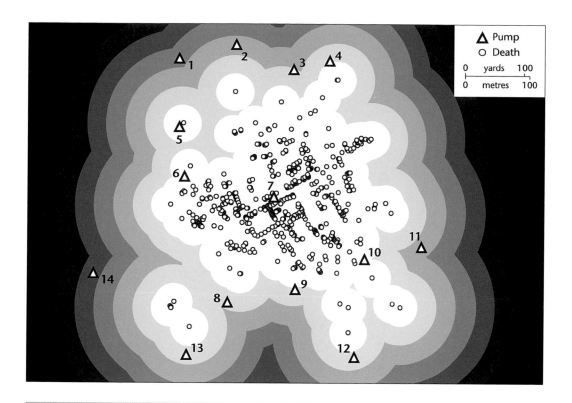

Figure 11.5 A GIS analysis of the Snow data using interlocking buffers around individual deaths to demonstrate the centrality of the Broad Street pump (number 7) and to define the spatial parameters of the area outbreak.

Source: Courtesy of Koch and Denike.

By creating nondissolving, proximate buffers around not the deaths but the pumps themselves, a more focused map can be drawn. The radius of the buffer is manually selected as half the distance between Broad Street (number 7) and its nearest neighbor, the Marlboro pump (number 5). On the resulting surface not only is the Broad Street pump central but also the densest cluster of all deaths is clearly centered on that pump alone. The buffers, easily drawn with almost any GIS program, confirm Snow's observation. To quantify the observation requires only that deaths in each buffer be counted (approximately a quarter of all deaths are in the Broad Street buffer) and their numbers be compared.

A more precise "cholera area" defined by proximity to the Broad Street pump can be drawn joining the set of fourteen pumps to those of all 578 deaths in a "nearest neighbor analysis." The result assigns the nearest pump to each death and simultaneously calculates the distance between each death and the pump nearest to it. With this approach 69 percent of all deaths (361)—the small, white circles in the map—are assigned to the Broad Street pump in a manner that creates a "cholera area" far more specific

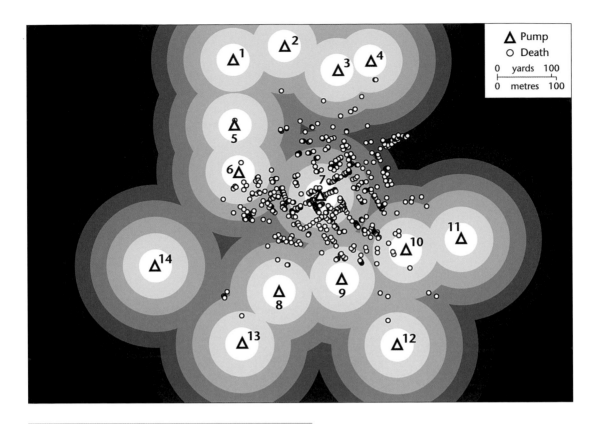

Figure 11.6 A set of four-ring buffers drawn around each of the pumps in the St. James, Soho, area of London demonstrates the centrality of the Broad Street pump (number 7) to the cholera outbreak of 1854. It complements and supports the conclusion of the buffer or contour map based on incidence of cholera deaths.

Source: Courtesy of Koch and Denike.

than those created by the buffering approach. As a boon, the resulting area is one similar to that of the Thiessen polygon in a Voronoi network that Cliff and Haggett described in the 1980s. Nor is this surprising. Polygon analysis is based on proximity and the nearest neighbor approach as well.

There are, however, several problems. Distance calculations are based on relative location and the deaths in the dataset are stacked, one upon each other, moving away from the street where multiple deaths occur at individual house locations. This will affect the calculations between some of the individual deaths and the members of the set of pumps. Indeed, it makes somewhat imprecise all the calculations—buffered and nearest neighbor—in the analysis. The CDC dataset therefore collected all deaths to a single, referenced location and projected the whole in a universal transverse Mercator projection (UTM) with latitude and longitude correctly assigned to the pumps and deaths.

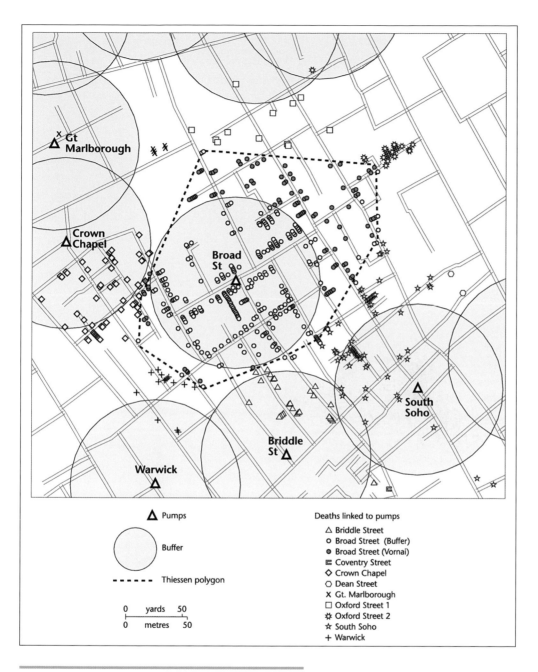

Figure 11.7 A nearest neighbor analysis for Soho study area with buffers is used here to generate a Thiessen polygon. In a color version of this map each death is clearly allocated to the nearest pump.

Source: Courtesy of Koch and Denike.

Alas, its database lacks not only topographic data (schools, etc.) but also a number of deaths recorded by Snow. The two can be normalized to create a dataset with all Snow's deaths and pumps in a map that is correctly projected and referenced. Different GIS use slightly different techniques for spatial adjustments of this kind. In most, common points between two maps are chosen and one is "warped" onto the other until, with at least four and often more than twelve, the one is bent to the other. In this case, the Cliff-and-Haggett-based dataset is bent to the CDC map so that the result will have correct latitude and longitude for each point. In the process, streets can be added to the CDC network, severely truncated, until the network mapped by Snow is recreated.

Drawn in ArcView 3.2 with a warping extension written in Avenue™ script, the result is less than satisfactory. It is difficult to read and the process of correction is arduous. And, frankly, why compare these when we can compare either with the originals? Because a GIS can project graphic images in

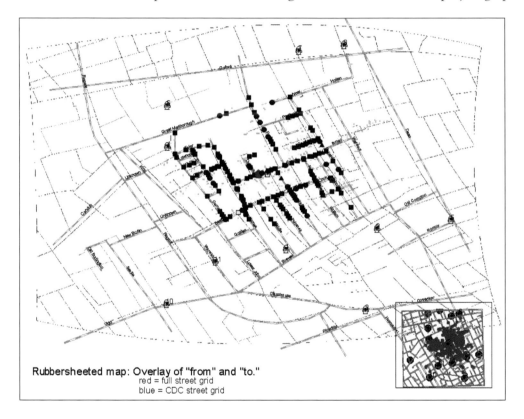

Rubbersheeted map: Overlay of "from" and "to."
red = full street grid
blue = CDC street grid

Figure 11.8 The Snow-based dataset "bent" to the CDC version of the Soho data to permit a complete and correctly referenced dataset for analysis. Gray streets are those in the CDC version. Red streets are those mapped by Snow. Green dots are the fuller set of deaths Snow collected while the black rectangles are locations from the CDC map.

Source: Courtesy of Cliff, Haggett, and Smallman-Raynor and reproduced by permission of Hodder Education.

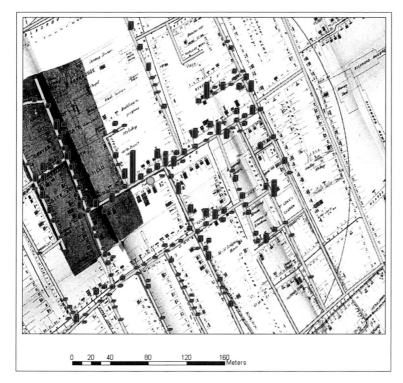

Figure 11.9 Spatial adjustment of CDC data and original map in ArcGIS 8.3 comparing Whitehead's map of the 1854 cholera outbreak with the abridged CDC version of the Snow study map. Light blue lines are those of the digital version bent onto the gray lines of a TIFF of the original map.

Source: Courtesy of the Center for Disease Control.

almost any format (.TIFFs, .GIFs, .JPEGs, etc.), the best approach may be to compare either a CDC or Snow-like version with either Snow's or Whitehead's original maps. As a boon, in the process, additional data, for example the location of sewer lines, can be added to the reconstructed electronic version of the dataset and of the map that results from its projection.

In the accompanying illustration the CDC dataset, with one symbol for each location where each death occurred, was adjusted to fit Whitehead's map of the 1854 outbreak. More precisely, the map was warped so it would overlie the correctly referenced CDC map to whose database data is in the process of being added. The process of correction was left incomplete for illustration purposes. The Broad Street pump is correctly located, as are the central streets. Others, New Street, for example, are yet to be bent to fit the CDC projection. Similarly, deaths occurring outside the primary study area—to the map's northeast, for example, have yet to be included.

Because the resulting electronic database aggregates deaths by house location to permit more precise locational comparison and aggregation, the number of deaths per unit is symbolized, here, not horizontally but vertically. Those homes that were the site of multiple deaths are symbolized with a horizontal bar whose height is defined by the number of deaths at a specific location. Because the locations are correctly located with precise latitude and longitude, the result permits precise measures of incidence (density at a location), distance, and centrality.

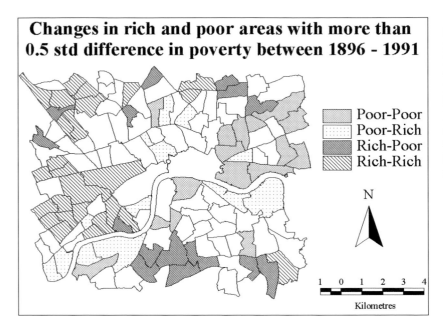

Changes in rich and poor areas with more than 0.5 std difference in poverty between 1896 - 1991

Poor-Poor
Poor-Rich
Rich-Poor
Rich-Rich

N

1 0 1 2 3 4
Kilometres

Figure 11.10 Orford map of relative poverty in London. Orford et al. (2002) regularized boundaries used in Booth's map of poverty in London with contemporary census data to compare relative poverty in 1891 and 1991.

Source: Courtesy of Scott Orford.

Historical epidemiology

The process of spatial adjustment, and more generally, of comparing varying datasets with different perspectives and different data is common in historical studies using mapping. Earlier mapped studies can be evaluated, their data transformed to a modern, mapped surface and studied using modern analytic tools (Knowles 2002). The practical utility of this kind of work to contemporary epidemiology and public health has been shown at one scale of research by Duncan (2003), who used maps to locate the gravesites of those who died during the 1918 influenza epidemic and whose bodies might have been preserved in permafrost graves.

The ability to regularize maps from different periods using different systems of referencing has other advantages, however. Significant among them is the ability to map changes between historical and contemporary states. Orford et al. (2002), for example, used Charles Booth's famous map of poverty in London as the basis for a study of the degree to which relative poverty has changed in London over the last one hundred years. The project required contemporary parish boundaries and street locations and those used by Booth to be regularized in a manner that permitted comparison.

The 1991 United Kingdom census provided the data required to create a contemporary index of poverty that would be compatible with the one Booth used in his map. The result was a discouraging map of then and now. Its general conclusion was that "although the overall standard of living had increased, the geography of poverty at the end of the nineteenth century was very similar to that at the end of the twentieth century. Moreover, the geography of all causes of death for people over the age of 65 was more strongly related to the geography of poverty in the late nineteenth century than

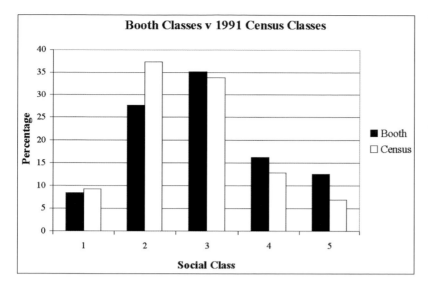

Figure 11.11 Changes in relative percentage of rich and poor in London study based on Booth's study and 1991 census data. The basic distribution remains relatively constant across the one-hundred-year period.

Source: Courtesy of Scott Orford.

contemporary patterns of poverty. This relationship was also true for mortality for specific diseases that are related to deprivation in early life" (Orford et al. 2002).

The map distills this argument nicely. So, too, do the stark bar graphs of relative poverty, then and now, the aggregated statistical argument of the map itself. The choropleth map makes what is in fact a complex and arduous task look simple, almost commonplace. Spatially, regularizing boundaries is a time-consuming pursuit requiring careful analytics if the areas of spatial aggregation of a century ago (the parish district) and those of today are to be correctly compared. Similarly, current census statistics provide a wealth of poverty-related indices that were unavailable to Booth in his study. That contemporary data must be ordered, however, to assure accurate and meaningful mapped comparisons. In the argument and its final distillation, maps and statistics served interdependently. The result is statistical and graphic at once, each medium informing the other as the analysis progressed.

Salmonella

Historical studies of health and the determinants of disease are not ends in themselves. They also serve in the development of analytic approaches to recurrent problem classes that retain a contemporary relevance. *Contra* by Monmonier, a GIS exploration of the Snow dataset, is a useful exercise whose utility is contemporary and real. Modern spatial epidemiology retains the basic concerns Snow and his colleagues expressed: Where is a disease outbreak clustered and what possible sites of contamination are those clusters close to? How can we understand an epidemic's progression at the scale of the state or province, the region, the nation, or the world? Tobler's famous law still holds as a starting point: Everything is related to everything and closer things are more related than distant ones.

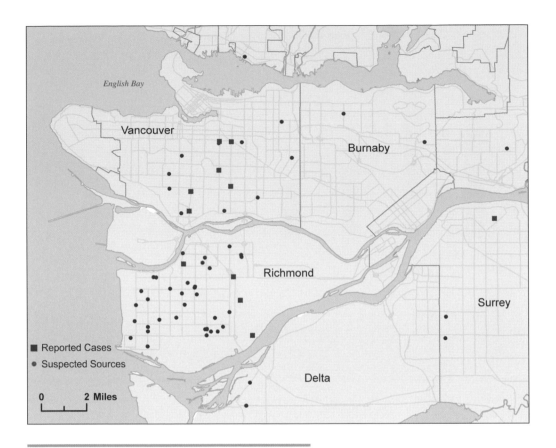

Figure 11.12 Map of 2000 salmonella outbreak in Greater Vancouver. Reported cases, symbolized with red diamonds, and suspected sources, symbolized with green diamonds, are randomized from epidemiological data to assure privacy. The result is illustrative but not reflective of the outbreak.

Source: Koch. Data courtesy of B.C. Centre for Disease Control.

Consider, for example, the analysis of a relatively recent salmonella outbreak in Greater Vancouver, Canada, in 2000, the type of mundane disease outbreak faced by epidemiologists and public health experts everywhere. Sixty-two cases of food poisoning were reported in the Greater Vancouver Regional District (GVRD), a collection of urban and suburban municipalities with a combined population of about 2.1 million persons. A preliminary investigation revealed those affected had eaten at one or more of twenty-one restaurants in the region.

Data on the outbreak was made available for teaching purposes by the B.C. Center for Disease Control. Locational data was randomized to a two-city block by the BCCDC to protect both the privacy of people affected by the outbreak and that of the owners of suspect restaurants. The accompanying illustrations therefore represent not the epidemiological dataset but one modified for illustrative and teaching purposes. Two datasets modified in this fashion were used for this analysis. The first was a set of twenty-one food outlets at which sixty-two people who were treated for food poisoning had eaten or purchased food within the previous three days. The second included the randomized home addresses of persons treated for salmonella during the outbreak. Both were considered within a general database of major metropolitan roads similar to those available for most North American cities.

To map the outbreak, the individual cases and suspected restaurants had to be individually referenced, matched from the database to locations on the street map and then converted into a map file of cases and another of suspected sources. The transformation is largely automated in contemporary GIS programs, each of which handles the process a bit differently.

Once correctly referenced and projected, there appeared to be two general clusters of cases, the larger lying south of the Fraser River in the suburb of Richmond and the other, smaller cluster above it. The first, and more concentrated, extends westward while the second, smaller concentration north of the river appears more contained and less dense. Similar congregations of suspected restaurants are also shown south and north of the river. At a more precise scale of analysis they can be seen to exist along major streets in both municipalities.

No one source leaps out from the map in a Picklesian, "Aha!" moment. A range of techniques used first here in the Snow analysis will serve, however, to consider the data and the attempt to locate the source likely responsible for the outbreak. Assuming that a restaurant or food store closest to the most cases is likely complicit, the goal is to discover which restaurant or restaurants is closest to the largest number of salmonella cases. This requires a spatial join of suspected restaurants to the set of salmonella victims in a manner that assigns to each case a restaurant and the distance from the patient's home to the restaurant. In the GIS, a new database is generated of restaurants nearer to one or more case of food poisoning. One restaurant in Richmond was the nearest to nineteen cases while another two blocks from it was most proximate to fifteen cases. Together these two restaurants accounted for slightly more than one-half of the salmonella cases.

To test their centrality, and seek confirmation of their likely complicity, overlapping buffers around all suspected sources were drawn and their intersect areas then abstracted into a new layer. These intersects served as the locus of a second generation of new, nonoverlapping buffers whose relative importance was determined by calculating the number of cases each contained. A second iteration of the process used only the circles created from the two most southerly intersects, those with by far the greatest number of cases. The eventual result was a single buffer centered approximately between the two restaurants that the nearest neighbor analysis identified as together accounting for thirty-four cases, more than half the total.

Hägerstrand's MIF searched across the gridded surface of his mapped data, testing every square, to consider the probability of innovation adoption based on location and proximity. Openshaw's GIM similarly searched across his study surface in a systematic fashion to find the circles that represented

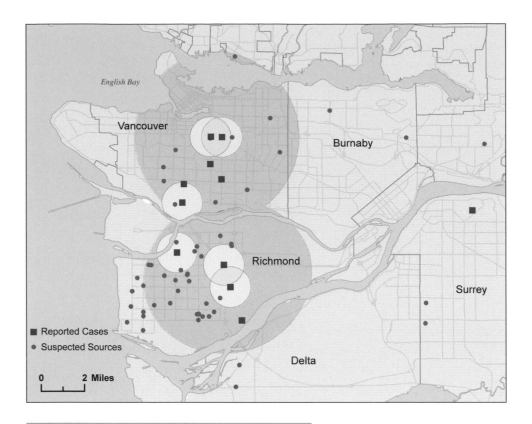

Figure 11.13 Map of salmonella outbreak using buffers and intersects. Light green intersects of buffers drawn around suspected sources in a salmonella epidemic become the loci of buffers used to determine the centrality of clusters of disease. Data, altered to protect privacy, is for illustrative purposes only.

Source: Koch. Courtesy of B.C. Centre for Disease Control.

a likely relation between childhood leukemia and proximity to nuclear reactors. To do this, he overlaid the surface of the map with interlocking circles, choosing the ones that his simulation showed would be significant. In this example, only those areas in which concentrations of salmonella cases are found in relative proximity to suspected sites of infection are tested with buffers centered on those suspected sites. In each iteration, those with no cases within the buffer, or a minimal number of cases, are rejected until a single, central buffer identifies the epicenter of the outbreak. It is a crude, almost clumsy, but in the end effective approach to the problem.

In the end, not one but three restaurants, all near each other, were returned by these approaches. No "Aha!" and no simple, "it's the water!" The mapping helped, and although it did not perfectly identify the real source, it did identify the area and narrow the field geographically to a small set of suspects.

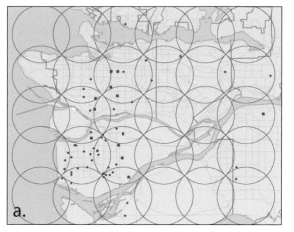

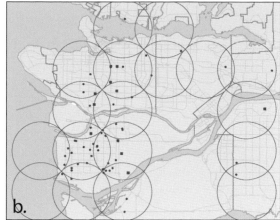

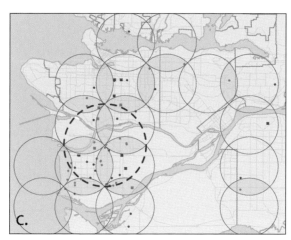

Figure 11.14 Buffers maps of disease outbreak. In 11.14a, the whole surface of the map is tested for disease occurrence. In 11.14b, testing is restricted only to those areas where the disease has occurred. In 11.14c, buffers are drawn only around sites of suspected disease diffusion. New buffers are then drawn around overlapping intersects, colored green in this illustration. A second-generation buffer results, show here with a dotted line.

Source: Data courtesy of B.C. Centre for Disease Control.

This argues not any limits inherent in the approach but the simple fact that in the analysis of a new outbreak sometimes the best answer is a partial one focusing bacterial or viral testing on a few members of a larger set of suspect sources. A clue to the nature of this outbreak, one that distinguishes it from simple point-source outbreaks like the one in Soho's Broad Street, lies in the pattern of the cases of reported salmonella and of the restaurants themselves. In the Broad Street example, the incidents and the pumps are clustered while here they are strung out along the roads. Using a deviational ellipse to measure the angle of incidence of the cases, and the direction of that ellipse, reveals an extended, north-south oval bisected by major local roads in the salmonella case and an almost perfect circle with no similarly revealing directionality in the Broad Street case. The former is typical of an outbreak whose source is distributed along roads from a single distributor, the latter of a single-source outbreak. These ellipses are not simple to calculate by hand, but the algorithm for their generation has been embedded into several programs, including a script for ArcView 3.2 and the Spatial Analyst extension of ArcGIS 9.1.

Public health

Through the 1990s and into the first decade of the twenty-first century the emphasis on mapping in public health studies has been by medical geographers more familiar with mapping and spatial analytics than issues of epidemiology and public health. Slowly, the utility of mapping using GIS systems also has begun to reenter the greater field of epidemiology and public health. The old is become new and a spate of articles on GIS-based approaches to public health has begun to appear in both more general journals (Higgs 2002) as well as those dedicated to epidemiology and public health. Much of this work has been about health economics, the planning of health service areas and designing of health practice catchment areas (see, for example, Gordon and Womersley 1997). Increasingly, however, it has been about the study of disease occurrence and spread in environments that humans have prepared for bacterial or viral engagement. The gradual return of mapping to these disciplines returns as well a focus on spatiality as well as temporality, the former much harder to model than the latter for epidemiologists and public health experts.

Gould's critique has taken root and spatio-temporal analysis, with spatiality a full partner, has become a recognized goal. "Of the three core epidemiologic variables of time, place, and person, place has always been the most difficult and time-consuming to analyze and depict" (Melnick 2002, 3). In his *Introduction to Geographical Information Systems in Public Health*, Melnick argues the benefits of using GIS in public health, of applying its spatial analytics to specific problems. So, too, do Cromley and McLafferty in their *GIS and Public Health* (Cromley and McLafferty 2002). The authors of both books review recent work done with GIS and offer suggestions on where a GIS approach might be better integrated into contemporary health studies.

Perhaps the best examples of that potential lie not in map of disease incidence and possible sites of causation but in the mapping of potential health dangers. Recent work by Johnson and Thota (2003) show the manner in which concern for environmental contamination—of foul air and the ground—is sometimes best carried out in a GIS environment permitting rigorous statistics and GIS-based graphic approaches. The two environmental consultants evaluated underground contamination at a former petroleum refinery and processing facility in the United States. This required an understanding of the nature of non-aqueous phase liquid (NAPL), a distinct oil phase, whose effect is specific to soil, groundwater, and volume of a specific hydrocarbon contaminant. To understand the extent of contamination and its potential risk required not only that areas with NAPL be identified but also that the liquid's degree of mobility, the degree to which the contaminant was static, localized, and easily addressed, be calculated. Low mobility would present less of a danger to the soil and water table than

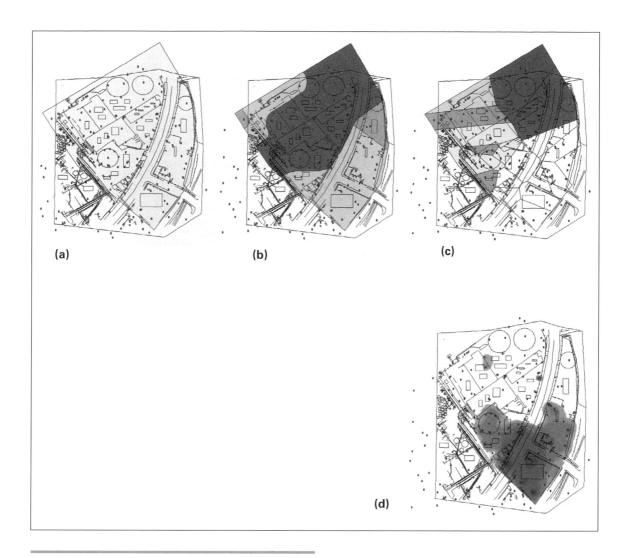

(a)

(b)

(c)

(d)

Figure 11.15 Map of NAPL contamination example. Clockwise the maps describe (a) NAPL test sites (red representing wells where NAPL was present), (b) distribution of soils across the test site (c), viscosity distributions of subsurface oils across the test site, and (d) soil saturation levels. In each, the characteristic is fused by spatial coordinate to the site. In each, data is summarized across the well and boring locations. Together the maps serve to quantify and distill the elements of an equation for potential mobility of the subsurface contaminants.

Source: Courtesy of Jeffrey Johnson and Pramod Thota.

$$M_o = \frac{\dfrac{\rho_{ro}}{\eta_{ro}} \displaystyle\int_{Z_l}^{Z_u} k_{ro} K_{sw}\, dZ}{\displaystyle\int_{Z_l}^{Z_u} \phi S_{of}\, dZ}$$

Figure 11.16 NAPL mobility quantitatively expressed where ϕ is porosity, S_{of} is the oil saturation, Z is the product elevation, n_{ro} is the oil viscosity ratio, K_{sw} is the saturated hydraulic conductivity of water, K_{ro} is the oil relative permeability, and Z_u and Z_1 are the upper and lower elevations where free oil occurs.

Source: Courtesy of Jeffrey Johnson and Pramod Thota.

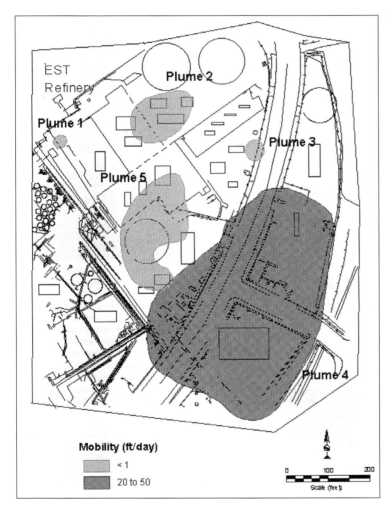

Figure 11.17 Map of NAPL mobility based on oil viscosity, soil type, saturation levels determined at well and test boring sample sites. The result combines statistical and graphic analysis in a single process that is numerical and graphical at once.

Source: Courtesy of Jeffrey Johnson and Pramod Thota.

high mobility. Mobility, however, is a complex outcome whose equation is based on the dynamic relation of elevation, oil saturation, soil composition, and viscosity of the petroleum liquid.

In an attempt to determine NAPL mobility and extent the researchers needed to draw samples from test sites, fifty oil borings and thirty-five groundwater wells. The result revealed NAPL plumes of different types varying from fuel oil to diesel fuel at a thickness ranging from .025 feet to more than eight feet in an area whose water table varied in height daily based on tidal fluctuations in a nearby inlet.

The test sites were fused into an area map and the resulting test surface was considered in relation to other variables contributing to mobility, the potential of the contaminant to spread through the subsoil area. Sequential maps each considered individual variables that together determine NAPL mobility. Each map represented, in other words, a part of the problem. Each argued a spatial and statistical relation between an individual variable joined to the location of the soil borings and existing wells.

The result *(Figure 11.17)* is a "map of maps" in which one subsurface area is shown to have greater mobility resulting from elements individually mapped in Figure 11.15. Figure 11.17 is a graphic and statistical conclusion of the earlier series in which higher levels of (d) saturation centered in a (b) permeable soil type where the (c) specific viscosity of the petroleum products was identified in (a) individual well and test boring sites. The final map in the series solves the equation defining mobility of NAPL by summing the attributes of the individual maps based on data collected. Practically, among the sites that need to be cleaned up, clearly the one with the greatest mobility, and thus the greatest danger of migration into the human habitat, is the one that must first be addressed.

The example seems specialized, unrepresentative. It is, however, precisely the type of example both Farr and Snow would have understood. After all, the focus is the potential contamination of the water table whose importantance lies in its use as the principal source of water for area homes, shops, and agriculture. While the approach is used here in a geological example, similar procedures, perhaps more typically, serve in studies of atmospheric pollution. In the ground or in the air, the basic approach to mapped analysis using precise calculations is the same.

Organ transplantation[6]

The potential of GIS mapping to meld statistical and graphical thinking about states of health and disease is typically argued in just such a way and at this level of analysis. In some cases, however, very simple, basic mapping opens new avenues of thinking, perspectives other than those returned by narrowly focused statistical studies. Exploratory mapping may lead to new arguments, new perspectives that, to be accepted, must be rigorously considered by all available means. In these cases, mapping opens the door, signaling the approach that advances a distinct argument.

The debate in the late 1990s over the best way for the United States to organize its graft organ transplantation system is an example. In a February 1998 letter to Congress, Department of Health and Human Services Secretary Donna Shalala announced proposed changes to the U.S. system of graft organ distribution because the system in place was unfair. "We have not achieved equitable distribution to those with greatest medical need," she told Congress. Since fairness and equal treatment are principles enshrined in the 1984 National Organ Transplant Act (NOTA), this was clearly unacceptable. The "Final Rule," as she called it, would redress inequalities inherent in the system.

The problem, Shalala said, was that "in some areas of our nation, patients wait five times longer or more for an organ than in other areas... in the worst case, patients die in areas where waiting times are long while at the same time organs are being made available to less-ill patients in areas with shorter waiting times." The result was an unacceptable inequality based in part on a system of regional organ collection and distribution that would have to be changed because "transplant patients are best served by an allocation system that functions equitably on a nationwide basis" (Shalala 1998). The thrust of the argument was clearly geographic. Regional variations in graft organ transplantation violated the spirit if not the labor of the government law by creating inequalities between patients based on their location. As importantly, the different waiting times directly impacted patient care and, as she pointed out elsewhere, patient survival.

The organization charged with supervising organ distribution and collection, the United Network for Organ Sharing (UNOS), mounted an intense lobbying effort against the Shalala directive.

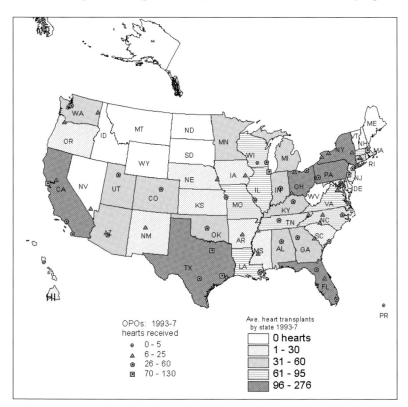

Figure 11.18 Map of heart transplant performance in the United States, 1993–1997, showing the inequality of distribution in a system that promises equality of treatment.

Source: Reproduced with permission of Greenwood Publishing Group, Inc. Westport Connecticut.

In March 1998, for example, its executive director, Walter Graham, wrote its members urging all to lobby against the proposed changes. "It is imperative that patients, donor family members, and transplant professionals at transplant centers, OPOs (Organ Provider Organizations), laboratories, and associations around the country, speak [against the Final Rule] to their lawmakers and to the public."

Defense of the then-existing system by UNOS and its experts spoke less to the systems fairness and equality than it did to issues of efficiency, of maximizing the use of available organs (Pritsker 1998). Equality and fairness were at the bottom of the modeler's list of important variables, minor factors in his calculations. In 1998, I began to consider the issue of geographical inequality and its possible effect on both graft organ collection and distribution. For this project, I decided to focus on the distribution of donor hearts within the existing system of eleven UNOS regions in which 164 transplant-performing hospitals were accredited. In addition, there were a total of sixty-six Organ Provider Organizations (OPO's), administration centers within the regions charged with supervising transplantation. If UNOS was correct, then the location of transplant services should roughly reflect the population distribution of U.S. citizens in their various citizens and towns. If geographical equality was absent, there would be large holes in the coverage. Whether these holes would be large enough to affect organ distribution or timely collection was, at the onset, unclear. Because of the perishability of graft organs—hearts could survive, in 1998, a maximum of four to five hours outside a host—inequalities of distribution would result, I argued, in service inequalities.

The result at a state level was that twelve states and Puerto Rico (the site of an OPO) were wholly without heart transplant-performing hospitals. In states where at least one heart transplant-performing hospital existed, the number of transplants being performed at individual sites varied extremely. Analysis of these differences broadened Shalala's description of waiting times from livers, the organ she focused on, to hearts. As well, it helped explain in part the vastly different waiting times she had described. Geographical inequalities appeared to be directly correlated with increasing waiting times. Calculating performance by state and OPO for the years 1993–1997, the results were clear. Some states had no service and their citizens became transplant emigrants, traveling elsewhere in search of service. Where transplant-performing hospitals existed, service levels were highly unequal.

Using first a simple buffer analysis and then a more rigorous nearest neighbor analysis, I then calculated the distance patients would have to travel from cities with populations above ten thousand people (3,149 towns and cities) to where they might receive a heart transplant.[7] Given the four-to-five hour window of viability for hearts, I used a 180-mile, three-hour drive time measure to analyze the result. The effect was startling; a clear inequity emerged placing some people far away from the centers that were supposed to be equitably and equally shared by all. I later quantified the differences based on air travel time, assuming patients who could not drive might fly instead if flights were available. Too often, they are not.

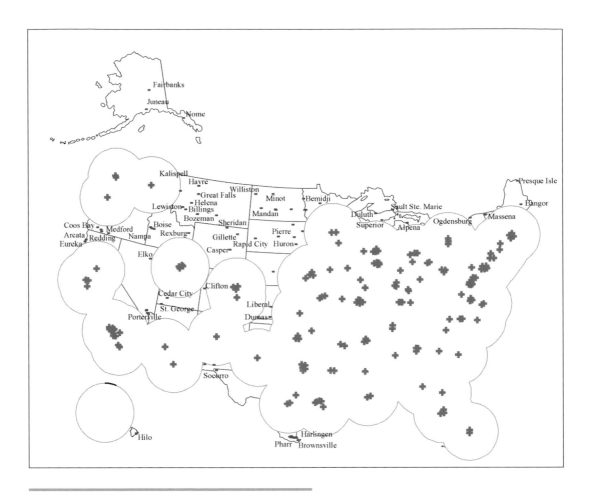

Figure 11.19 Buffer showing cities outside a three-hour, 180-mile drive time range of transplant-performing hospitals. Distance inhibits rapid service for patients from outlying areas and collection of organs from distanced areas.

Source: Reproduced with permission of Greenwood Publishing Group, Inc. Westport Connecticut.

Other studies considered the efficiency of the system in terms of graft organs already collected. The mapped approach chosen in this study focused on the availability of transplant service to people based on location. This mapped perspective permitted the question to emerge: If patients cannot get to a heart-transplant-performing hospital within the four-to-five hour ischemic window before a donated heart spoils, then can hearts collected in outlying areas get to hospitals where patients living nearby are waiting? The mapped analysis suggested one reason for the chronic shortage of organs—and the high spoilage rate of those that are donated but not transplanted—was the structure of the system itself, its concentration in large cities. Holes in the network, areas without service, created populations in which arguments for donation were less powerful. And even if local people did contribute, the likelihood of organ spoilage increased on the basis of distance and the time required to recover and then transport the organ on commercial airplanes to cities with transplant facilities.

Since the beginning of nonexperimental transplantation in the 1980s, supply has always been a limiting factor preventing all those who might benefit from organ donation from receiving one in a timely fashion. Historically, African and Hispanic Americans have been less likely to donate than Caucasian citizens. The reason typically given for this is either African and Hispanic religious affiliations (although religious leaders typically favor transplantation), or fear and ignorance concerning transplantation. The answer, therefore, was to speak of the benefits to society as a whole, to instruct them in their duty as beneficent citizens.

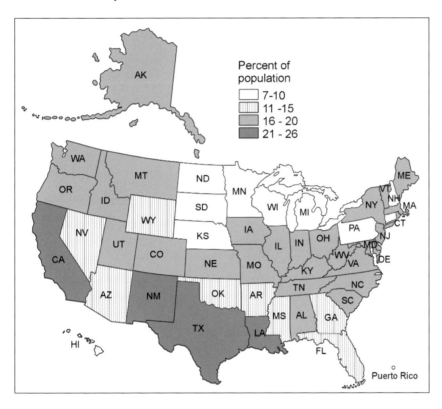

Figure 11.20 Variable rates of health insurance in the United States by state. Darker colors represent higher percentages of persons without health insurance. Rates are especially high in states with high African and Hispanic-American populations.

Source: Reproduced with permission of Greenwood Publishing Group, Inc. Westport Connecticut.

Even preliminary evidence of a range of socioeconomic data argued, however, a very different explanation. African and Hispanic citizens were less likely statistically to have jobs and, therefore, health insurance. By almost every index, African and Hispanic Americans, who tend to be less wealthy than their Caucasian counterparts, also tend to live in less healthy environments, to be sicker, less well educated, and, across a range of conditions (including transplantation), are treated less rapidly than their Caucasian counterparts. Here was the reverse of Gould's AIDS-space in which citizens were closer than geographical distance suggested *(figures 10.18-20)*. In transplant space people of color living in cities with transplant facilities were effectively distanced from service by a lack of financial and health resources. As one article on the problem was titled by editors, "They might as well be in Bolivia" (Koch 1999c).

African and Hispanic Americans therefore represent, by this analysis, a class of people who, even if they live near a heart transplant-performing hospital, are more likely than Caucasians to be disquali-

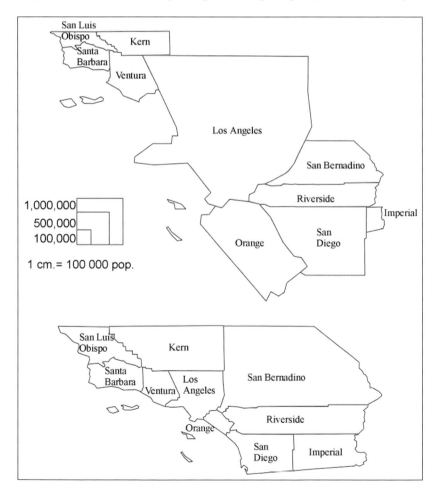

Figure 11.21 Cartogram showing effect of non-insurance on potential donation pools in southern California by county. The most populated county, Los Angeles, is significantly reduced by this indicator.

Source: Koch. U.S. Census data.

Cartographies of Disease

fied from organ receipt because of lack of health insurance because they are unemployed and they lack money for transplantation and aftercare. The likelihood of chronic illnesses resulting from poverty and lack of care is greater, and these may serve to disqualify on medical grounds from transplant service. The lower rates of graft organ donation, therefore, are less likely to result from religious bias or ignorance (most religious leaders in fact encourage donation) than from a well-founded mistrust of a system that seeks organ donation without assuring equal opportunity for transplantation. Put another way, the study concluded inequalities in health care, coverage and insurance create a class of people less likely to receive a heart (they're poorer and sicker) and, therefore, a class of people less likely to donate.

An unexpected consequence of this conclusion was the likelihood that failure to provide adequate health and social service results in a diminished pool of potential donors, exacerbating the chronic shortage in graft organs. To calculate the potential effect of these inequalities, I chose Southern California, an area whose Hispanic population is in some areas 50 percent. Knowing the percentage of people uninsured by race in the USA (Hispanic, African American, Asian, and so on), I calculated the effect of noninsurance for each county in Southern California. To illustrate the result I used a cartogram to redraw the target districts of potential donors based on census data. The largest pool of donors by population—Los Angeles County—shrinks by more than fifty percent because of the county's large non-Caucasian population and the greater likelihood they will not be covered by health insurance.

Papers based on this mapped analysis led to an occasionally furious debate. For example, Alan Pritsker, the simulation modeler who worked as a consultant for UNOS (Pritsker and Koch 1999), reacted strongly to this argument's presentation in the journal *OR/MS Today*. And while praised by some, this study contradicted the conclusions reached by the National Institute of Medicine (Institute of Medicine 1999). In a special report at the request of the U.S. Congress, it found the UNOS System equitable if not "optimal." That its authors found "the system is equitable for women and minorities once they are listed" is not surprising (Gibbons et al. 2000). The critical issue of equitability rested with those not listed because of a lack of health insurance and regular medical care. Those who become ill because they can't afford regular physical exams or are too poor to afford healthcare insurance are not going to be considered at all. They are, however, precisely the people whose families and friends will be asked to donate by a transplant nurse or doctor in the hospital. The mapped analysis drew attention precisely to those who by dint of residential location, ill health, or poverty were desired as donors but off the National Institute of Medicine authors' charts, and likely off the registry of UNOS, too.

Third-world mapping

It is easy to forget that the wealth of data contemporary researchers assume will be available is unavailable in much of the world. We who live in the richest nations swim in a sea of publicly available data, much of it now digital and online, from which information can be culled through a range of analytics based on that extraordinary wealth. Census data for the United States—by county and city block—is available online. The ubiquitous street and topographic maps, and accumulated health registries so common to contemporary health studies, are there, too. These collections are the result of years of investment in a library of data and an infrastructure that permits widespread, ready access to the materials stored online. Neither the data itself nor the infrastructure that provides it is necessarily available in the many under-developed and developing nations of the world whose health challenges are exigent, and as nineteenth-century researchers discovered, pertinent to our own health concerns. It is in these regions, where data and infrastructure to deliver it are both scarce, where GIS mapping may have the greatest impact on studies of health and disease through the enablement of local physicians and local health authorities. Two recent studies suggest the importance of mapping in areas where the information infrastructure is less developed.

Thailand: AIDS

The epidemic mapped so brilliantly in the United States by Gould and his colleagues has spread around the globe. In the developed countries of Europe and North America, the resources for addressing the pandemic are more evident than in poorer nations with neither the medical expertise nor the resources to analyze and then address the problem. In many ways, researchers are like their nineteenth-century counterparts, facing health crises with neither the medical nor the knowledge infrastructure that western countries bring to these problems.

AIDS in Thailand is an example (Anderson et al. 2002). The disease reached that country in 1984 and spread rapidly in subsequent years. By the early 1990s, it was epidemic and the government began an aggressive campaign to slow its spread. This included a public information campaign, distribution of free condoms, the closing of many commercial sex establishments, and counseling for commercial sex workers who were required to use condoms. What was required was both a clear portrait of the extent of the problem and a measurement of the success of the anti-AIDS campaign. Beginning in 1991, the Royal Thailand Army began testing all army inductees called up for national service for virus antibodies. And so, like Malgaigne in 1840s France, Thai researchers quickly gained a wealth of data based upon army inductees from every province and district in the country. While maps of HIV+ incidence at the provincial level were drawn in the mid–1990s, what was needed was a finer scale of analysis, one involving district-level data, to assess the course of AIDS and prevention programs.

These were developed as the result of collaboration between U.S. Army Medical Corps Lt. Col. Arthur E. Brown and Royal Thailand Army Col. Kalyanee Torugsa. Scott W. Anderson, a college friend of Col. Brown's, brought the two men together. Anderson had served in Thailand first as a civilian researcher investigating leprosy and malaria and later as a medical officer attached to the U.S. Armed Forces Research Institute of Medical Sciences. Torugasa collected data while Anderson worked to assure its statistical relevance. This meant refiguring provincial data files to permit a district level

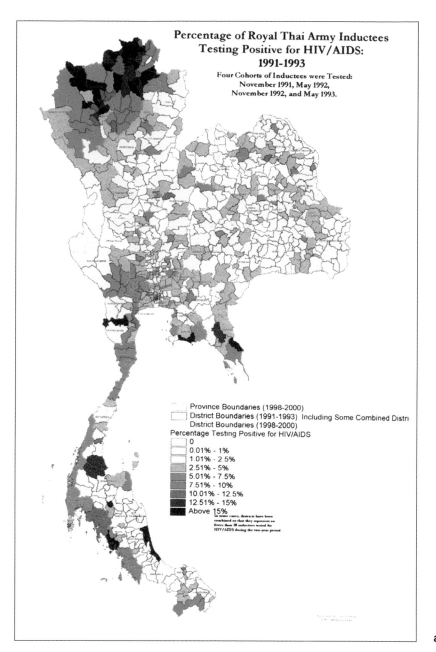

Percentage of Royal Thai Army Inductees
Testing Positive for HIV/AIDS:
1991-1993

Four Cohorts of Inductees were Tested:
November 1991, May 1992,
November 1992, and May 1993.

Province Boundaries (1998-2000)
District Boundaries (1991-1993) Including Some Combined Distri
District Boundaries (1998-2000)

Percentage Testing Positive for HIV/AIDS
0
0.01% - 1%
1.01% - 2.5%
2.51% - 5%
5.01% - 7.5%
7.51% - 10%
10.01% - 12.5%
12.51% - 15%
Above 15%

a

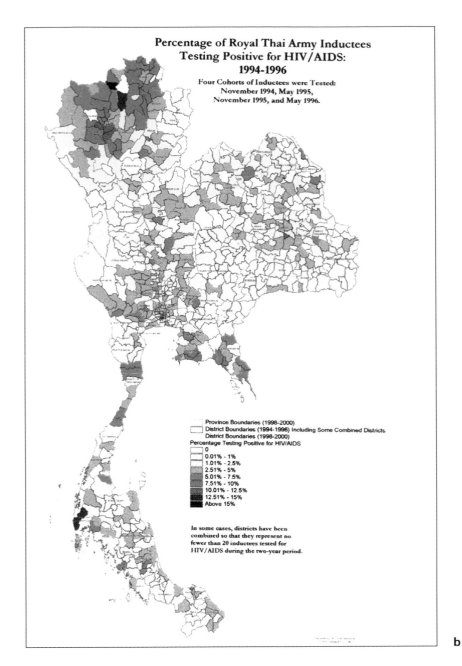

**Percentage of Royal Thai Army Inductees
Testing Positive for HIV/AIDS:
1994-1996**

Four Cohorts of Inductees were Tested:
November 1994, May 1995,
November 1995, and May 1996.

Province Boundaries (1998-2000)
District Boundaries (1994-1996) Including Some Combined Districts
District Boundaries (1998-2000)
Percentage Testing Positive for HIV/AIDS
0
0.01% - 1%
1.01% - 2.5%
2.51% - 5%
5.01% - 7.5%
7.51% - 10%
10.01% - 12.5%
12.51% - 15%
Above 15%

In some cases, districts have been
combined so that they represent no
fewer than 20 inductees tested for
HIV/AIDS during the two-year period.

b

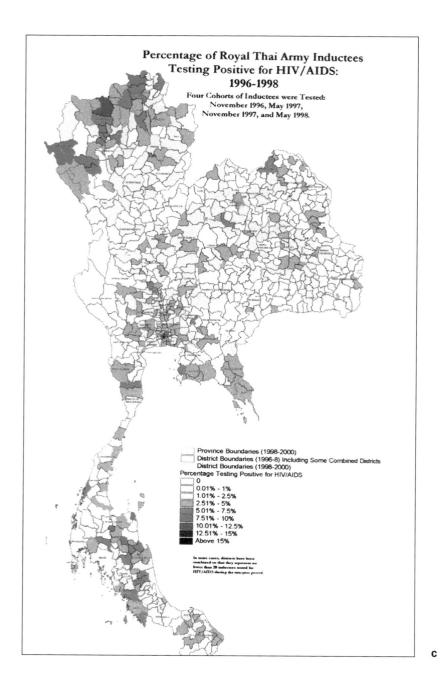

Percentage of Royal Thai Army Inductees
Testing Positive for HIV/AIDS:
1996-1998

Four Cohorts of Inductees were Tested:
November 1996, May 1997,
November 1997, and May 1998.

c

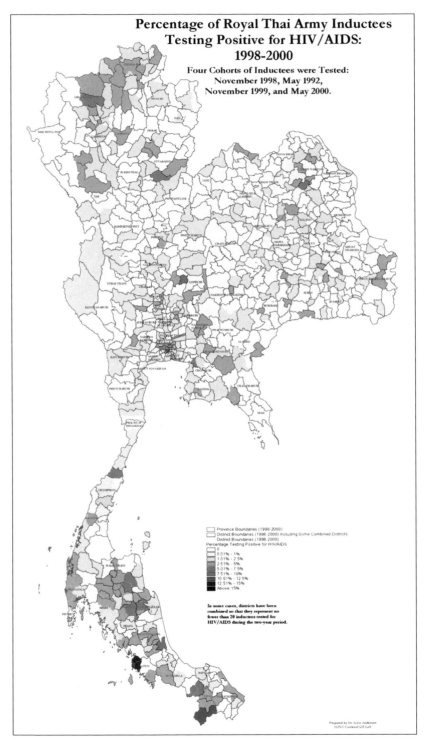

Figure 11.22a–d Map of incidence of AIDS among Thai military inductees by population district, 1991–1993(a), 1994–1996(b), and 1996–1998(c). The maps demonstrate the success of public campaigns in slowing the progress of the disease.

Source: "GIS Assists Public Health Campaign in Thailand" by Dr. S. Anderson, Col. K. Trugsa, Col. S. Nitayapan, Lt. Col. A. Brown, and Maj. Grn. S. Sangkharomya appeared in July–September 2002 issue of *ArcUser*. Courtesy of the authors.

d

of analysis. That, in turn, meant correcting for incidence of AIDS as a percentage of district population. Because some were too small to easily permit calculation at this level, some districts with small populations were collapsed to assure adequate sampling. This required, in turn, the redrawing of the maps based on a sufficient population size and army inductee sample. And because the issue was the course of the disease over nearly ten years of AIDS awareness and prevention campaigns, the maps had to be temporally explicit as well as spatially precise.

Here the resemblance to Malgaigne ends. A ten-year data sampling based on military inductees not by province but by district requires a wealth of data that nineteenth-century researchers could not have handled and would have found nearly impossible to collect. And, today, statistical sampling relevance is a far more precise tool than it was in mid-nineteenth century France, the assessment of data more stringent. So, too, mapping has become more precise and its use in such programs better defined. An advantage of modernity emphasized by this study was the ease with which the electronic data and the elements of the maps themselves could be shared. Data from Thailand was mailed in Microsoft Excel files to U.S. research partners who worked electronically with their Thai associates in the district mapping.

The apparently simple choropleth maps that resulted were, in the end, anything but simple. It took local researchers six months to collect basic data for the nine hundred Thai districts from which inductees were drafted. It took months longer, and several meetings, before problems with data could be addressed and the issue of population per district considered. What results, however, is not simply a portrait of the diffusion of AIDS in Thailand and the especially virulent outbreak of AIDS in the northern provinces. What results as well from these maps is a confirmation of the proposition that public information, counseling of sex workers, and the distribution of condoms over time may help to slow if not arrest the spread of the disease.

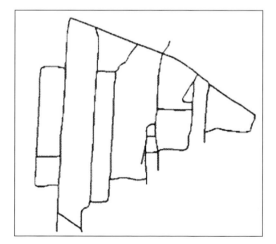

Figure 11.23a Map of streets of Pennathur, India, drawn with a GPS and handheld GIS program.

Source: © 2001–2004. CHAD/Community Health, Christian Medical College, Vellore.

India: Dengue fever

In most of the world one cannot assume that the city, state, or national maps that westerns take for granted will be available. In the 1790s, New York began to build its investment in commercial city maps, one that would later be mirrored by other cities. In the 1860s, McClellan was able to use for his mapping of cholera simple maps of a majority of the major cities on the Mississippi River. But it was not until the twentieth century and the automobile, perhaps, that city maps became commonplace instruments of every level of government and of individual travel. Nor are maps of every village a constant in the world today.

A recent report on studies in India by Dr. Jay Devasundaram, an Indian-born physician who has worked as a consultant for ESRI, offers an example of the problem of disease mapping and study in an

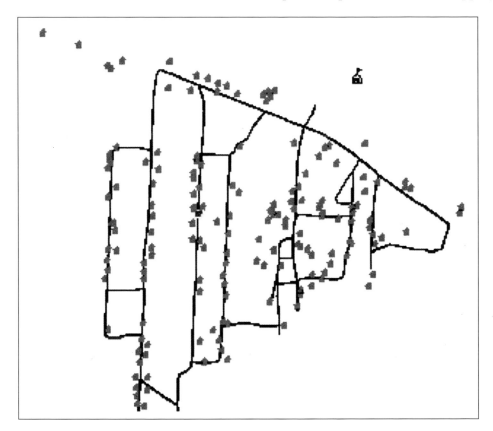

Figure 11.23b Map of streets and houses of Pennathur village, India. Red dots symbolize homes where high fever related to dengue fever was found. Blue dots are those where it was not found.

Source: © 2001–2004. CHAD/Community Health, Christian Medical College, Vellore.

environment that is not map rich (Pratt 2003). In 2001, a man with a high fever from Pennathur village visited a Community Health and Development (CHAD) site for treatment. Fever means something different in India, where dengue fever (and dengue hemorrhagic fever) are common, than it does in the United States, Canada, or Great Britain.

One problem was that there were no good health statistics on these fevers among the population, no database that might help physicians and officials combat outbreaks. Similarly unavailable were maps of the city and its structures, the houses in which the patients lived and the local stores at which they shopped. Devasundaram happened to be in the area on a family visit and decided to address the problem by developing a database for the village. With the assistance of local students from his old college, Devasundaram used a handheld GPS device linked to a computer to create a rough street map of the village and then to map the homes along each street. With his students he then began to build an epidemiological database for the village, one whose data would include basic population facts (how many people in each house of which age and what sex) as well as data pertinent to the residents' experience with serious fevers. Based on that work, a sample population was tested for dengue fever.

The result was startling: of the 989 people living in the village, 301 were found to have contracted the disease. The results strongly argued for proactive mosquito control programs and for a more comprehensive system that would permit a careful surveillance and tracking of the population's health status and needs. As part of this program Dr. Devasundaram, with the assistance of friends at ESRI, developed a 2 x 2 contingency table based on the fever data returned in his house-to-house survey and data from the local health census conducted at the same time. This was later incorporated into the ArcGIS software to permit ease of calculation and simultaneous mapping of the relative risk based on local elements in a manner permitting greater risk to be highlighted.

Contingency tables are a basic tool of epidemiology, a first step in the analysis of many health problems.[8] What they do is compare persons exposed to a variable and those unexposed to the same variable within a specific population. In a basic epidemiology text Rothman (2000, 56–88) explains the idea, albeit for a simple risk table rather than contingency, using data from Snow's South London study. In the table, cholera deaths of those whose water came from the Southwark and Vauxhall water

	Water companies	
	Southwark and Vauxhall	Lambeth
Cholera deaths	4,093	461
Population	266,516	173748
Risk	0.0154	0.0027

Figure 11.24 Risk table using data from John Snow's South London study.
Source: Koch.

company were compared to cholera deaths from the Lambeth water company based on the total populations served in South London by one or the other. In effect, it's what Snow wanted, to demonstrate overwhelmingly greater risk for those supplied by one company when compared to those supplied by the other. It is used here only as an example.

For Snow it was simple: this water company or another. In many cases, however, one needs to consider a range of risk factors in an analysis. A better, more realistic computation of the effect of exposure on disease incidence is typically more complex (see, for example Rothman 2002, 139–140). In the Indian example the real question was whether some local factor made some persons more likely to be bitten by virus carrying *Aedes aegypti* mosquitoes than others in their community. Might, for example, thatched roof houses be a better breeding ground than tin roof houses, making those in the former more likely to be bitten than inhabitants of the latter? By configuring the GIS to visually report not simply disease incidence but potential risk factors within that population, those factors became part of the landscape, lighting up as the analysis proceeded. The tool, which permits varying risk factors to be sequentially considered in a contingency table is now under development by ESRI as part of a suite of health-related GIS-based tools.

Modern epidemiologists may view the joining of the contingency table to the map as a relatively simple if not trivial advance. In developing nations without basic tools it can be significant, however. The result permits rapid calculation of the relation between disease incidence and a range of potentially complicit exposure factors: thatched versus tin huts, well water versus water from a purified source, and so on. For each, the relation or its lack is located in the map within the set of houses on the streets of the study, compared with each mapped iteration with the homes of those who have clinical symptoms of the disease under consideration. The whole is concrete and practical, graphically demonstrable and statistically grounded. It thus provides a first, visual tool of relative importance of potentially contributing factors that then can be quantified for a precise definition of the visual relation exposed in the map.[9]

The Pennathur village study broke no epidemiological ground and advanced no scientific frontier. All it did was make it easier to do modern epidemiology and public health medicine in a village whose resources and links to the national health care system are minimal by Western standards. The plates on which Seaman and Pascalis worked, the maps that Snow and Whitehead used in their studies, represent a social wealth whose availability is dependent on years of surveying and socioeconomic development. In those communities where such wealth has yet to accumulate, the simple map represents a technological boon that is not ubiquitous, not generally available. For Devasundaram and his local associates, the evolving GIS technology provided a medium for analysis for the accumulation and analysis of basic but critical health data. In the database and the maps that resulted, treatment plans for the fever outbreaks, and more generally, data pertinent to community health, were developed, considered, and shared among the community of those affected.

Endnotes

1. In the mid-1990s Clark University's IDRISI program was perhaps the one most frequently taught in universities. By the end of the 1990s, however, ArcView, and its successor the ArcGIS suite, had become the default for academic instruction and arguably for GIS-based analysis. Consideration of the relative merits of different GIS systems, or their technical evolution as a class, is a subject outside the scope of this work. ArcView and ArcGIS are offered here in part because of the software's dominance in the contemporary market place and secondarily because of my own familiarity with them. No argument is made for their inherent superiority over other mapping programs or systems, however. The point is the mapping, not the software that is emphasized across this history.

2. The story raises a range of interesting questions about the nature of the news in general and of its coverage of medical issues. These are questions I have treated at some length elsewhere, both in a book on the form of the news (Koch 1990) and on the relation of report, subject, and electronic data (Koch 1991). The continuing transformation of digital data suggests the need for a return to the subjects considered in those works as electronic data was becoming, for the first time, generally available.

3. Koch and Denike (2004) present an outline of this approach to teaching John Snow in a multidisciplinary setting. The self-conscious goal was to teach the "map thinking" using GIS to analyze the basic approach to local outbreaks pioneered by Snow. The program it describes was developed for an undergraduate geography class at the University of British Columbia, "Spatial data analysis using GIS."

4. The idea of using the intersections of buffers in this type of analysis was contributed by Ken Denike as we worked with undergraduates on analyzing this local outbreak. While the intent was pedagogic, teaching the idea behind types of sampling and cluster analysis, the result was a useful, first-order analysis in itself.

5. Surprisingly, the use of the deviational ellipse as a diagnostic for outbreaks like the ones described here is rarely, if ever, considered. Several epidemiologists and health experts to whom I proposed this situation were either unfamiliar with the ellipses and their generation or simply had not considered their potential utility as a diagnostic tool. One reason may be that until recently their calculation was cumbersome and difficult to map, a problem diminished by the more recent analytic programs.

6. Material for this section is drawn from a number of papers and a book detailing the argument. The broad argument is necessarily condensed here. For a more detailed consideration of the argument see, *Scarce Goods: Justice, Fairness, and Organ Transplantation* (Koch, T. 2001).

7. Later analysis showed the locational inequalities based on transplant performing hospital were greater than the original UNOS list of hospitals would have suggested. Many transplant-performing hospitals listed on the UNOS Web site were "non-performing," receiving no organs over several years while a number of other hospitals received only one or two hearts a year, not enough by official standards to qualify their personnel as suitably trained for this procedure.

8. For an introduction to contingency tables see *Epidemiology: An Introduction* (Rothman 2002, 134–140).

9. Work in Pennathur village continued after the departure of Dr. Devasundaram, first for the United States and later for another position in international health. Developers at ESRI continued to work on the project as well, developing the more sophisticated contingency table tool described here. I am greatly obliged to ESRI application prototype specialist Tanya Costain for making a copy of the new contingency tool available for my review.

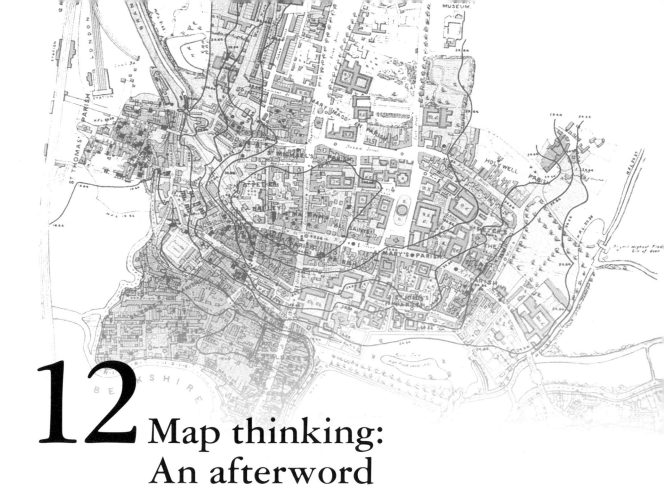

12 Map thinking: An afterword

Maps are the battlefields on which health scientists have contested. For more than three hundred years maps have permitted the graphic expression of relational propositions whose arguments are the essence of map thinking and the mapping that results. Some of those propositions were, in retrospect, as foolish as the presumed relation of olive oil use to the incidence of hernias. Others—Chadwick's correlation of poverty and infectious disease in Leeds, for example—are as contemporary as the incidence of AIDS in Haiti or tuberculosis in the prison camps of Russia (Farmer 2003).

It was in the map as much as the table and graph that the Paris School of statisticians fought first to understand health in the aggregate and then to test theories of causation. Maps anchored both Snow's complex topography and Farr's correlation of altitude and health evidenced in Acland's wonderful study. It was through his maps that McClellan transformed the local reports of individual respondents into a deeper study of cholera's pathways of diffusion along the Mississippi River. And it was in the mapping that Verghese came to understand the relation of his small Tennessee practice to the social patterns of the greater society as Gould fought to map the process of AIDS diffusion at the scale of the nation itself.

Across the three hundred years that this volume surveys, clinical and analytic tools slowly developed in power and sophistication. Mapping no less than microscopy offers evidence of this transformation. Copperplate gave way to lithography, lithography to more modern print processes and eventually to the current digital systems of data storage, manipulation, and presentation. Each step advanced, improved, changed the marriage of improving mapping technology and scientific thinking. The paucity of representative symbols that Seaman lamented is replaced by the rich symbol sets of modern GIS. The graphic palette of personal computers and commercial printers today resolve Snow's problems with coloration in his South London map. So, too, the problems of graded symbolization that frustrated the mapping of Howe and Hopps is now almost effortlessly resolved in the graded circles and coloration of Smallman-Raynor's computer-based maps of cumulative AIDS cases in U.S. cities.

None of this is important in and of itself. It is only important because the increasing sophistication of the medium has influenced and been influenced by increasingly sophisticated research. The ability to create a shaded, black-and-white cholorpleth map of a nation or province in the 1820s came into being as crude population statistics were first being employed. Hand coloration improved Chadwick's map of Leeds and, later, Booth's mapping of poverty and affluence in late nineteenth-century London. Computers permitted the realignment of complex mathematics with a deeper understanding of inter-urban relations and diffusion over time in space.

GIS technologies introduced in the last decades of the twentieth century are the current step in the continuing transformation of our knowing. Technically, they provide an expanded palette of colors and symbols at a time in which the cost of color printing has decreased, enabling ever-greater visual presentations enhanced as well by 3D presentations and animation. Within the GIS, alone or in tandem with statistical programs, data mapped onto the GIS surface is ever-more rigorously concerned in its relation to location, population characteristics, and environmental constraints. What has not changed is the relational proposition inherent in the map, the calculus of relation that mapping has always presented and that assures a necessary attention is paid not to disease incidence *in vitrio*, abstracted to a table or a model alone, but *en vivo*, in relation to the geographic and social aspects of the community whose practices and policies inhibit or promote the environments in which diseases are encouraged or discouraged.

The whole potentially transforms through the clarity of its presentation and the sophistication of its elements a tradition whose essence—relational and ecological—remains constant. From the start, mapping provided a medium for the distillation and presentation of data on the incidence of disease and the communities affected by those diseases. That was the message of Arrieta's maps of plague containment, the location within the society of Bari and the methods of its containment in the space of the towns and countryside of the province. At least since the early decades of the nineteenth century, social theories have been considered through statistical analysis just as those theories created the need for statistics (like Booth's poverty index) as a tool for the consideration of phenomena to be mapped. At every step the idea has been to test in this or that place a theory or hypothesis (Can we locate cholera outbreaks along the rivers of cities affected?), each testing defined by better calculation, each calculation distilled into a better map.

The history of mapping and the science it considered cannot be disassociated. Nor can the history of the technologies of production and distribution be ignored. The now-lost map Finke prepared for his text on medical geography was never printed; the process was just too expensive for inclusion in his text. The Bari plague map is a rarity not because others of Arrieta's era made no maps but because so few were printed and preserved. It remains for us today a tantalizing hint of map thinking in an era in which the technology of mapmaking was sufficiently cumbersome to restrict map reproduction, in which the economies as well as the technologies of printing limited the dissemination of both official and public texts. Advances in printing technology slowly changed the equation of cost and benefit, thus increasing the potential of the maps themselves. The result encouraged the increased production and distribution of maps in both official and popular publications whose market lay among the scientific elite and the increasingly educated, expanding middle classes of the evolving city and nation.

Every map is a selected knowing, a limited proposition about the world. Our theories determine the elements of any problem we map, graph, or chart and then argue before the world. Seaman did not map the incidence of yellow fever on ships in New York City harbor because he did not think those cases were important. Snow did not map the Craven Hill plague pit because he assumed, unlike his contemporaries, that it could not be complicit in the cholera outbreak in St. James, Soho, in 1854. Gould did not map the individual cases in his study of AIDS diffusion, just as Verghese's simple map was all about cases, about the people he knew and cared for. He came to understand AIDS general pattern as he unpacked the map, its distillation of the life experiences of his patients. For his part, Gould saw in his study of diffusion at the national level the lives of the students he taught and whose health he worried about.

That health and its determinants are rarely mapped across this history is a result of our historical assumption that science is dedicated not to understanding normalcy but aberration. Health is the default, a blank space on our maps of epidemic and endemic disease. It is the inverse of our researchers' focus. It doesn't have to be that way, of course. In the nineteenth century, for example, Rudolf Virchow argued that the basis of understanding disease is in the study of how it distorts normal structure, and normal function (Nuland 1989, 312). The implication was we needed to understand normalcy in order to distinguish the conditions that destroyed it, opening the door to epidemic disease.

Of course, one could think as deeply about healthy normalcy as diseased dysfunction, map the constituents of health as easily as the contributors to disease. A lesson of this history is each is the inverse of the other; both are elements of a single concern. To understand disease one has to understand health of both the humans who become ill and the vectors of the disease that haunt our population. But the essence of the science and social history distilled in the maps studied in this book focuses our attention not on promoting health, however it is defined, but on understanding this or that serious disease that has taken hold in our communities and our world.

Some talk of GIS as if it was the science rather than one method by which thinking about specific things in certain ways occurs. Medical mapping is not medical science, however, but the mapping of elements of a medical problem. It is a tool of investigation and the maps that result are the traces of arguments about the nature of this or that disease in a village or city, a state or province or nation. Each map is bounded by the author's point of view and the cultures, social and technological, in which the mapper struggles. We map data based on theories that raise questions that can be first framed cogently and then considered graphically or statistically. The results are limited by the theories we present, as restricted as the ideas that propel the studies whose results are distilled in graphic form.

In this history, the maps speak to the chronic inadequacy of changing scientific perspectives over time, the historical boundaries of our knowing and our attempts to extend them. This is as true of Acland and his research as it is of Snow and his, of course. It is only our own, contemporary prejudice that insists we forget the former while mythologizing the latter. The result is necessarily incomplete, one half of the historical argument. It denies the hard work of science, "a practical, goal-oriented and goal-revising dialectic of resistance and accommodation" (Pickering 1994, 22–23), rewriting it as a simple, linear tale of knowledge advanced rather than of knowing transformed in unexpected, unpredictable ways. But it is precisely in the tension between resistance and accommodation, between contending theories represented here by contrasting maps, that the real learning takes place. To speak of Snow while dismissing Acland and Farr, to extol Gould's work while ignoring Verghese's, or vice versa, is to tell only half the tale, a limited perspective that misses the point.

Because every study presents at best a limited perspective, bound by theory and restricted by the analytic tools at hand, even the best work is necessarily incomplete. Good ideas unsupported today may be, with new tools and new perspectives, returned to as tomorrow's breakthrough. "The most basic of the principles that underlie the hunting-rules of those who would track down Nature's secrets: [is that] an idea must never be presented before its time" (Nuland 1989, 239). We return again and again to older arguments and historic cases to seek and transform those rough ideas whose time has come, to find through the lens of advancing modernity and its maturing tools a new perspective on old, often discarded theories. Pyle's understanding of rank-order informed anew the nineteenth-century studies of cholera diffusion in the United States, and thus of the relation between urban structure and disease diffusion generally. Issues of rank-order informed, in turn, the geography that powered Gould's application of geographical theories of diffusion to AIDS.

History's importance therefore lies not in a simple cataloging of past experiences but in their potential applicability to contemporary problems and future trends. That is why we return to the past, constructing and reconstructing it, generation by generation, in search of new approaches to our own, immediate crises. In this process of review and reformation, the past we think we understand is transformed in the present by new perspectives informed by new data argued through improved technologies. The result adds complexity to the tale we earlier told, making historical studies and old, discarded theories contemporary once again.

By replacing the idea of John Snow as the far seeing, lone investigator who single handedly transformed medical mapping (and epidemiology and public health) for the real, collegial Snow we gain immensely, for example. In the mid-1850s Snow and his contemporaries were trading data, assisting each other, comparing results and arguing theories. Snow, for example, drew on not only work done in Great Britain but also research from the United States and from Europe. He was not opposed by Farr but assisted by him despite their differences of operation and theory. The story is not simply more complex, but more real and its lessons more relevant to the modern context.

It is not simply that modern epidemiology and medical geography and public health texts teach Snow's work as a first example. Rather in Snow's story we have the model of people with different perspectives and different theories assisting each other in their respective studies and then arguing the results. The plethora of maps and charts, the growth of medical mapping and statistics, was the direct result. This collegial sharing demanded papers whose maps and statistics advanced not only the subject of their analysis but also the modes of investigation themselves. More work by people of different perspectives means better criticism, and potentially, better ideas as a result.

Today, as local and regional data is not simply nationalized, but made internationally available in an electronic fashion, this is a critical lesson. Writing from Vancouver, Canada, I can review the work of the researcher in Pennathur, India. Using the GIS program on my computer I can replicate his work, his map, and perhaps advance it with a better one of my own. The move to electronic data and standardized forms of graphic and statistical presentation invites this type of comparison by researchers otherwise locked into less expansive perspectives. Mapping is both a tool of that comparison (I can see the data even if I can't pronounce the name of the village) and of that international focus. Its relational perspective insists we consider avenues otherwise unexplored, as did my mapping of the U.S. graft organ transplantation data. The result should be not simply a flood of data but an increase in information, in the means by which data is understood.

This is important and necessary because we are again facing international health challenges that demand concerted effort. In the first decade of the twenty-first century epidemic as well as endemic disease is again an urgent contemporary challenge. Old ideas of disease ecology and medical geography are being reborn in an ever-more detailed understanding of the way "anthropogenic land-use changes drive a range of infectious disease outbreaks and emergence events and modify the transmission of endemic infections" (Patz et al. 2004, 1092). "These changes, including deforestation, pollution, poverty, and human migration cause a cascade of factors that exacerbate infectious disease emergence."

The new work, detailed and highly specific, is the descendent of the more general studies in the 1950s of May, Rosenwaldt and Jursatz, itself built upon that of earlier, nineteenth-century medical geographers, whose disease ecology considered not just the simple vector of this or that disease but as well the environmental determinants—physical and social—that promoted it. Deforestation, house form, and urban settlement patterns were as much a part of the story May and his contemporaries told as were the precise boundaries of a mosquito's niche or the habitat of a specific tick. Together they mapped both the local environments complicit in individual diseases, or at a different scale, the global processes of human activity that assured their spread. Similarly, sanitarians from Seaman and Pascalis to Chadwick and Snow considered the urban environment not as a passive location, a set of coordinators, but as an active contributor to the diseases and states of impoverished ill health they studied.

The weight of the maps that inform this history argues a conclusion that is stark. We are the ecological engine that assures the propagation and diffusion of the diseases we fear. From the plague Arrieta mapped to the cholera in London to the dengue fever study of Devasundaram, one thing is clear: *We are the primary vectors of the diseases that hunt us.* In war wagons and sailing vessels, in airplanes, automobiles and trucks, we carry the rats, mites, and mosquitoes that harbor the bacteria and viruses that afflict our populations. In the inequality of our cities, and our failure to assure adequate housing, nutrition, and sanitation, we create environments in which those vectors flourish, the fields in which bacteria and virus will best evolve.

It was to impede human travel and the plague it facilitated that Arrieta deployed troops to halt costal shipping and stop land-based travel in the province of Bari, Italy at the end of the seventeenth century. Cholera's arrival in Sunderland, England, in 1831 was an inevitable outcome of travel and trade patterns linking India and England through land and sea routes of travel and trade. Officials had watched the disease's progression until it was not a question of if but when, what month it would arrive and which port population would be first struck. British officials tried local quarantines as a tool of disease containment but found it both ineffectual and unpopular. It interfered with the trade that was by the nineteenth century the lifeblood of every town and of the nation. And, to be fair, localized containment would serve perhaps to slow but not to stop the importation of pandemic disease. There were too many ports of entry, too many pathways for transmission for it to be effective without halting the process of exchange that had become the lifeblood of the evolving mercantile nation.

Time and again—from plague to AIDS—the conclusion has been the same: *Global trade promotes global illness.* We have resisted the equation at least since Seaman and then Pascalis rejected the idea that ships in the New York City docklands were a source of yellow fever. It was not simply outdated Hippocratic medicine theories but a modern resistance to the association of trade and disease that led the medical officers in New Orleans to insist that cholera was not an imported epidemic but a local, miasmatic constant. To argue otherwise was to agree with those who saw in the spread of epidemic disease a human agency encouraged by poverty and the failure of cities to assure an infrastructure that would diminish the likelihood of new infections, new epidemics taking root.

Saying that says not half enough because trade may provide the vector of transmission but does not assure the environment that will make of a population a favorable habitat for this or that bacterium or virus. Here we are again learning the hard lesson of the degree to which income inequalities and the inequities they create prepare an environment that assures a fertile field for illness. In recent years the manner by which elements of social organization and its inequalities contribute to disease has been renamed, "social epidemiology" (Kawachi 2002), the study of "our bodies and the body politic" (Krieger 2001), of how patterns of social organization and settlement contribute to the incidence of disease. In this, social epidemiologists are the modern inheritors of the nineteenth-century tradition that began with men like Chadwick, Booth, Snow, and Wilde.

It is not simply that humans are the vectors of disease but that in structuring our societies and cities to permit and perhaps promote inequalities (Wallace and Wallace 1998) we prepare the environments that promote the evolution and spread of bacterial and viral communities. We do this primarily through the failure to create healthy infrastructures that will inhibit their spread and promote health. Trade is the vector of diseases that lodge in our cities, environments prepared by social patterns of urban structure that embed disparities, thus promoting the risk of ill health. Chadwick saw the relation in the greater incidence of contagious disease among the poor in mid-nineteenth century London, a pattern Snow detailed in his study of the relation between cholera and professional status.

None of this is to suggest modern researchers are nineteenth-century retreads. The theories they argue are more sophisticated, the data they consider more complete than that of their predecessors. So, too, are the tools at their disposal. The study of deforestation and its positive effect on insect habitation has satellite imaging, soil sampling, detailed weather records, and the computer to analyze and map the result. Computerized records of local, regional, national, and international disease states provide a range and type of data that permit more rigorous theories to be argued statistically and graphically with a specificity and complexity that was previously impossible. The bar of our knowing is raised as better data promotes new theories argued through more powerful technologies of knowledge. And so we return with a new perspective on old arguments, sometimes with surprising results.

A lesson of this history is not simply our complicity in the construction of epidemic and endemic illness, the anthropogenic contribution to disease ecologies, but the intense spatiality of that ecology. Here maps by their very nature are critical reminders that diseases evolve in environments we create. Argued in this history and these maps is the necessity of attention to spatiality across the interrelated disciplines of disease studies and health promotion. If states of disease and health are to be fully understood they must be considered in the relation of people in place and at a specific time. "It is people who structure spaces: by their technology, by their movements, and by their very presence. And so if various pathogens—bacteria and viruses—need people as suitable ecological niches to exist and reproduce,

John Snow: Incidence of cholera by profession		
Profession	No. of Deaths	Ratio (death/total professional population)
Agents	12	1 in 40
Bricklayers	14	1 in 39
Dairymen, milkmen	8	1 in 20
Egg merchants	8	1 in 6
Fishmongers	11	1 in 20
Livery-stable keepers	5	1 in 37
Papermakers	2	1 in 15
Poulterers	3	1 in 32
Sail-makers	2	1 in 30
Ballast-heavers	7	1 in 24
Coal heavers and porters	53	1 in 32
Dustmen and scavengers	6	1 in 39
Founders	10	1 in 12
Hawkers	67	1 in 22
Lithographers	3	1 in 48
Modelers	3	1 in 41
Polishers	4	1 in 36
Sailors	299	1 in 24
Tanners	22	1 in 39
Weavers	102	1 in 36
Physicians and surgeons	16	1 in 265
Magistrates, barristers, and solicitors	13	1 in 375
Merchants	11	1 in 348
Auctioneers	1	1 in 266
Saddlers	1	1 in 250
Brass-finishers	3	1 in 318
Coach-makers	16	1 in 262
Cork-cutters	2	1 in 279
Footmen and man servants	25	1 in 1,572
Jewelers, goldsmiths, and silversmiths	6	1 in 583
Undertakers	2	1 in 325

Figure 12.1 Snow's correlation of employment and cholera incidence in the 1854 epidemic. An example of early social epidemiology shows that members of the working poor were more likely to be attacked by cholera than middle-class professionals whose living conditions and water supplies were better (based on Snow 1855c, table XIV, 123).

Source: Koch, based on Snow's 1854 study.

we are really talking about 'disease spaces,' enormously complex spaces that control the movement of viruses in much the same way that the hills and valleys of the familiar topographic map control the flow of water" (Gould 1999, 196).

Mapping has served uniquely in the articulation of Gould's proposition because mapping is about relationships in space, about the processes we consider and the places in which they operate. It is not, as Petermann put it in 1948, that "a map will make visible to the eye the development and nature of any phenomenon in regard to its geographical distribution." What's important is that maps make clear to the mind the relations of things distributed in space. That was the point of the work of Seaman and Pascalis. It was what the mapped disease ecology of the 1950s did, identifying the niches that the vectors of bacterial disease inhabited in a world infected by the result. It was the thinking in the maps that in the 1970s and 1980s laid bare the human pathways of bacterial and viral diffusion. In these histories mapping and the maps that resulted from it served intellectually and rhetorically, first presenting and then testing propositions and their arguments in a way that was compelling, comprehensible, and concise.

Individually and as a class, the maps that resulted were artifacts of thinking and therefore bounded by each individual researcher's background and point of view. Snow was a physician focused on his practice and the clinical lessons it forced him to consider. The registrar Farr was an early statistician interested in the broad pattern the records he collected argued. Gould was a geographer interested in spatial process, Verghese a clinician who understood the world, or at least the nation, through the lens of his patients' experience. To say their maps, and the science they enabled, were limited does them no disservice, however. History is never complete; no study encompasses the world. The study of "disease spaces," or any other space, are neither more nor less than the traces of the things we deem important enough to calculate and map.

References

Acland, H. W. 1856. *Memoir of the cholera at Oxford, in the year 1854, with considerations suggested by the epidemic*. London: J. Churchill.

Allen-Price, E. D. 1960. Uneven distribution of cancer in West Devon with particular reference to the divers water-supplies. *The Lancet* June 4: 1235–1238.

American Medical Association. 1855. Minutes of the 8th annual meeting of the AMA. Transactions of the American Medical Association 8, 9–12.

Anderson, S., K. Torugsa, S. Nitayapan, A. Brown, and S. Sangkharomya. 2002. GIS assists public health campaign in Thailand. *ArcUser* July-September: 18–21.

Arbona, S., and S. C. Crum. 1996. Medical geography and cholera in Peru. *The Geographer's Craft Project, Department of Geography, The University of Colorado at Boulder.* www.colorado.edu/ geography/gcraft/warmup/cholera/cholera.html

Arbona, S., and S. Crum. 1996. Medical geography and cholera in Peru. www.colorado.edu/ geography/gcraft/warmup/cholera/cholera.html

Arrieta, F. 1694. *Raggualio historico del contagio occorso della provincia de Bari negli anni 1690, 1691 e 1692.* Napoli: Dom. Ant. Parrino e Michele Luigi Mutii.

Associated Press. 2004. Las Vegas officials fed up with stink emanating from downtown storm sewers. August 1, 2004. www.azcentral.com/arizonarepublic/local/articles/0801backpagefiller01.htm

Athenaeum, The. 1844. Reviews: Census of the population of Ireland in 1841. No. 846. London, 13 January, 29.

Badcock, B. 2002. Making sense of cities: A geographical survey. London: Arnold, 184.

Bailey, T. C., and A. C. Gatrell. 1995. *Interactive spatial data analysis.* London: Longman Scientific and Technical, Longman Group Ltd.

Barrett, F. A. 2000a. August Hirsch: As critic of, and contributor to, Geographical medicine and medical geography. In *Medical geography in historical perspective (Medical History, Supplement No. 20)* edited by N. A. Rupke. London: Wellcome Trust, 98–190.

———. 2000b. Finke's 1792 map of human diseases, the first world disease map? *Social Science and Medicine* 50(7): 915–921. Elsevier Science.

———. 2000c. *Disease and geography: The history of an idea.* York University Department of Geography Monograph 23. Toronto: Atkinson College, 300, 301.

Barry, J. M. 2004. *The great influenza: The epic story of the deadliest plague in history.* New York: Viking.

Barthes, R. 1983. Myth today. In *A Barthes reader* edited by S. Sontag. New York: Hill and Wang, 93–149.

———. 1982. The plates of the encyclopedia. In *Barthes: Selected writings* edited by S. Sontag. Glasgow: Fontana Press, 218–219.

———. 1972. *Mythologies.* New York: Hill and Wang, 104, 105.

Beck, R. J., and D. Wood. 1976. Cognitive transformation of information from urban geographic fields to mental maps. *Environment and Behavior* 8(2): 199–238.

Berghaus, Heinrich and Hermann. 1838–1848. Physikalisch atlas oder sammlung von karten, 2 vols. Gotha: Justus Perthes.

Berry, J. K. 1999. Beyond mapping: Extending spatial dependency to maps. *GIS Today.* www.geoplace.com

Best, J. 2001. *Damned lies and statistics: Untangling numbers from the media, politicans, and activists.* Berkeley: University of California Press.

Bhattacharya, S. 2003. From foe to friend: Geographical and environmental factors and the control and eradication of smallpox in India. *History and Philosophy of the Life Sciences* 25:3, 299–317.

Binding, P. 2003. *Imagined corners: Exploring the world's first atlas.* London: Review.

Board of Health. 1878. *Annual report.* Map showing the sources of some of the odiferous odors perceived in Boston, 1878. Boston: City of Boston Archives.

Boyd, R. 1999. *The coming of the spirit of pestilence: Introduced infectious diseases and population decline among Northwest Coast Indians*, 1774–1874. Seattle: Washington Press.

Brigham, A. 1832. *A treatise on epidemic cholera: Including an historical account of its origin and progress, to the present period.* Hartford: H. and F. J. Huntington.

Brody, H., M. R. Rip, P. Vinten-Johansen, et al. 2000. Map-making and myth-making in Broad Street: The London cholera epidemic, 1854. *Lancet* 356: 64–68.

Brunn, S. D., S. L. Cutter, and J. W. Harrington, Jr., eds. *Geography and technology.* Dordrect: Kluwer Academic Publishers. 81–108.

Burkitt, D. N. 1962a. A tumour safari in east and central Africa. *British Journal of Cancer* 16: 379–386.

Burkitt, D. N. 1962b. Determining the climatic limitations of a children's cancer common in Africa. *British Medical Journal* October: 1019–1023.

Camerini, J. 2000. Henrich Bernhaus's map of human diseases. In *Medical geography in historical perspective* (*Medical History*, Supplement No. 20), edited by N. A. Rupke. London: Wellcome Trust, 186–210.

Campbell, F. R. 1885. The relation of meteorology to disease. *Buffalo Medical and Surgical Journal* 26: 193–214.

CDC. 2004. Cholera epidemic associated with raw vegetables—Lusaka, Zambia, 2003–2004 (CDC Editorial note). *Journal of the American Medical Association* 202 (17): 2077–2078.

———. 2000a. *Weekly Epidemiological Record 31* (4. Aug.), *Cholera*, 1999. Geneva: World Health Organization, 249–256.

———. 2000b. *Epi Info.* Washington, D.C.: U.S. Department of Health and Human Services. www.cdc.gov/epiinfo

Chadwick, E. 1842. *Report on the sanitary condition of the labouring population of Great Britain to the poor law commissioners* 26: map page 160.

Christie, J. 1876. *Cholera epidemics in East Africa.* London: MacMillan, 174, 457, 476.

Churchill, R. R., and S. J. Slarsky. 2004. Mapping September 11, 2001: Cartographic narrative in the print media. *Cartographic Perspectives* 47: 13–27.

Clemow, F. G. 1903. *The geography of disease.* Cambridge: University Press.

Cliff, A. D., and P. Haggett. 2003. The geography of disease distributions. In *A century of British geography* edited by R. Johnston and M. Williams. Oxford: Oxford University Press for the British Academy, 11, 12, 521–543.

———. 1988. *Atlas of disease distributions: Analytic approaches to epidemiological data.* London: Blackwell. 53–55.

Cliff, A. D., P. Haggett, and M. Smallman-Raynor. 2004. *World atlas of epidemic diseases.* London: Arnold, 88, 89, 120–122.

Cockerill, M. 2003. Data mining: Open access research. *The Scientist* (17) 17: A2–3.

Cooper, E. 1854. *Report on an enquiry and examination into the state of the drainage of the homes situate in that part of the Parish of St. James, Westminster.* 22 Sept. Metropolitan Commission of Sewers 478/21. London Metropolitan Archives, 1, 2, 6.

Coswell, C. 1849. On the propagation [sic] of cholera by contagion. *Medical Times and Gazette* 44 (Nov 2): 752–754.

Crampton, J. W. 2002. Maps, politics, and history: An interview with Mark Monmonier. *Environment and Planning* D: Society and Space 20: 637–646.

Cromley, E. K., and S. L. McLafferty. 2002. *GIS and public health.* New York: Guilford Press.

Croner, Charles M. 2004. Public health GIS and the Internet. Journal of Map and Geography Libraries 1 (1): 105–135. www.cdc.gov/nchs/data/gis/GIS_AND_THE_INTERNET.pdf

Dartmouth Atlas of Health Care. 1998. Chicago: American Hospital Association. www.dartmouthatlas.org/atalslinks/98atlas.php

Davidson, A. 1892. *Geographical pathology: An inquiry into the geographical distribution of infectious and climatic diseases*, 2 vol. London.

Davies, J. N. P. 1957. James Christie and the cholera epidemics in East Africa. *East African Medical Journal* 36 (1): 1–6.

Dimenstein, I. B. 2003. Upfront: Letter. *The Scientist* 17 (17): 14.

Dorling, D., and D. Fairbairn. 1997. *Mapping: Ways of representing the world.* Essex, United Kingdom: Addison Wesley Longman, Ltd.

Dotto, L. 2003. Outbreak: The climate connection. *Toronto Globe and Mail.* 30 (August): F7.

Drake, D. 1850. *A systematic treatise, historical, etiological, and practical, on the principal disease of the interior valley of North America.* Cincinnati: Winthrop B. Smith.

Duncan, K. 2003. Hunting the 1918 *Flu: One scientist's search for a killer virus.* Toronto: University of Toronto Press.

Dunham, L. J., and J. C. Bailar, 1968. World maps of cancer mortality rates and frequency rations. *Journal of the National Cancer Institute* 41 (1): 155–203.

Farmer, P. 2003. Pathologies of power: Health, human rights, and the new war on the poor. Berkeley: University of California Press.

Farr, W. 1866. Report on the cholera epidemic of 1866 in England. *Medical Times and Gazette*, 8 September. UK Parliament Session Papers 1867–1868, vol. 37.

———. 1855. *Letter of the President of the General Board of Health to the Right Honorable Viscount Palmerston accompanying a report from Dr. Sutherland on epidemic cholera in the metropolis in 1854.* London: George E. Eyre and William Spottiswoode.

Finke, L. L. 1792. *Versuch einer allgemeinen medicinisch-praktishcen Geographie*, 3 vols. Leipzig.

Firby, P.A. and C.F. Gardiner. 1982. *Surface topology.* New York: John Wiley and Sons.

Forry, S. 1842. *The climate of the United States and its endemic influences.* New York: J & H. G. Landley.

———. 1841. Statistical researches elucidating the climate of the United States and its relation with diseases of malarial origin, based on the records of the medical department and the adjutant general's office. *American Journal of the Medical Sciences* 1: 13-46.

Fotheringham, A. S., and F. B. Zhan. 1996. A comparison of three exploratory methods for cluster detection in spatial point patterns. *Geographical Analysis* 28 (3): 200–218.

Fremlin, G., and A. H. Robinson. 1998. Maps as mediated seeing. *Cartographica* 35 (1 and 2): monograph 51.

French, W. S., and E. O. Shakespeare. 1885. *Report upon the epidemic of typhoid fever at Plymouth, Luzerne County,* PA. Philadelphia: Ledger Job Print. 9, 10.

Gattrel, A.C. 1983. *Distance and space: A geographical perspective.* Oxford: Oxford University Press.

General Board of Health (Medical Council). 1855. Appendix to report of the committee for scientific inquires in relation to the cholera-epidemic of 1854. London: George E. Eyre and William Spottiswoode.

General Register Office (GRO). 1853. *Weekly return of births and deaths in London* November 19 supplement.

Gibbons, R. D., D. Meltzer, N. Duan, et al. 2000. Waiting for organ transplantation. *Science* 287 (January 14): 237, 238, 549, 550.

Gibson, A., S. Asthana, P. Brigham, G. Moon, and J. Dicker. 2002. Geographies of need and the new NHS methodological issues in the definition and measurement of the health needs of local populations. *Health and Place* 8 (1): 47–60.

Gilbert, E. W. 1958. Pioneer maps of health and disease in England. *Geographical Journal* 124: 172–183.

Girtz, J. L. 1972. Simple chronic bronchitis and urban ecological structure. In *Medical geography: Techniques and field studies* edited by N. D. McGlashen. London: Methuen and Co., Ltd.

Godfrey, C. M. 1968. *The cholera epidemics in Upper Canada*, 1832-1866. Toronto: Seecombe House.

Goodchild, M. 1994. GIS and geographic research. In *Ground truth: The social implications of geographical information systems*, edited by J. Pickles, 31–50. New York: Guilford.

Gordon, A., and J. Womersley. 1997. The use of mapping in public health and planning health services. *Journal of Public Health Medicine* 19 (2): 139–147.

Gould, P. 1999. *Becoming a geographer.* Syracuse, New York: Syracuse University Press.

———. 1993. *The slow plague: A geography of the AIDS pandemic.* Cambridge, Massachusetts and Oxford, United Kingdom: Blackwell Publishing.

———., J. Kabel, W. Gorr, and A. Golub. 1991. AIDS: Predicting the next map. *Interfaces* 21 (3): 80–92.

Grainger. 1850. *Report of the General Board of Health on the epidemic cholera of 1858 and 1859: Appendix B.* Parliamentary papers. Session 1850, vol. 21. 199.

Guillet, E. C. 1963. *The great migration: The Atlantic crossing by sailing-ship since 1770.* 2nd ed. Toronto: University of Toronto Press.

Gundersen, L. 2000. Mapping it out: Using atlases to detect patterns in health care, disease, and mortality. *Annals of International Medicine* 133 (2): 161-164.

Hage, P., and F. Harary. 1983. *Structural models in anthropology.* New York: Cambridge University Press.

Hägerstrand, T. 1975. Survival and arena: On the life-history of individuals in relation to their geographical environment. *The Monadnock* 49 (June): 9–29.

———. 1969. Innovation diffusion as a spatial process, trans. A. Pred. Chicago: University of Chicago Press.

Haggett, P. 2000. *The geographical structure of epidemics.* Oxford: Clarendon Press.

———. 1966. Locational analysis in human geography. New York: St. Martin's Press.

Haglund, K. 2002. *Inventing the Charles River.* Cambridge, Massachusetts: MIT Press.

Hall, E. 2003. Reading maps of the genes: interpreting the spatiality of genetic knowledge. *Health and Place* 9: 151–161.

Hansen, M. L. 1961. *The Atlantic migration: 1607–1860.* 2nd ed. New York: Harper Torchbooks.

Harrison, M. 2000. Differences of degree: Representations of India in British medical topography, 1820-c.1870. In *Medical geography in historical perspective* (*Medical History*, Supplement No. 20) edited by N. A. Rupke. London: Wellcome Trust, 51–69.

Haviland, A. 1892. *The geographical distribution of disease in Great Britain.* 2nd ed. London: Swan Sonneschein and Co. vii.

Heersink, P. 2001. Review, Life of the land: The secret life of maps. Carlucci A., and P. Barber, eds. London: British Library Board 2001. *Cartographica* 38 (1): 136–137.

Higgs, G. 2002. Researching applications of geographical information systems in health: An introduction. *Health and Place* 8: 1–2.

Hillary, W. 1763. *Observation on the changes of the air and the concomitant epidemiological disease in the island of Barbados. To which is added a treatise on the putrid bilious fever, commonly called the yellow fever; and such other diseases as are indigenous or endemial in the West India islands, or in the torrid zone.* London: C. Hitch and L. Hawes.

Hirsch, A. 1883-1886. *A handbook of geographical and historical pathology*, 3 vols. London: Trans. Charles Creighton. 2.

Holling, C. 1992. Cross-scale morphology, geometry, and dynamics of ecostystems. *Ecological Monographs* 62: 447–493.

Hopps, H. C. 1969. Computerized mapping of disease and environmental data. In *The mapping of disease* edited by F. J. Spencer. *SLA Bulletin: Geography and Map Division* 79: 24–30.

Howe, G. M. 1969. The national atlas of disease mortality in the United Kingdom, 2nd ed. *SLA Bulletin: Geography and Map Division* 78: 16–18.

———. 1963. The national atlas of disease mortality in the United Kingdom, 2nd ed. London: Thomas Nelson and Sons, Ltd. 1, 7.

———. 1963. The national atlas of disease mortality in the United Kingdom. London: Thomas Nelson and Sons, Ltd. 7–10.

Huff, D. 1993. *How to lie with Statistics.* Rev. ed. New York: W. W. Norton.

Hunter, J. M., and J. Young. 1971. Diffusion of influenza in England and Wales. *Annals of the Association of American Geographers* 61: 637–653.

Ingold, T. 2000. *The perception of the environment: Essays on livelihood, dwelling, and skill.* London and New York: Routledge. 223–235.

Institute of Medicine. 1999. *Organ procurement and transplantation: Assessing current policies and the potential impact of the DHHS Final Rule.* Washington, D.C.: National Academy Press.

Jacob, J. 2003. Editorial: Home rules. *Transactions of the Institute of British Geographers* 28: 259-263.

Jarcho, S. 1974. Trans. An early medicostatistical map (Malgaigne, 1840). *Bulletin, New York Academy of Medicine* 40 (1).

———. 1970. Yellow fever, cholera, and the beginnings of medical cartography. *Journal of the History of Medicine and Allied Sciences* 25: 131–142.

———. 1969. The contributions of Heinrich and Hermann Berghaus to medical cartography. *Journal of the History of Medicine and Allied Sciences* 24: 412–415.

Jenkins, S. 2001. Maps that charted the distortions of time. *The Times of London*, August 30.

Johnson, J., and P. R. Thota. 2003. NAPL contamination evaluation using GIS. *ArcUser* 6 (3): 24–25.

Johnston, A. K. 1856. *The physical atlas of natural phenomena.* Edinburgh: W. Blackwood.

Jones, G. E. 1995. *How to lie with charts.* New York: Sybex.

Jusatz, H. J. 1977. Cholera. In *A world geography of human diseases* edited by G. M. Howe. London: Academic Press.

———. 1969. In *The mapping of disease: Medical mapping as a contribution to human ecology* edited by F. J. Spencer. SLA Bulletin no. 78: 19–23.

Kaiser, W. L., D. Wood, and R. Abramms. 2005. Afterward. *Seeing through maps.* 2nd ed. Amherst, Massachusetts: ODT, Inc.

Kawachi, I. 2002. Editorial: What is social epidemiology? *Social Science and Medicine* 54: 1739–1741.

Kitchin, R. 2002. Participatory mapping of disabled access. *Cartographic Perspectives* 50–60.

Knowles, A. K. 2002. *Past time, past place: GIS for history.* Redlands, Calif.: ESRI Press.

Koch, T. In press. The map as intent: Variations on the theme of John Snow. *Cartographica.*

———. 2005. Response to Mark Monmonier. *Cartographica*, In Press.

———. 2004. The map as intent: Variations on the theme of John Snow. *Cartographia* 39 (4): 1–14.

————. 2003. *The wreck of the William Brown.* Vancouver, Canada: Douglas and McIntyre Publishers.

————. 2002. *Scarce goods: Justice, fairness, and organ transplantation.* Westport: Praeger Publishing.

————. 1999a. Mapping the ORMS world. *ORMS Today* 26 (4): 26–30.

————. 1999b. The organ transplantation dilemma. *ORMS Today* February: 22–31.

————. 1999c. They might as well be in Bolivia: Race, ethnicity and the problem of solid organ donation. *Theoretical Medicine and Bioethics* 20 (6): 563–474.

————. 1998. *The limits of principle: Deciding who lives and what dies.* Westport, Conn.: Praeger Publishing.

————. 1994. *Watersheds: Stories of crisis and renewal in everyday life.* Toronto: Lester Books. 176-198.

————. 1991. *Journalism for the 21st Century: Online libraries, databases, and the News.* Westport, Conn.: Praeger Publishing.

————.1990. *The news as myth: Fact and context in journalism.* Westport, Conn.: Praeger Publishing. 26.

Koch, T., and K. Denike. 2004. Medical mapping: The revolution in teaching—and using—maps for the analysis of medical issues. *Journal of Geography* 103 (2): 76–85.

————. 2001. GIS approaches to the problem of disease clusters: a Brief Commentary. *Social Science and Medicine* 51: 151–154.

Kohli, S., H. Noorland Brage, and O. Löfman. 2000. Childhood leukemia in areas with different radon levels: A spatial and temporally analysis using GIS. *Journal of Epidemiology and Community Health* 54: 822–826.

Krieger, A., and D. Cobb, eds. 2001. *Mapping Boston.* Cambridge, Mass.: MIT Press.

Krieger, N. 2001. Historical roots of social epidemiology: socioeconomic gradients in health and context analysis. *International Journal of Epidemiology* 30: 899–903.

————. 2001. Glossary for social epidemiology. *Journal of Epidemiology and Community Health* 55: 693–700.

Krim, A. 2002. Review: Mapping Boston. *The Professional Geographer* 54 (3): 472–473.

Lancet. 1849. Reviews. *Lancet.* 2: 317.

Lang, L. 2000. *GIS for health organizations.* Redlands, Calif.: ESRI Press.

Langlands, B. W. 1969. Maps and medicine in East Asia. In *The mapping of disease. SLA Geography and Map Bulletin Number* 78: 9-15.

Learmonth, A. T. A. 1988. *Disease ecology: An introduction.* London: Blackwell Publishing.

————. 1957. Some contrasts in the regional geography of malaria in India and Pakistan. *Transactions of the Institute of British Geographers* 23: 37–59.

Lederberg, J. 2003. Getting in tune with the enemy—microbes. *The Scientist* 17 (16): 20–21.

Lee, R. 2002. Nice maps, shame about the theory? Thinking geographically about the economic. *Progress in Human Geography* 26 (3): 333–356.

Lefebvre, H. 1974. *The Production of space.* Oxford: Blackwell Publishing.

Lemann, N. 2001. Atlas shrugs: The new geography argues that maps have shaped the world. *New Yorker* April 9: 131–134.

Lewis, R. 2004. Devious and deadly: Influenza through the ages. *The Scientist* 18 (1): 19.

Lewontin R. C. 1992. *Biology as ideology: The doctrine of DNA.* New York: Harper-Collins.

Lind, J. 1771. *An essay on diseases incidental to Europeans in hot climates, with the method of preventing their fatal consequences.* London.

Lombard, H. C. 1877-1880. *Traité de climatologie medicale, comprenant la meteorology médicale et l etude des influences physiologques, patholoqgiques, prophylactiques et thérapeutiques du climat sur la santée,* 4 vol. Paris.

Longley, P. A., and M. Batty, eds. 2003. *Advanced spatial analysis.* Redlands, Calif.: ESRI Press.

Lyons, R. D. 1859. [Parliamentary] *Report on the pathology, therapeutics, and general aitiology of the epidemic of yellow fever which prevailed at Lisbon during the latter half of the year 1857.* London: George Edward Eyre and William Spottiswoode.

Malgaigne, J. F. 1840. Recherches sur le fréquence des hernies selon les sexes, les ages, et relativement à la population. *Annales d'Hygiène et de Médecine Légale* (July 1840): 1–50.

Marriott, E. 2003. *The plague race: A tale of fear, science, and heroism.* London: Picador.

Martin, D., H. Wrigley, S. Barnett, and P. Roderick. 2002. Increasing the sophistication of access measurement in a rural health care study. *Health and Place* 8 (1): 3–13.

Maturana, H., and F. Varela. 1992. *The tree of knowledge: The biological roots of human understanding.* Rev. ed. Boston: Shambhala.

May, J. M. 1950. Medical geography: Its methods and objectives. *The Geographical Review* 50: 10–41.

————. 1961. Introduction. In *Studies in disease ecology* edited by J. M. May. New York: Hafner Publishing.

————. 1965 or 1955?. World atlas of diseases. American Geographical Society.

Mayer, J. D. 1996. The political ecology of disease as one new focus for medical geography. *Progress in Human Geography* 20 (4): 441–456.

McGlashan, N. D. 1977. Viral hepatitis in Tasmania. *Social Science and Medicine* 11: 731–744.

————. 1972. *Medical geography: Techniques and field studies.* London: Methuen and Company, Ltd. 135.

McGlashan, N. D., and J. R. Blunden. 1983. *Geographical aspects of health: Essays in honor of Andrew Learmonth.* London: Academic Press. 85.

McLeod, K. 2000. Our sense of Snow: The myth of John Snow in medical geography. *Social Science and Medicine* 7 and 8 (February): 923–936.

McNeill, W. H. 1976. *Plagues and people.* New York: Anchor Press, Doubleday.

Medical Times and Gazette. 1866. The East London Water Company. September 8.

Melnick, A. L. 2002. *Introduction to geographic information systems in public health.* Gaithersburg, Md.: Aspen Publishing. 2, 3.

Melosi, M. 2000. *The sanitary city: Urban infrastructure in America from colonial times to the present.* Baltimore and London: Johns Hopkins University Press. 46.

Mitman, G., and R. L. Numbers. 2003. From miasma to asthma: The changing fortunes of medical geography in America. *History and Philosophy of the Life Sciences* 25 (3): 391–412.

Monmonier, M. and T. Koch. 2005. Mark Monmonier's rejoinder and Tom Koch's response to the article: Koch, Tom. 2004. The map as intent: Variations on the theme of John Snow. *Cartographica* 39 (4):1–14.

Monmonier, M. 1999. *Air apparent.* Chicago: University of Chicago Press.

————. 1997. *Cartographies of danger.* Chicago: University of Chicago Press. 263.

————. 1996. *How to lie with maps.* 2nd ed. Chicago: University of Chicago Press. 158, 159.

————. 1989. Maps with the news: The development of American journalistic cartography. Chicago: University of Chicago Press.

Morris, R. J. 1976. Cholera 1832: *The social response to an epidemic.* London: Croom Helm.

Morse, S. S. 1999. Factors in the emergence of infective or infectious? Diseases. *Emerging Infectious Diseases* 1 (2). www.cdc.gov/ncidod/eid/vol1no2/wilsom.htm

Mühry, A. 1856. *Thesaurus Grundzüge der Noso-Geographie oder geordnete Samlung noso-geographischer Berichte, mit Hinzugefugten Commentation.* Leizig and Heidelberg: C.F. Winter.

New York Board of Health. 1821. *A statement of facts relative to the late fever which appeared in Bancker Street and its vicinity.* New York: Bliss.

Nuland, S. B. 1989. *Doctors: The biography of medicine.* New York: Vintage Books. 239.

Numbers, R. A. 2000. Reflections on the history of medical geography. In *Medical geography in historical perspective (Medical History*, Supplement No. 20) edited by N. A. Rupke. London: Wellcome Trust. 219.

O'Connor, E. 2000. *Raw material: Producing pathology in Victorian culture.* Durham: Duke University Press. 11.

O'Sullivan, D. and Unwin, D. J. 2003. *Geographic information analysis.* Hoboken, N.J.: John Wiley and Sons, Inc.

Openshaw, S., M. Charlton, and A. Craft. 1988. Searching for leukemia clusters using a geographical analysis engine. *Papers of the Regional Science Association* 64: 95–106.

Openshaw, S., M. Charlton, C. Wymer, and A. Craft. 1987. A Mark 1 Geographical Analysis Machine for the automated analysis of point data sets. *International Journal of Geographical Information Systems* 1 (4): 335–358.

Orford, S., D. Dorling, R. Mitchell, M. Shaw, and G. D. Smith. 2002. Life and death of the people of London: A historical GIS of Charles Booth's inquiry. *Health and Place* 8 (1): 25–35.

Parks, E. 1855. Review: Mode of communication of cholera by John Snow. *British and Foreign Medico-Chiurgical Review* 15: 449–456.

Pascalis-Ouvière, Felix. 1796. *Medio-chymical dissertations on the cause of the epidemic called yellow fever, and on the preparation of the best antinomial preparations for the use of the medicine.* Philadelphia: Snowden and M'Corkle.

———. 1819. *A statement of the occurrences of a malignant yellow fever, in the city of New-York, in the summer and autumnal months of 1819; and of the check given to its progress, by the measures adopted by the Board of Health. With a list of cases and names of sick persons; and a map of their places of residence within the infected and proscribed limits: with a view of ascertaining, by comparative arguments, whether the distemper was engendered by domestic causes, or communicated by human contagion from foreign ports.* New York: W. A. Mercein. 17, 19, 241.

———. 1820. A statement of the occurrences during a malignant yellow fever in the city of New York. *Medical Repository.* 229–256.

Patz, J. A., P. Daszak, G. M. Tabor et al. 2004. Unhealthy landscapes: Policy recommendations on land use change and infectious disease emergence. *Environmental Health Perspectives* 112 (10): 1092–1098.

Petermann, A. 1848. Statistical notes to the cholera map of the British Isles showing the districts attacked in 1831, 1832, and 1833. London: John Betts.

Pickering, A. 1995. *The mangle of practice: Time, agency, and science.* Chicago: University of Chicago Press.

Pickles, J. 1997. Tool or science? GIS, technoscience, and the theoretical turn. *Annals of the Association of American Geographers* 87 (2): 363–372.

Porter, D. H. 1998. *The Thames embankment: Environment, technology, and society in Victorian London.* Akron: University of Akron Press. 22.

Porter, R. 1998. *The greatest benefit to mankind: A medical history of humanity.* New York: W.W. Norton. 56, 58.

Pratt, M. 2003. Down-to-earth approach jumpstarts GIS. *ArcUser*, January-March: 68–69.

Pray, L. A. 2004. Viroids, viruses, and RNA silencing. *The Scientist* 18 (16): 23.

Pred, Alan. Trans. for Torsten Hägerstrand, *Innovation Diffusion as a Spatial Process.*

Pritsker, A., and T. Koch. 1999. Organ debate transplanted to pages of *OR/MS Today*. June, 16–18.

Pritsker, A. 1998. Life and Death Decisions: Organ transplant allocation policy analysis. OR/MS Today 25 (4): 22-28.

Punch, or the London Charivari 1847. Modern Streetology. 12 (January to June): 265.

———. 1846. London Leaving Town. 11 (July to December): 32.

———.1845. The Battle of the Streets. 8 (January to June): 63.

Pyle, G. F. 1986. *The diffusion of influenza: Patterns and paradigms.* Lanham, Md.: Rowman and Littlefield.

———. 1979. *Applied medical geography.* Washington, D.C.: Winston and Sons. 81-83, 98.

———. 1976. Introduction: Foundations to medical geography. *Economic Geography* 52 (2): 95–102.

———. 1969. The diffusion of cholera in the United States in the nineteenth century. *Geographical Analysis* 1 (1): 59–75.

Pyle, G. F. and P. H. Rees. 1971. Modeling patterns of death and disease in Chicago. *Economic Geography* (October): 475–488.

Reeder, M. 2002. Burkett's lymphoma. Tropical Medicine Center Resource. tmcr.usuhs.mil/tmcr/chapter41/clinical.htm

ReVelle, C. 1993. Facility siting and integer-friendly programming. *European Journal of Operational Research* 65: 147–158.

Richardson, B. W. 1936. Introduction. *Snow on cholera: Being a reprint of two papers by John Snow, M.D.,* edited by W. H. Frost. New York: The Commonwealth Fund.

Robinson, A. H. 1982. *Early thematic mapping in the history of cartography.* Chicago: University of Chicago Press.

Robinson, A. H., and B. B. Petchenik. 1986. *The nature of maps: Essays towards understanding maps and mapping.* Chicago: University of Chicago Press. xv, 156, 170, 171, 180, 181, 183, 184.

Rodenwaldt , E., R. E. Bader, and H. J. Jusatz. 1952-1961.*Welt Seuchen Atlas: Weltatlas der Seuchenverbreitung und Seuchenbewegung.* Hamburg: Falk-Verlag.

Rogers, E. 1962. *Diffusion of innovation.* New York: Free Press.

Rothenberg, J. N. 1836. *Die cholera-epidemie des jahres 1832 in Hamburg.* Hamburg: Perthes and Besser.

Rothman, K. J. 2002. *Epidemiology: An introduction.* New York: Oxford University Press.

Rupke, N. A. 2000. Adolf Mühry (1810-1888): Göttingen's Humboldtian medical geography. In *Medical geography in historical perspective* (*Medical History*, Supp. No. 20) edited by N. A. Rupke. London: Wellcome Trust. 86–97.

Rush, B. 1794. An account of the bilious remitting yellow fever as it appeared in the city of Philadelphia in the year 1793. T. Dobson.

Russell, R. C. 1987. Survival of insects in the wheel bays of a Boeing 747B aircraft on flights between tropical and temperate airports. *Bulletin*, World Health Organization 65: 659–662.

Sapolsky, R. M. 2004. Of mice, men, and genes. *Natural History* (May): 21–31.

Schurmann, N. 1999. Critical GIS: Theorizing an emerging science. *Cartographica* 36 (4): monograph 53.

Scott, W. 1824. *Report on the epidemic cholera as it appeared in the territories subject to the presidency of Fort St. George.* Madras: Asylum Press.

Seaman, V. 1798. Inquiry into the cause of the prevalence of yellow fever in New York. *Medical Repository* 1 (3): 314–332.

———. 1796a. *An account of the epidemic yellow fever, as it appeared in the city of New York in the year 1795.* New York: Hopkins, Webb, and Company.

———. 1796b. An account of the epidemic yellow fever as it appeared in the city of New York in the year 1795. In *A collection of papers on the subject of bilious fevers* edited by N. Webster, 1–52.

Sedgwick, W. T. 1911. *Principles of sanitary science and the public health, with special reference to the causation and prevention of infectious diseases.* 4th ed. New York: MacMillan.

Shalala, D. 1998. Letter from the Secretary of Health and Human Services to members of Congress. (February 26.)

Shannon, G. W. 1981. Disease mapping and early theories of yellow fever. *Professional Geographer* 33 (2): 221–227.

Shapin, S., and S. Schaffer. 1985. *Leviathan and the air-pump: Hobbes, Boyle, and the experimental life.* Princeton: Princeton University Press.

Shapter, Thomas. 1849. *The history of cholera in 1832 in Exeter.* London: John Churchill; Exeter: Adam Holden. 2, 24, 44–45.

Smallman-Raynor, M., A. D. Cliff, and P. Haggett. 1992. *London international atlas of AIDS.* Oxford: Blackwell Publishing.

Snow, J. 1858. Drainage and water supply in connection with the public health. *Medical Times and Gazette.* February 13: 16-17; February 20: 223–224.

———. 1856. Cholera and the water supply of the south districts of London in 1854. *Journal of Public Health* 2: 239–257.

———. 1855a. Dr. Snow's Report. In *Report of the cholera outbreak in the parish of St. James, Westminster, during the autumn of 1854.* London: Churchill. 97–120.

———.. 1855b. On the comparative mortality of large towns and rural districts, and the causes by which it is influenced. *Journal of Public Health, and Sanitary Review* 1: 16–24.

———. 1855c. *On the mode of communication of cholera,* 2nd ed. London: Churchill. Reprinted in *Snow on Cholera: Being a reprint of two papers by John Snow, M.D.,* ed. W. H. Frost, 1936. New York: The Commonwealth Fund.

———. 1854a. Communication of cholera by Thames water (letter). *Medical Times and Gazette* 9 (September 2): 247–248.

————. 1854b. The cholera near Golden-square and at Deptford. *Medical Times* 9: 321–322.

————. 1851. On the mode of propagation of cholera. *Medical Times and Gazette* 24: 559–562; 610–612.

————. 1849a. On the pathology and mode of transmission of cholera. *Medical Times and Gazette* 44 (November 2): 745–752.

————. 1849b. On the pathology and mode of transmission of cholera. *Medical Times and Gazette* 44 (November 30): 923–929.

————. 1849c. *On the mode of transmission of cholera.* London: Churchill.

————. 1847. *On the inhalation of the vapour of ether in surgical operations: Containing a description of the various stages of etherization and a statement of the result of nearly eighty operations . . . .* London: Churchill.

Sontag, S. 1978. *Illness as metaphor.* New York: Vintage Books.

Spencer, F. J. 1969. Woodworth's tome: A biblio-geographical contribution to medical history. In *The mapping of disease: A special issue* edited by F. J. Spencer. *SLA Bulletin* 78: 2–8

Spielman, A., and M. D'Antonio. 2001. *Mosquito: A natural history of our most persistent and deadly foe.* New York: Hyperion.

Stamp. L. D. 1964. Some aspects of medical geographpy. London: Oxford University Press. 163, 146.

Stevenson, L. G. 1965. Putting disease on the map: The early use of spot maps in the study of Yellow Fever. *Journal of the History of Medicine and Allied Sciences* 20: 226–261.

Sui, D. and R. Morrill. 2004. Computers and geography: From automated geography to ditigal earth. In, Brunn, Cutter, and Harrington, eds. *Geography and technology* edited by Brunn, Cutter, and Harrington, 81–108.

Sutherland, W. 1865. [Parliamentary] Report of the sanitary condition of MALTA and GOZO with reference to the Epidemic Cholera in the year 1865. London: George E. Eyre and William Spottiswoode.

Tan, D., H. S. Upshur, E. G. Ross, and N. Ford. 2003. Global plagues and the global fund: Challenges in the fight against HIV, TB, and malaria. *BMC International Health and Human Rights 3.2.* www.biomedcentral.com

Taylor, L. H. 1886. First annual report, State Board of Health and Vital Statistics of Pennsylvania. Harrisburg, Penn. 176–195.

Thomas, L. T. 1983. *The youngest science: Notes of a medicine-watcher.* New York: Viking Press.

Tomalin, C. 2002. *Samuel Pepys: The unequalled self.* New York: Penguin Books.

Torsten Hägerstrand. *Innovation diffusion as a spatial process,* trans. Alan Pred.

Tropical Medicine Central Resource. Burkitt's lymphoma. 2003. tmcr.usuhs.mil/tmcr/chapter41/clinical.htm

Tufte, E. 1983. *The visual display of quantitative information.* Cheshire, Conn.: Graphics Press.

———. 1997. *Visual explanations: Images and quantities, evidence, and narrative.* Cheshire, Conn: Graphic Press. 27–37.

Turner, S. 1991. Social construction and social theory. *Sociological Theory* 9 (1): 22–33.

Twigg, G. 1984. *The black death: A biological reappraisal.* London: Batsford Academic and Educational Publishers. 186, 187.

U.S. Department of Health and Human Resources. 1997. *Atlas of the U.S. mortality.* Washington, D.C.: National Center for Health Statistics.

Valenčius, Conevery B. 2000. The geography of health and the making of the American West: Arkansas and Missouri, 1800-1860. In *Medical geography in historical perspective* (*Medical History*, Supplement No. 20) edited by N. A. Rupke. London: Wellcome Trust, 121–145.

Vergano, D. 2000. The operation you get often depends on where you are. *USA Today* (September 19): 1–2A.

Verghese, A. 1995. My own country: A doctor's story. New York: Vintage Books.

Verghese, A., S. L. Berk, and F. Sarubbi. 1989. *Urbs in Rure*: Human immunodeficiency virus infections in rural Tennessee. *Journal of Infectious Diseases* 160 (6): 1051–1055.

Vinten-Johansen, P., H. Brody, N. Paneth, S. Rachman, M. Rip, and D. Zuck. 2003. *Cholera, choloroform, and the science of medicine: A life of John Snow.* New York: Oxford University Press.

Wackers, G. L. 1994. *Constructivist medicine.* Maastricht: Universitaire Pers Maastricht.

Wakley, T. 1855. Editorial. *Lancet* 1: 635.

Walden, M. M. 1991. Spreading stain. *Science* 29 (March): 1022.

Wallace, D., and R. Wallace. 1998. *A plague on your houses.* New York: Verso Press.

———. 1997. Community marginalization and the diffusion of disease and disorder in the United States. *British Medical Journal* 314 (May): 1341–1345.

————. 1995. U.S. Apartheid and the spread of AIDS to the suburbs: A multi-city analysis of the political economy of spatial epidemic threshold. *Social Science and Medicine* 41(3): 333–345.

Wallace, R., D. Wallace, H. Andrews, R. Fullilove, and M. Fullilove. 1995. The spatiotemporal dynamics of AIDS and TB in the New York metropolitan region from a sociogeographic perspective: understanding the linkages of central city and suburbs. *Environment and Planning* A (27): 1085–1108.

Wallace, R., Y. Huang, P. Gould, and D. Wallace. 1997. The hierarchical diffusion of AIDS and violent crime among U.S. metropolitan regions: Inner-city decay, stochastic resonance and reversal of the mortality transition. *Social Science and Medicine* 44 (7): 935–947.

Ward, R. D. 1897. The teaching of climatology in medical schools. *Boston Medical and Surgical Journal* 136: 103–106.

————. 1908. *Climate: Considered especially in relation to man.* New York: G. P. Putnam's Sons. 181.

Weed, L. 1942. John Tyndall and his contribution to the theory of spontaneous generation. *Annals of Medical History* 4 (1): 55–62.

Whitehead, H. 1855. Mr. Whitehead's report, In *Parish, St. James. Report of the cholera outbreak in the parish of St. James, Westminster, during the autumn of 1854.* London: Churchill. 120–167.

Wilde, W. R. 1843. *Report upon the tables of deaths, part V. Special sanitary report on Dublin City: Part 4 of the Census of Ireland,* 68–75.

Wilson, J. E. 1942. An early Baltimore physician and his medical library. *Annals of Medical History* 4 (1): 63–80.

Wilson, M. E. 1999. Travel and the emergence of infectious disease. *Emerging Infectious Diseases* 1 (2). www.cdc.gov/ncidod/eid/vol1no2/wilsom.htm

Winterton, W. R. 1980. The Soho cholera epidemic in 1854. *History of Medicine* 8 (2): 11–20.

Wood, D. 2004a. Five billion years of global change: A history of the land. New York: Guilford Press.

————. 2004b. Cartography is dead (Thank God!). *Cartographic Perspectives* 45 (Spring): 4–7.

————. 2003. Thinking about maps as propositions instead of pictures. NACIS Annual Meeting, Jacksonville, Florida.

————. 2002. Thinking about maps as propositions instead of pictures. NACIS Annual Meeting, Jacksonville, Florida.

————. 1993a. What makes a map a map? *Cartographica* 30 (2 and 3): 55–60.

————. 1993b. The fine line between mapping and mapmaking. *Cartogaphica* 30 (4): 50–60.

————. 1992a. *The power of maps.* New York: Guilford Press.

————. 1992b. How maps work. *Cartographica* 29 (3 and 4): 66–74.

Woodworth, J. M. 1875. *The cholera epidemic of 1873 in the United States.* House of Representatives. Washington, D.C.: Government Printing Office. 43d Cong. 2d Session, House Ex. Doc. No. 95.

World Health Organization. 1996. Fact Sheet N107. Geneva: World Health Organization. www. who.int/mediacentre/factsheets

————. 2000. *Weekly epidemiological record* 31 (75): 249–256.

Wright, D. J., M. F. Goodchild, and J. D. Proctor. 1997. Demystifying the persistent ambiguity of GIS as a "tool" versus "science." *Annals of the Association of American Geographers* 87 (2): 346–362.

Yeo, E., and E. P. Thompson. 1971. The unknown mayhew. New York: Schocken Books.

York, J. 1855. Mr. York's Report. In *Report of the cholera outbreak in the parish of St. James, Westminster, during the autumn of 1854.* London: Churchill, 168-172.

Young, T. C., A. E. Richmond, and G. R. Brendish. 1926. Sandflies and sandfly fever in the Peshwar District. *Indian Journal of Medical Research* 13: 961-1021.

Zeiler, M. 1999. *Modeling our world: ESRI guide to geodatabase design.* Redlands, Calif.: ESRI Press.

Index

A

B

D

E

East Africa, cholera epidemics in, 180–184
East London detail of Booth's poverty map, 64
East Riding of Yorkshire, impact of influenza on, 251–252
EBV (Epstein-Barr virus), 242, 247
education, Gould's position on, 270
Edward R. Tufte
    The Visual Display of Quantitative Information, 145
    Visual Display of Communication, 146
    Visual Explanations, 146
eighteenth century
    mapping in, 24–26
    yellow fever in, 26–33
ellipses, measuring angle of incidence with, 305, 325
emigration and immigration, relationship to disease, 16
endemic diseases
    in eighteenth century, 26
    spread of, 16
Endnotes
    for Chapter 1, "Mapping and Making," 3, 5, 6, 7, 8, 12–13
    for Chapter 2, "Medical Mapping: Early Histories," 16, 21, 26, 27, 28, 33, 34, 39
    for Chapter 3, "Mapping and Statistics: 1830-1849," 41–42, 44, 47–48, 49–50, 54–55, 60, 63, 65, 72–74
    for Chapter 4, "John Snow: The London Epidemics," 75, 79, 85, 92, 95, 102–103
    for Chapter 5, "The Cholera Debate," 110, 118, 123, 126–127
    for Chapter 6, "Map as Intent: Variations on John Snow," 132, 133, 148, 149, 150, 151, 154–155
    for Chapter 7, "Mapping Legacy," 159, 160, 170, 176, 181, 185, 189, 191–192
    for Chapter 8, "Public Health: The Divorce," 200, 205, 208, 214
    for Chapter 9, "Disease Ecologies: Disease Atlases," 230, 233, 237, 242, 243, 246–247
    for Chapter 10, "Complex Processes: Diffusion and Structure," 250, 254, 258, 267, 269, 281–282
    for Chapter 11, "GIS and Medical Mapping," 285, 291, 293, 309, 323, 324, 325–326
England
    appearance of cholera in 1849, 82–90
    appearance of measles in Cornwall, 262, 264
    cancer in, 266
    cholera deaths in, 42
    diffusion of influenza in, 250
    male death rates in (1958–1962), 228
    plague epidemic in, 207
    reappearance of cholera in 1853, 90
    spread of cholera in, 159
ENIAC computer, completion of, 229
environmental contamination, using GIS-based graphic approaches with, 306
environments
    impact on health, 4, 32
    relationship to disease incidence, 224
    role in British bronchitis study by Girtz, 258
epidemic disease
    analyzing outbreaks of, 304
    bi-directionality of, 172

K

L

M

N

O

P

UNOS (United Nations work for Organ Sharing), 310, 311, 326
urban areas. *See* cities
urban structure, perception by Chicago School, 256
urban theory, application by Girtz, 257–258
urban waste versus cholera, 84
USA Today story on mapping surgeries, 291, 292
U.S. CDC (Center for Disease Control). *See* CDC (Center for Disease Control)
USGS National Atlas of the United States, 289
U.S. SMSAs (Standard Metropolitan Statistical Areas), cumulative AIDS in, 287, 288

V

Vancouver, Canada
    premature births in, 4, 6, 12
    salmonella outbreak in, 301–305
Varela and Maturana (structural coupling), 7, 13
vectors for yellow fever, 33
Verghese, Abraham, xv–xvi
    AIDS research done by, 276–281
    and map thinking, 327–328, 329, 335
vertical versus horizontal perspective, 33–38, 57, 62
Vibrio cholerae, xv, 114, 139, 142
Vienna conference of 1874, authority of, 160–161
Vinten-Johansen (cholera maps between 1832-1855), 44–45
Virchow, Rudolf (normalcy versus disease), 329
Visual Display of Communication (Tufte), 146
The Visual Display of Quantitative Information (Tufte), 145–146
Visual Explanations by Edward R. Tufte, 146
von Andree, Karl *(Geographie des Weltandels)*, 208
von Pettenkofer, Max (scientist), 114
Voronoi network, significance of, 139–140

W

Wakley, Thomas versus John Snow, 114–115
Wales
    cholera deaths in, 42
    diffusion of influenza in, 250
    male death rates in (1958–1962), 228
Warburton, John and John Snow, 76
Ward, Robert Decourcy, 186–187
water closets, complicity of, 133, 155
water supply
    as factor in London cholera epidemic (Snow), 93, 94
    role in spread of cholera, 88–89, 90–91, 92
    role in typhoid fever in Plymouth, Pennsylvania (1885), 195–196
"The Water We Drink" report (1866), 172
Watson, John and John Snow, 76
Web sites
    for graft organ retrieval and use, 286
    of online atlases, 289

Z